INHALED PARTICLES

IV

PART 2

ORGANIZING COMMITTEE

Chairman:	Dr J. S. McLintock	*Chief Medical Officer, National Coal Board, London.*
	Dr A. Critchlow	*Health and Safety Executive, Safety in Mines Research Establishment, Sheffield.*
	Dr J. C. Gilson	*Director, Pneumoconiosis Unit, Medical Research Council, Penarth.*
	Mr G. A. Hedgecock	*Group Occupational Hygienist, Pilkington Brothers Limited, St Helens.*
	Dr S. Holmes	*Secretary, Asbestosis Research Council.*
	Mr S. Luxon	*Deputy Chief Inspector of Factories, Health and Safety Executive, London.*
	Dr L. Magos	*Medical Research Council, Toxicology Unit, Carshalton.*
	Dr D. C. F. Muir	*Director, Institute of Occupational Medicine, Edinburgh.*
	Mr R. J. Sherwood	*Consultant Occupational Hygienist, United Nations Development Organization.*
	Mr W. H. Walton	*Deputy Director, Institute of Occupational Medicine, Edinburgh.*
Organizing Secretaries:	Dr J. Burns	*Institute of Occupational Medicine, Edinburgh.*
	Mr J. Dodgson	*Institute of Occupational Medicine, Edinburgh.*

INHALED PARTICLES IV

(IN TWO PARTS)

Proceedings of an International Symposium organized by The British Occupational Hygiene Society, Edinburgh, 22–26 September 1975

Edited by

W. H. WALTON

Hon. Editor-in-Chief, *Annals of Occupational Hygiene*
Institute of Occupational Medicine, Roxburgh Place, Edinburgh

assisted by

BRENDA McGOVERN

Editorial Assistant, *Annals of Occupational Hygiene*

PART 2

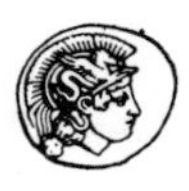

PERGAMON PRESS

OXFORD . NEW YORK . TORONTO . SYDNEY . PARIS . FRANKFURT

U.K.	Pergamon Press Ltd., Headington Hill Hall, Oxford OX3 0BW, England
U.S.A.	Pergamon Press Inc., Maxwell House, Fairview Park, Elmsford, New York 10523, U.S.A.
CANADA	Pergamon of Canada Ltd., 75 The East Mall, Toronto, Ontario, Canada
AUSTRALIA	Pergamon Press (Aust.) Pty. Ltd., 19a Boundary Street, Rushcutters Bay, N.S.W. 2011, Australia
FRANCE	Pergamon Press SARL, 24 rue des Ecoles, 75240 Paris, Cedex 05, France
FEDERAL REPUBLIC OF GERMANY	Pergamon Press GmbH, 6242 Kronberg-Taunus, Pferdstrasse 1, Federal Republic of Germany

First edition 1977

Reprinted 1978

Library of Congress Cataloging in Publication Data

Main entry under title:
Inhaled particles IV.
1. Lungs—Dust diseases—Etiology—Congresses.
2. Dust—Physiological effect—Congresses.
3. Lungs—Dust diseases—Congresses.
4. Coal-miners—Diseases and hygiene—Congresses.
I. Walton, W. H.
II. British Occupational Hygiene Society.
RC773.I55 1977 616.2'44 76-55009

ISBN 0-08-020560-7

Printed in Great Britain by Biddles Ltd., Guildford, Surrey

CONTENTS

SESSION 3. DEPOSITION AND CLEARANCE

SESSION 4A. FACTORS AFFECTING CLEARANCE

Contents

SESSION 4B. BIOLOGICAL REACTIONS TO DUST (1)

PART 2

SESSION 5. BIOLOGICAL REACTIONS TO DUST (2)

SESSION 6. BIOLOGICAL REACTIONS TO DUST (3)

Contents

SESSION 9. EPIDEMIOLOGICAL STUDIES (1)

SESSION 10. EPIDEMIOLOGICAL STUDIES (2)

SESSION 5

Wednesday, 24th September

BIOLOGICAL REACTIONS TO DUST (2)

THE EFFECTS OF INHALED SILICA AND CHRYSOTILE ON THE ELASTIC PROPERTIES OF RAT LUNGS; PHYSIOLOGICAL, PHYSICAL AND BIOCHEMICAL STUDIES OF LUNG SURFACTANT

M. McDERMOTT, J. C. WAGNER

Medical Research Council, Pneumoconiosis Unit, Llandough Hospital, Penarth, Wales

T. TETLEY, J. HARWOOD and R. J. RICHARDS

Department of Biochemistry, University College, Cardiff, Wales

Abstract—When rats breathed air containing approximately 70 mg m^{-3} of respirable crystalline silica 7 h daily for 10 days (5000 mg m^{-3} h) the surface tension forces of the alveolar lining film were reduced. This was shown both by surface tension measurements on lung extracts and by pressure–volume studies with air and saline filling of excised lungs. Larger quantities of inhaled silica produced similar effects. Chrysotile inhalation caused an even more marked decrease in the surface tension forces. In the chrysotile studies these findings were supported by biochemical estimations of the quantity of surfactant in the lungs, which was increased 10-fold by an inhalation of 6500 mg m^{-3} h.

Electron microscopy showed an increased number of the Type II alveolar cells which produce surfactant and of free phospholipid lattices in the air spaces of the lungs of rats exposed to chrysotile and silica.

Both the surface tension and biochemical estimations on a control group of rats suggest that there is an increase in the amount of surfactant in the lungs up to about 12 months of age.

INTRODUCTION

The alveoli of the mammalian lung are lined with a non-cellular liquid film. This surfactant film has the property that during compression and expansion such as occurs in respiration, the surface tension of the film varies with its area. At the end of expiration when the alveolar area is minimal the surface tension decreases almost to zero, increasing again during inspiration. The surface tension properties of the film are responsible for two-thirds of the total lung elasticity, whereas the lung tissue accounts for only one-third. The film consists mainly of phospholipids, in particular, dipalmitoyl lecithin which is 60/80% of the total lipid (KING and CLEMENTS, 1972a; 1972b). Proteins, regarded by some workers as an important determinant of the surface tension properties of the film, form 8–18% of the total surfactant (KING, 1974; TIERNEY, 1974). The phospholipids are synthesized by the Type II cells lining the alveolar wall and also possibly by the Clara cells in the terminal bronchioles (SMITH *et al.*, 1974).

The surfactant film has at least three functions:

1. A low surface tension, by reducing the pressures required to inflate and deflate the lung, minimizes the work of breathing compared with that needed if the film had surface properties similar to fluids such as saline or blood.
2. A surface tension which varies with area helps to maintain alveolar stability by equalizing the pressures between small and large alveoli.
3. The surfactant film may play a part in preventing the transudation of liquid from the capillaries into the alveolar spaces.

Little is known of the effect of changes in the properties of the surface-lining film on function apart from extreme cases such as respiratory distress syndrome when the film is absent.

The alveolar wall including the Type II cells, the surfactant film and the alveolar macrophages are all in direct physical contact with dusts and inhaled irritants entering the lung. It seems therefore likely that one of the first responses of the lungs could be a change in the properties of the surfactant film. In 1960 Marks and Marasas showed that when guinea pigs inhaled silica there was an increase in lung phospholipid and lecithin. Heppleston *et al.*, in 1974, showed that rats who had inhaled silica developed a pulmonary disease similar to alveolar lipoproteinosis in man. The total lipid was greatly increased, with dipalmitoyl lecithin being affected to the greatest degree. In an experiment in our laboratory (McDermott *et al.*, 1973) we showed that in rats a small quantity of inhaled silica produced a change in the surface tension properties of the lining film.

This paper reviews the results of several inhalation experiments in rats using crystalline silica (Min–U–Sil) and some preliminary work using U.I.C.C. Rhodesian chrysotile.

MATERIALS AND METHODS

The methods used to estimate the effects of inhaled silica and chrysotile included:

1. Measurement of lung elasticity in excised lungs by recording pressure–volume relationships during air and saline inflation and deflation. The air curve gives the sum of the tissue elasticity plus that due to the surfactant film, whilst the saline curve is affected by the tissue component alone provided the structure of the lung is not altered by areas of consolidation. Gross tissue changes will cause a different distribution of forces within the lung during the air and saline inflations.
2. Surface tension measurements on an extract made from lung tissue minced in saline (Sekulic *et al.*, 1968).
3. Estimation of surfactant in lung washings in the chrysotile dusted animals only.
4. Light and electron microscope studies.

Table 1 lists the dusting data for four experiments with silica and two with Rhodesian chrysotile.

All the rats were male Wistar Specific Pathogen Free (SPF) and with the exception of the group exposed to 25 000 mg m^{-3} h of respirable silica they were dusted at the Pneumoconiosis Unit for 7 h a day until the required dose had been achieved. The

TABLE 1. DUST EXPOSURE OF RATS USED FOR SURFACE TENSION AND PRESSURE–VOLUME MEASUREMENTS

Dust	No. of rats	Dust concn. (mg m $^{-3}$)	Period of dusting (days)	Period of dusting (h/day)	Dust dose (mg m $^{-3}$ h)	Survival after exposure (months)	Age at death (months)
	6 + 6	70	10	(7)	5000 (A)	0	6.5
Silica	6 + 6	70	10	(7)	5000 (B)	7	13.5
(Min–U–Sil)[a]	4	35	42	(7)	10 000	14.5	17–21
	12				25 000	7.5	14–21
Rhodesian	4	12	80	(7)	6500	0	5
chrysotile	4	12	130	(7)	11 000	0	8–9
(U.I.C.C.)							

[a] See text for details of experiment.

25 000 mg m $^{-3}$ h silica group were dusted for between 7 and 20 h a day, some at the Pneumoconiosis Unit and some at the University of Newcastle upon Tyne (HEPPLESTON *et al.*, 1975). For each exposed group there was a corresponding control group. Surface tension, pressure–volume measurements and light and electron microscope studies were made on all groups.

The details of the exposure of rats to Rhodesian chrysotile on which the biochemical study was carried out are shown in Table 2. A single estimation of surfactant was made

TABLE 2. DUST EXPOSURE OF RATS USED IN BIOCHEMICAL STUDIES
Rhodesian chrysotile, concentration 12.5 mg m $^{-3}$ for 7 h per day

No. of rats	Control or treated	Period of dusting (days)	Dust dose (mg m $^{-3}$ h)	Survival after exposure (months)	Sex + age at death (months)
4	C				♂3.0, ♂7.5, ♂7.5, ♀7.5
4	T	33	3000	0	♂5.0, ♂7.5, ♀7.5, ♀7.5
4	C				♂5.0, ♂9.0, ♂9.0, ♀9.0
3	T			0	♂5.0, ♂9.0, ♀9.0
5	C				♂8.5, ♂12.5, ♂12.5, ♀12.5, ♀12.5
3	T	73	6500	3.5	♂8.5, ♂12.5, ♀12.5
3	C				♂15.0, ♂17.0, ♂17.0
3	T			8	♂17.0, ♂17.0, ♂17.0

on pooled lung washings from between three and five rats which included both male and female rats. No biochemical studies were made on the silica dusted rats as such studies have already been carried out by HEPPLESTON *et al.* (1974).

Measurement of Pressure–Volume Curves

The rats were killed by intraperitoneal pentobarbital anaesthesia and exsanguination. The trachea was cannulated, the thorax opened and the lungs and heart removed *en bloc*. The lungs were degassed and attached to a pressure transducer and syringe system for determination of the pressure–volume curves. Air was added to the system in 1-ml steps and 2 min allowed for pressure equilibration after each addition of air. The lungs were inflated to 3 kN m^{-2} (approximately 30 cm H_2O) and then deflated in 1-ml steps to residual volume. The lungs were degassed again, suspended in a bath of saline and inflated with saline to the maximum lung volume used with air, and again deflated. In the experiments with a silica exposure of 5000 mg m^{-3} h the lungs were inflated to a constant volume of 16 ml rather than a constant pressure. Pressure readings were corrected for the volume of air in the system during the air inflation and deflation and for changes in the liquid level in the bath during the saline measurements.

The indices of the pressure–volume curves discussed in this paper are:

1. The difference between the pressures measured with air and saline filling as a function of the percentage of the lung volume at 3 kN m^{-2} (per cent maximum lung volume). This index measures the elastic component due to the surface tension of the alveolar lining layer after the tissue elastic component has been removed. The use of per cent maximum lung volume compensates for differences in lung size. Only the *deflation* curves are used to measure the lung elastic properties as the inflation curve represents mainly sequential opening of alveolar spaces rather than the surface tension properties of the alveolar lining.
2. The saline *deflation* curves which measure tissue elasticity.

Measurement of Surface Tension

Surface tension area loops from minced lung extracts were obtained with a modified Langmuir Wilhelmy balance (BROWN *et al.*, 1959). After the pressure–volume curves were completed, the lungs were inflated several times with air, then minced with sharp scissors in 10 ml of saline. More saline was added to make up 50 ml and the mixture placed in the Teflon trough of the surface tension balance. The extract was allowed to stand 30 min for a film of surfactant to form. The surface of the film was contained within a tape boundary kept taut and moved in such a way that the film area was decreased to 20% of its original area and then re-expanded without the film moving outside the boundary. The surface tension of the film was recorded throughout the change of area. The compression and re-expansion took 13 min and cycling continued for at least 3 h. Measurements were made on the cycle with the lowest minimum surface tension, and the indices used in this paper are the maximum surface tension (σ_{max}), minimum surface tension (σ_{min}) and the stability index:

$$2\frac{(\sigma_{max} - \sigma_{min})}{(\sigma_{max} + \sigma_{min})}.$$

In the experiments with a silica exposure of 5000 mg m^{-3} h the rats were killed in pairs and the minced lung extract used for surface tension measurements included two left lungs and one right lung. In all but this group the surface tension measurements were made in an air-conditioned room at 20–22°C.

Measurement of Surfactant

Pulmonary surfactant was obtained by a modification of the method of ABRAMS (1966). After lung lavage with isotonic saline, which was repeated 10 times, the free cell population was removed by centrifugation at 300*g* for 20 min. The supernatant was centrifuged at 1000*g* for 60 min and the pellet resuspended in 21 % (w/v) NaCl. Further centrifugation at 1500*g* for 20 min resulted in a three-phase separation into an insoluble floating fraction (surfactant pellicle), a soluble fraction (soluble surfactant) and a small precipitate at the bottom of the tube. The surfactant pellicle fraction was dialysed against millimolar tris buffer (pH 7.4) for 48 h (DESAI *et al.*, 1975). All the above procedures were carried out at 4°C. The pellicle surfactant was freeze dried and weighed, and the amount of surfactant per animal calculated.

RESULTS

Surface Tension Measurements

The surface tension results for the experiments with silica are shown in Table 3. The wet weight of the rat lungs appears abnormally high as it includes the weight of saline which cannot be completely recovered at the end of the pressure–volume curves. The heart was not removed earlier for the lungs to be weighed as to do so might have caused pleural damage.

In the 5000 (A) mg m^{-3} h exposure group on whom measurements were made within a few days of the end of inhalation the lung weight was 1.9 g compared with 1.5 g in the controls. In group 5000 (B) which was killed 7 months after dusting, the increase in weight was greater suggesting that changes continued after removal from the dust.

In the groups with dust exposures of 10 000 and 25 000 mg m^{-3} h the weight of the lungs was increased many fold and ranged from 8.2 to 15.5 g. To the eye the lungs appeared grossly enlarged with deposits in the alveoli.

In the 5000 mg m^{-3} h groups the minimum surface tension was significantly reduced both immediately after ($P < 0.05$) and in the rats killed 7 months after ($P < 0.002$) the end of dusting compared with the controls. There was only a slight decrease in the maximum surface tension. In the control rats aged 13.5 months the minimum surface tension was 3.6 compared with 6.6 mN m^{-1} for those aged 6.5 months. The stability index was increased in the older group.

A significant decrease in the minimum surface tension ($P < 0.05$) occurred in the rats dusted at 10 000 mg m^{-3} h, compared with the controls although not in the mean value for the 25 000 mg m^{-3} h group. However, if in this latter group the four values greater than 10 are excluded, a mean value of 3.6 mN m^{-1} is obtained. These four high minimum surface tensions were probably due to the alveolar deposits preventing the formation of a stable film in the surface tension trough (HEPPLESTON *et al.*, 1975).

The stability index in all dusted groups was increased if these four rats are excluded.

TABLE 3. SURFACE TENSION MEASUREMENTS ON RATS EXPOSED TO SILICA

Dust dose	Wet wt. of lungs (g)		σ_{min}(mN m^{-1})		σ_{max}(mN m^{-1})		Stability index	
(mg m^{-3} h)	Control	Treated	Control	Treated	Control	Treated	Control	Treated
5000 (A)[a]	1.2	1.1	4.5	5.8	33.5	33.0	1.53	1.40
	1.5	1.6	6.5	3.8	34.0	33.0	1.36	1.59
	—	2.2	6.7	3.1	39.0	34.2	1.41	1.67
	1.6	1.8	9.8	3.6	33.6	36.3	1.10	1.64
	1.5	2.9	8.3	3.7	34.5	40.0	1.22	1.66
	1.9	1.6	4.0	5.0	45.0	38.5	1.67	1.54
Mean	1.5	1.9	6.6	4.2	36.6	35.8	1.38	1.58
5000 (B)[b]	1.3	—	5.0	1.2	35.5	35.8	1.51	1.87
	1.4	3.8	3.5	1.4	43.9	37.7	1.70	1.86
	1.2	2.2	4.7	1.8	36.0	37.8	1.54	1.82
	1.8	1.8	3.8	1.0	32.3	33.0	1.58	1.88
	1.7	1.8	2.8	1.9	34.7	30.0	1.70	1.76
	1.1	2.5	2.0	1.5	34.3	34.8	1.78	1.83
Mean	1.4	2.4	3.6	1.5	36.1	34.8	1.64	1.84
10,000	1.9	15.2	5.0	2.9	37.4	38.5	1.53	1.72
	2.0	10.0	5.7	3.0	43.0	39.1	1.53	1.71
	1.8	9.5	8.2	2.6	33.6	39.3	1.22	1.75
	1.7	8.2	4.9	4.7	39.0	37.0	1.55	1.55
Mean	1.8	10.7	6.0	3.3	38.2	38.5	1.46	1.68
25,000	1.9	10.4	5.0	6.2	37.4	38.8.	1.53	1.45
	2.0	11.5	5.7	4.6	43.0	42.0	1.53	1.61
	1.8	12.8	8.2	2.0	33.6	34.8	1.22	1.78
	1.7	12.1	4.9	12.9*	39.0	31.9	1.55	0.84*
	1.5	10.8	4.6	3.0	38.6	35.8	1.57	1.69
	2.3	8.8	5.0	2.5	34.6	37.8	1.50	1.75
	2.5	11.5	4.4	12.0*	36.9	37.7	1.57	1.03*
	1.9	13.5	8.2	3.0	44.6	39.0	1.38	1.71
	2.5	9.8	5.3	3.7	39.5	32.2	1.53	1.59
	1.4	15.5	5.2	12.3*	35.3	32.0	1.49	0.89*
	1.9	11.8	3.9	3.5	43.6	34.5	1.67	1.63
	1.6	10.2	5.2	10.5*	42.3	38.9	1.56	1.15*
Mean	1.9	11.6	5.5	6.4	39.0	36.3	1.51	1.43
Mean excluding*				3.6				1.65

[a] The rats were killed at the end of dusting, aged 6.5 months.
[b] The rats were killed 7 months after the end of dusting, aged 13.5 months.

The surface tension results for the experiments with chrysotile are shown in Table 4.

TABLE 4. SURFACE TENSION MEASUREMENTS ON RATS EXPOSED TO CHRYSOTILE

Dust dose	Wet wt. of lungs (g)		Surface tension ($mN\ m^{-1}$) Min		Max		Stability index	
($mg\ m^{-3}\ h$)	Control	Treated	Control	Treated	Control	Treated	Control	Treated
6500[a]	1.4	2.4	9.2	5.3	45.0	38.0	1.32	1.51
	2.2	2.1	13.5	5.2	46.0	45.5	1.09	1.59
	1.9	2.7	5.5	3.9	45.0	41.0	1.56	1.65
	1.6	2.4	11.5	5.1	45.5	40.0	1.19	1.55
Mean	1.8	2.4	9.9	4.9	45.4	41.1	1.29	1.58
	1.8		4.9		43.6		1.60	
	2.0	2.6	4.9	1.8	50.0	46.0	1.64	1.85
11,000[b]	1.7	2.3	5.5	2.0	45.2	41.0	1.57	1.81
	2.5	3.2	6.0	0.8	46.9	40.0	1.55	1.92
	2.0	2.4	5.3	1.8	50.0	48.0	1.62	1.86
Mean	2.0	2.6	5.3	1.6	47.1	43.8	1.60	1.86

[a] The rats were killed at aged 5 months.
[b] The rats were killed at aged 8–9 months.

The increase in wet lung weight for both the chrysotile exposed groups was similar to that for lowest dose of silica.

The minimum surface tension was again significantly lower in both the dusted groups compared with the controls ($P < 0.03$, $P < 0.01$ for the 6500 and 11 000 $mg\ m^{-3}\ h$ groups, respectively.) There was also a reduction in the maximum surface tension and an increase in the stability index. The maximum surface tensions were higher in the chrysotile than in the silica study, probably due to a technical improvement in the method by which the surfactant film was enclosed by the tape.

As with the silica control rats (5000 $mg\ m^{-3}\ h$ study) there was an apparent effect of age on the minimum surface tension, which was 5.3 $mN\ m^{-1}$ in the control group aged 8–9 months compared with 9.9 $mN\ m^{-1}$ in the rats aged 5 months. The stability index was also higher in the older controls. This age effect was only seen when both young and old rats had come from the same breeding.

Pressure–Volume Measurements

Figures 1 and 2 show the relationship between transpulmonary pressure (air minus saline) and lung volume during deflation for the silica- and chrysotile-dusted rats respectively. The whole of the curve is not shown as at small lung volumes the air and saline deflation pressures become very similar. The mean curve of the differences for

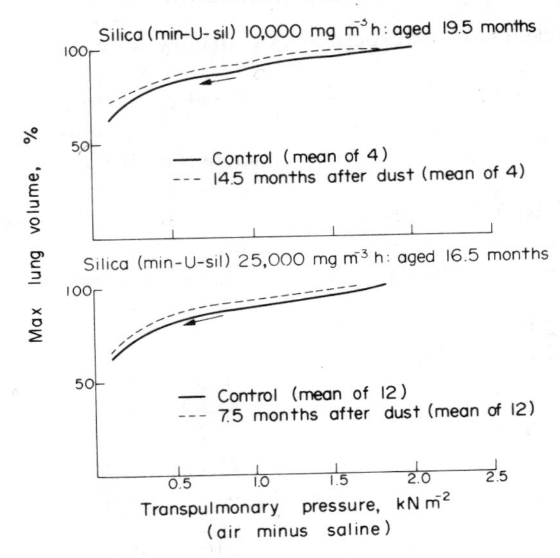

Fig. 1. Effect of silica (Min–U–Sil) on the surface tension component of lung elasticity.

several animals is therefore not informative. In the four groups illustrated the pressure at a given percentage of the maximum lung volume was lower in the dust exposed group than in the controls although the difference was considerably greater with chrysotile than with silica. As these curves reflect only the surface tension component of the lung elasticity this suggests that there is a reduction in the surface tension forces of the alveolar lining film in the lungs of the dusted rats. The curves for 5000 mg m^{-3} h silica exposure are not illustrated, but the change was in the same direction.

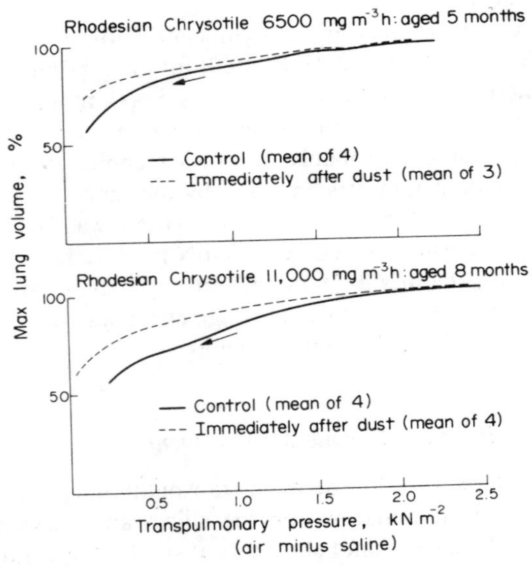

Fig. 2. Effect of Rhodesian chrysotile on the surface tension component of lung elasticity.

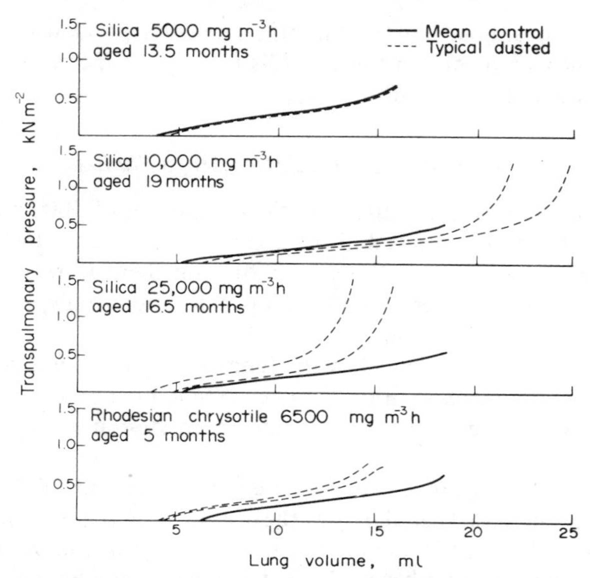

FIG. 3. Effect of Rhodesian chrysotile and silica on tissue elasticity.

Figure 3 shows the saline deflation curves for the three silica groups and one chrysotile group. With the lowest inhaled dose of silica there was little change, at 10 000 mg m^{-3} h the dusted curves differed mainly because the lungs were so much larger that a bigger volume was required for inflation. The results for silica inhalation at 25 000 mg m^{-3} h and chrysotile at 6 500 mg m^{-3} h show there was a larger pressure at any given lung volume which implies loss of tissue elasticity.

Biochemical Estimation of Surfactant

The biochemical estimations are shown in Table 5. At both levels of dust exposure the rats which inhaled chrysotile showed a large increase in the amount of surfactant per animal. The quantity of surfactant was highest immediately after the end of the

TABLE 5. ESTIMATION OF SURFACTANT IN LUNG WASHINGS FOR RATS EXPOSED TO CHRYSOTILE

Dust dose	Survival after exposure	Average age at death of controls	Amount of surfactant per animal (mg)	
(mg m^{-3} h)	(months)	(months)	Control	Treated
3000	0	6.5	0.42	0.77
6500	0	8	1.28	12.73
	3.5	11.5	2.28	5.27
	8	16.5	1.9	6.45

dusting, reducing to almost half 3.5 months later. As previously suggested by the surface tension measurements, in the controls there is an increase in surfactant with age up to approximately 12 months.

Light and Electron Microscope Studies

In the rats killed immediately after the silica exposure of 5000 mg m^{-3} h electron microscopy and histology showed little abnormality except dust in the alveolar macrophages. In rats killed 7 months after dusting there were some early silicotic nodules, foci of alveolar lipo-proteinosis and proliferation of Type II cells with many free phospholipid lattices in the air spaces.

With the high doses of inhaled silica the lungs showed varying degrees of alveolar lipo-proteinosis and an increase in the number of silicotic nodules. The ultrastructure features of the Newcastle exposed rats have been described by Heppleston and Young (1972).

In the chrysotile-dusted groups, immediately after the end of the 6500 mg m^{-3} h exposure there was increased cellularity of the area around the respiratory bronchioles. In the group exposed to 11 000 mg m^{-3} h the cellularity was more marked and there was a large increase in the number of Type II alveolar epithelial cells. In both groups the lungs contained chrysotile fibres mainly within the alveolar macrophages.

DISCUSSION

The biochemical studies show that the inhalation of chrysotile by SPF rats produces an increase in lung surfactant. Such an increase has previously been shown with silica. Electron micrographs confirm the chrysotile results.

These biochemical and electron microscope changes do not necessarily mean that the surface tension of the lung alveolar lining is decreased by the presence of the extra surfactant. It is possible that inhaled dusts might cause the release of substances which would interfere with the formation of the lining film, or that provided there is sufficient surfactant to produce a monomolecular layer any excess is unimportant (Scarpelli, 1968).

The pressure–volume studies, however, showed that the recoil pressure of the lungs of the dusted rats was reduced after allowing for the effect of changes in tissue elasticity caused by fibrosis. The surface tension estimates on the lung extracts were also in agreement with the biochemical and physiological results, with a reduction in the minimum surface tension and an increase in the stability index. Whether or not changes of this magnitude will affect respiration in the living animal has not yet been studied.

Other workers have looked at the effects of inhaled irritants. Kahana and Aronovitch (1966, 1968), using sulphur dioxide, and Rosenberg *et al.* (1962), using aluminium oxide, concluded that inhaled irritants decrease lung surface tension forces. Rhoades in 1972 found that inhaled carbon dust in rats produced an increase in phospholipid, but with only a slight difference in surface tension properties of extracts. Grunspan *et al.* (1973) showed that carborundum injected into rat lungs produced much less increase in phospholipids than did silica.

The significance, if any, of a decrease in the surface tension of the lung alveolar lining after the inhalation of irritants is not established. One possibility is that the increase in surfactant production caused by inhaled silica and chrysotile is a compensatory mechanism which helps counteract the high pressures which would otherwise be necessary to inflate fibrotic lungs.

Even though these are preliminary results, and the biochemical measurements are only one estimate on pooled lung washings for each group, the agreement between all the different measurements is such as to suggest that chrysotile may be even more potent in increasing surfactant in the lungs than is silica. This needs to be confirmed with larger numbers of animals and extended to other dusts which also produce fibrosis.

Further work is also needed to verify whether, as suggested by the biochemical results, the effect of inhaled chrysotile is reduced after a few months out of dust. In contrast, the surface tension results with silica suggest that the effect is progressive after the end of inhalation.

The possible decrease of the minimum surface tension and the increase of the stability index with age need further study in conjunction with biochemical estimations of surfactant on the same group of animals.

Acknowledgements—Mr J. W. Skidmore was responsible for the design of the dust inhalation equipment and the exposure of the animals. Mrs M. M. Bevan and Mr M. F. Clay made the physiological and surface tension measurements, and Mr R. Hill carried out the histology and electron microscopy. All are at the Pneumoconiosis Unit.

REFERENCES

ABRAMS, M. E. (1966) *J. appl. Physiol.* **21,** 718.
BROWN, E. S., JOHNSON, R. P. and CLEMENTS, J. A. (1959) *J. appl. Physiol.* **14,** 717.
DESAI, R., HEXT, P. and RICHARDS, R. (1975) *Life Sci.* **16,** 1931.
GRUNSPAN, M., ANTWEILER, H. and DEHNEN, W. (1973) *Br. J. ind. Med.* **30,** 74.
HEPPLESTON, A. G. and YOUNG, A. E. (1972) *J. Path.* **107,** 107.
HEPPLESTON, A. G., FLETCHER, K. and WYATT, I. (1974) *Br. J. exp. Path.* **55,** 384.
HEPPLESTON, A G., McDERMOTT, M. and COLLINS, M. M. (1975) *Br. J. exp. Path.* **56,** 444.
KAHANA, L. M. and ARONOVITCH, M. (1966) *Am. Rev. resp. Dis.* **94,** 201.
KAHANA, L. M. and ARONOVITCH, M. (1968) *Am. Rev. resp. Dis.* **98,** 311.
KING, R. J. (1974) *Fedn Proc. Fedn Am. Socs exp. Biol.* **33,** 2238.
KING, R. J. and CLEMENTS, J. A. (1972a) *Am. J. Physiol.* **223,** 707.
KING, R. J. and CLEMENTS, J. A. (1972b) *Am. J. Physiol.* **223,** 715.
McDERMOTT, M., COLLINS, M. M. and CLAY, M. F. (1973) *Bull. Physiopath. resp.* **9,** 1252.
MARKS, G. S. and MARASAS, L. W. (1960) *Br. J. ind. Med.* **17,** 31.
RHOADES, R. A. (1972) *Life Sci.* **11,** 33.
ROSENBERG, E., ALARIE, Y. and ROBILLARD, E. (1962) *Fedn Proc. Fedn Am. Socs exp. Biol.* **21,** 447.
SCARPELLI, E. M. (1968) *The Surfactant System of the Lung.* Lea and Febiger, Philadelphia.
SEKULIC, S. M., HAMLIN, J. T., ELLISON, R. G. and ELLISON, L. T. (1968) *Am. Rev. resp. Dis.* **97,** 131.
SMITH, P., HEATH, D. and MOOSAUI, H. (1974) *Thorax* **29,** 147.
TIERNEY, D. F. (1974) *A. Rev. Physiol.* **36,** 209.

DISCUSSION

A. G. Heppleston: May I amplify what has been said in regard to the biochemical and biophysical aspects of the silicotic reaction?

Lipids, notably phosphatides, figure early in the pulmonary response to quartz inhaled by SPF rats. This change is so pronounced as to reproduce with remarkable precision the human condition of alveolar lipo-proteinosis. The correspondence extends to ultrastructural and biochemical features, whilst metabolic tracer studies explain the pathogenesis of the disease as an imbalance between formation and removal of phospholipid. Concurrently hyaline silicotic nodules fail to form, though exceptionally focal cellular aggregations, including some reticulin, develop but remain small and scanty. Absence or gross limitation of silicotic fibrogenesis is attributable to isolation of quartz particles within the predominantly lipid alveolar material. Interaction of quartz and macrophages cannot then occur, with consequent failure to liberate the fibrogenic factor whose production depends on this interaction.

The principal biochemical finding is a massive accumulation of dipalmitoyl lecithin, one of the main components of lung surfactant. The physical behaviour of the intact lungs and of lung extracts, from rats affected by alveolar lipo-proteinosis as a consequence of high dose silica inhalation, was studied by means of pressure–volume relations and surface tension area loops in collaboration with Mrs McDermott.

Air inflation of diseased lungs occurred at a lower pressure and collapse was less on deflation than in control specimens, although there appeared to be little change in tissue elastic forces. When saline was used, dusted rat lungs showed at higher lung volumes a peculiar hysteresis effect which is attributable to consolidation of alveoli by the lipid material.

Extracts from affected lungs showed differences from controls in respect of maximum and minimum surface tensions and stability index, but all the values fell within the accepted limits of normal. However, with extracts from pathological lungs, the area of the hysteresis loop increased, the shape of the surface tension/area curve was abnormal, and the percentage compression required to reduce the surface tension to 120 μN/cm fell.

Extracts from diseased lungs depressed the maximum surface tension of normal lung extracts and increased the hysteresis area, but had little effect on the minimum tension, the stability index or the percent compression needed to achieve 120 μN/cm. The response was thus mainly that of an extract from a dusted rat. The surface activity of phospholipids may be affected by neutral lipid, cholesterol and the products of cell break-down, all of which are found in the alveolar material. The occurrence within the same lung of compounds which reduce surface tension and of others which modify this property suggests that their relative concentrations may determine the overall effectiveness of the lung lining.

I wonder, however, if Mrs McDermott's measurement of surfactant by protein estimation should be replaced by lipid determination, since these latter compounds include the important surface active elements, which may not be chemically bonded to protein. Moreover, the quantitative changes in lipids and protein are, in my experience with silica, grossly dissociated.

Mrs McDermott: Detailed analysis of the protein and lipid content of lung washings was made. The data discussed in this paper are for the quantity of solid material in lung washings which can be centrifuged out after removal of the free cell population.

D. J. Ferin: It has been shown that many inhalants, mainly oxidants, affect the Type I cell of the alveolar lining and the Type II cell acts as the source of replacement and regeneration—in this time missing Type I cells. I am wondering if when looking at your electromicroscopic studies you looked also at Type I cells and what your findings were?

Dr Wagner: We have observed the disappearance of the Type I cell after exposure to asbestos dust. There is proliferation of the Type II cell, which seems to replace the Type I cells. This proliferation becomes marked in the animals which have been exposed to asbestos dust for longer periods, leading eventually to the development of pulmonary adenomata.

Our experimental findings do not agree with those of Professor Heppleston. In our experience SPF rats exposed to quartz dust develop profuse foci of cellular dust reticulation in which collagenization is observed in animals surviving more than a year after the exposure to dust. Alveolar lipo-proteinosis is present but is more marked in the animals exposed for 20 h a day, than those receiving the same amount of dust over 8-h periods.

J. Bruch: We have found that the Type I cell ingests asbestos fibres after inhalation. The thickening of the alveolar walls is due in part to Type I cell proliferation. Very small amounts of quartz considerably increase the number of Type II cells. For instance, 6 h inhalation of quartz (40 mg/m^3) results in a significant rise of Type II cells. With reference to Professor Heppleston's remarks, lipo-proteinosis and Type II cell proliferation together with fibrosis can also be seen in conventional rats after inhalation of quartz dust. In our opinion, lipo-proteinosis is not a specific response of SPF rats to silica. We measured alveolar lipo-proteinosis after inhalation of quartz dust. We have considered the possibility that the change in surface tension may only be caused by the quantitative increase of phospholipids but also the qualitative change of phospholipid composition after inhalation of silica. Our unpublished data suggest that the biochemistry of the Type II cells is defective, morphometric measurement on E.M. photomicrographs show extremely extended mitochondrial surface and dilated cisternae of endoplasmatic reticulum.

A. G. HEPPLESTON: I should like an opportunity to reply—in the first place to Dr Wagner. I would assure him that I have exposed animals for 6 h as well as for 20 h. The results are exactly the same. To Professor Bruch, I have also used conventional as well as SPF rats. Our findings are essentially the same except that the silicotic lesions are not fully hyalinized.

Mrs McDERMOTT: We have studied rats exposed to silica by Professor Heppleston in Newcastle and by the Pneumoconiosis Unit. We find that in the Newcastle animals there is considerably more alveolar proteinosis with less silicotic nodulation than in the Pneumoconiosis Unit rats. The behaviour of the surfactant in our silica-dusted animals is far more similar to that which we see with chrysotile than is the case with the Newcastle rats.

E. P. RADFORD: I should like to make a comment with regard to the use of the difference between air and saline curves as indicative of the extent of energy dispersion in the surface alone. It is not a valid assumption that this difference reflects only surface forces. My second point is a question to the whole group. In a situation where you dust animals and develop rather massive cellular changes, would it not indeed be surprising if you did not find rather marked changes in the amount of the surfactant, either due to increased production or changes in the way the surfactant is lost from the lungs, perhaps through the mucociliary stream?

Mrs McDERMOTT: I would agree that the difference between the air inhalation and the saline inflation curve is not only dependent on the surface tension forces. Particularly in grossly abnormal lungs, the redistribution of forces during saline inflation invalidates this simple assumption. However, it was the best approximation we could get with our present experimental techniques.

Whether or not we would expect such changes depends on the quantity of irritant entering the lungs. The levels of dust with which we have been working have been really very small and have not been considered in the past to have much effect.

We are interested to find out what effect these surfactant changes may have on lung function, in particular on collateral ventilation channels, alveolar pores and the small airways. I accept that we do not know yet whether there is an increase in production or an abnormality of the system which destroys the surfactant. We are looking into this.

J. FERIN: You think that 70 mg m^{-3} of respirable silica dust is so low a concentration?

Mrs McDERMOTT: The silica was given for only 10 days. At the end of 7 months there was something like 1 or 2 mg of silica left in the rat lung. That is not very large compared with that retained by some people at the end of their working lives.

THE IMMUNOLOGY OF ASBESTOSIS*

E. KAGAN, I. WEBSTER, J. C. COCHRANE and K. MILLER

National Research Institute for Occupational Diseases of the South African Medical Research Council, Johannesburg

Abstract—Forty-one employees with varying degrees of asbestosis have been tested for any alteration in the immunological profile. Of these, twenty-two employees showed evidence of pleural thickening and nineteen parenchymal asbestotic fibrosis.

Those employees showing pleural thickening gave a strong reaction to different skin tests and a few of those with parenchymal asbestotic fibrosis showed depressed cutaneous reactivity. Lymphocytotoxic antibodies were present in the sera of 60% of those with pleural thickening and 94% of those with parenchymal asbestosis.

An immunological screening schedule is suggested for those employees who show pleural thickening.

THE pathological changes which occur after exposure to asbestos are well known but the exact pathogenesis of the different lesions which occur is far from clear.

It was in order to establish the manner in which the different lesions developed that we suggested the working hypothesis shown in Fig. 1.

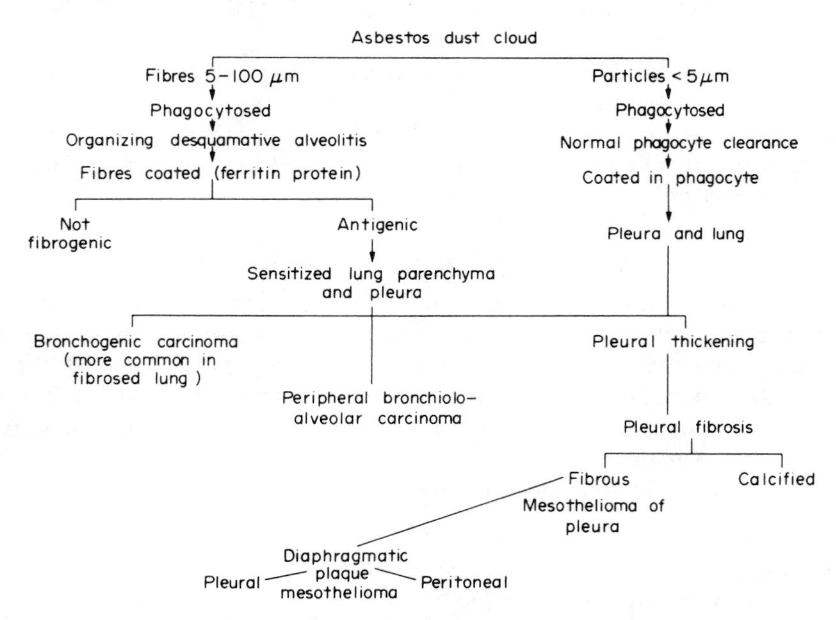

FIG. 1. Illustration of the working hypothesis.

* Presented by Dr. F. J. Wiles. See opening remarks to discussion, p. 433.

According to our hypothesis, fibres longer than 5μm enter the alveoli and cause a desquamative alveolitis, which becomes organized after lymphocytes enter the areas of alveolar desquamitis. In the macrophages or when the longer fibres become surrounded by macrophages, the fibres are coated with a ferritin protein complex. They are now no longer fibrogenic but with the coated material they may be capable of sensitizing the lung tissue to asbestos.

The particles which are less than 5 μm long are phagocytosed and coated but do not appear to damage the macrophage nor do they elicit a fibrogenic response. In the macrophages, however, they can move through the perivascular pathways of the lower respiratory tract and some are secreted into the junction of the terminal bronchioli and the respiratory bronchioli where they are further removed by ciliary action. Should the macrophage-clearing mechanism be blocked they will be found distributed in the perivascular tissue in the walls of the lower respiratory tract. The more peripheral macrophages move in the pleural lymphatics to the visceral and eventually to the parietal pleura where, if there is release of the coated small particles, an accentuated reaction will occur in the form of a localized fibrosis—the pleural plaque or areas of pleural thickening.

These foci of pleural thickening may calcify or remain fibrous. Should they remain fibrous in a few susceptible people a mesothelioma may develop.

There are indications that at least certain parts of this hypothesis are valid, as evidenced by morphologic studies in animals.

The desquamative alveolitis can be found in man but it is more evident in baboons exposed for a short period to asbestos dust. Organization of the alveolar spaces appears to be related to the presence of lymphocytes in the groups of cells in the alveoli.

The collagen which is laid down does not stain as normal collagen but has some of the staining characteristics of amyloid.

It is regretted that the full statistical analysis of the immunological tests is not available; however, it is hoped the information here presented will be of assistance to others working on similar lines.

MATERIALS AND METHODS

Three groups of individuals were examined clinically; they were also given lung function tests and a radiological examination including postero-anterior and oblique views. Delayed hypersensitivity skin tests were performed using purified protein derivative of *M. tuberculosis*, *Candida albicans* extract, streptokinase/streptodornase and 2, 4-dinitrochlorobenzene. A sensitizing dose of dinitrochlorobenzene in acetone was placed on the skin and allowed to dry.

Blood was taken for the following immunological assays:

1. Skin tests (CATALONA and CHRETIEN, 1973; KAGAN *et al.*, 1975).
2. Serum immunoglobulins (KAGAN *et al.*, 1975).
3. Secretory IgA (KAGAN *et al.*, 1975).
4. Percentage and absolute numbers of circulating T and B lymphocytes (BIANCO *et al.*, 1970; GAJL-PECZALSKA *et al.*, 1973; JONDAL *et al.*, 1972).
5. Lymphocyte transformation studies (SCHELLEKENS and EIJSVOOGEL, 1968).

6. Cytotoxicity of radiolabelled chicken erythrocytes and lymphoid cells (activated lymphoid killing (SHERWOOD and BLAESE, 1973).
7. Lymphocytotoxic antibodies in serum (DAUSSET *et al.*, 1968).
8. Anti-nuclear and rheumatoid factors in serum (VALKENBURG, 1963).

The patients tested were:

(a) *Forty-five controls*—the radiograph of the chest was normal and as far as could be ascertained there was no history of asbestos exposure. High kV X-rays were taken.

(b) *Twenty-two with pleural thickening* (*plaques*) with varying degrees of exposure to asbestos.

(c) *Nineteen with radiological evidence of parenchymal asbestosis*, again with varying degrees of asbestos exposure.

(d) *Cases of mesothelioma*—limited testing was carried out because it was necessary to start treatment (see p. 433, first item of Discussion).

IMMUNOLOGICAL RESULTS

Skin Tests

The reactions to purified protein derivative (PPD), *Candida albicans* extract and streptokinase/streptodornase (SK/SD) were strongly positive in those patients with pleural plaques but depressed in patients with parenchymal asbestosis. In the few cases of mesothelioma tested, the skin reactions were either negative or weakly positive.

In some patients with plaques the sensitizing dose of dinitrochlorobenzene (DNCB) gave a markedly positive result and in those in which the second application was required the reaction was strongly positive. However, there was a weaker reaction in those with parenchymal asbestosis.

Immunoglobulins

The average levels in the control group, those with plaques and those with parenchymal asbestosis are shown in Table 1. There is a significant increase in the levels of the immunoglobulins in parenchymal asbestosis which is not evident in the group with pleural plaques.

Although the percentage of B lymphocytes did not show any significant difference, the T lymphocytes showed a slight reduction in those cases with plaques and the cases of parenchymal asbestosis when the results were compared with the control group. The total lymphocyte count was lower in the parenchymal asbestosis than it was in those cases with pleural plaques. The PHA Transformation Assay was significantly lower in the groups with plaques than in the control and asbestotic groups.

Antibodies cytotoxic for lymphocytes were found in the sera of 94% of those patients with parenchymal asbestosis and in some 60% of those with pleural plaques.

Only an occasional positive result was found when the Human Erythrocyte Agglutination Test was carried out and a similar result was obtained with the Latex Test.

TABLE 1. IMMUNOGLOBULINS

		Plaques		Group controls		Asbestosis
		n=22		n=45		n=19
IgA	m	196.76		246.49		479.58
	s.d.	69.62		98.80		202.03
	P	←	0.05 (−)	→ ←	0.001 (+)	→
		←		0.001 (+)		→
IgG	m	1088.04		1290.73		1917.22
	s.d.	221.81		333.43		372.13
	P	←	0.05 (−)	→ ←	0.001 (+)	→
		←		0.001 (+)		→
IgM	m	146.44		149.27		216.94
	s.d.	61.63		56.15		83.84
	P	←	n.s.	→ ←	0.01 (+)	→
		←		0.01 (+)		→
IgA Secretory	m	14.50		12.07		24.11
	s.d.	10.05		6.53		11.67
	P	←	n.s.	→ ←	0.001 (+)	→
		←		0.01 (+)		→

n = number, m = mean, s.d. = standard deviation, P = probability, n.s. = not significant.

The preliminary results of these immunological studies indicate that the inhalation of asbestos causes a change in the immunological profile of the individual. Further work is required before the relationship of these changes to the different pathological manifestations of asbestos inhalation can be assessed.

REFERENCES

BIANCO, C., PATRICK, R. and NUSSENZWEIG, V. (1970) *J. exp. Med.* **132,** 702–720.

CATALONA, W. J. and CHRETIEN, P. B. (1973) *Cancer* **31,** 353–356.

DAUSSET, J., KOURILSKY, F., LEGRAND, L. and IVANYI, P. (1968) in *Manual of Tissue Typing Techniques*, pp. 1–2. Transplantation Immunology Branch, Collaborative Research, National Institute of Allergy and Infectious Diseases, National Institutes of Health, Bethesda, Maryland.

GAJL-PECZALSKA, K. J., LIM, S. D., JACOBSON, R. R. and GOOD, R. A. (1973) *New Engl. J. Med.* **288,** 1033–1035.

JONDAL, M., HOLM, G. and WIGZELL, H. (1972) *J. exp. Med.* **136,** 207–215.

KAGAN, E., SOSKOLNE, C. L., ZWI, S., HURWITZ, S., MAIER, G. M. G., IPP, T. and RABSON, A. R. (1975) *Am. Rev. resp. Dis.* **111,** 441–451.

SCHELLEKENS, P. TH. A. and EIJSVOOGEL, V. P. (1968) *Clin. exp. Immunol.* **3,** 571–584.

SHERWOOD, G. and BLAESE, R. M. (1973) *Clin. exp. Immunol.* **13,** 515–520.

VALKENBURG, H. A. (1963) in *The Epidemiology of Chronic Rheumatism* (edited by KELLGREN, J. H., JEFFREY, M. R. and BALL, J.), Vol. 1, pp. 330–333, 337–339. Blackwell, Oxford.

DISCUSSION

Dr Wiles: Professor Webster, who regrets that he was not able to present the paper himself, intended to add the following remarks: "The prognosis in cases of mesothelioma is so bleak that we felt the need to attempt some programme of treatment. It appears that with mesothelioma, even when the tumour load is probably insufficient to cause immunological depression, the skin reactions are weak or negative and there are other indications of a depressed immune state. This theory is the basis of a course of treatment using cytotoxic drugs as well as BCG with the aim of raising the level of the immune response. Ten cases have been treated so far, but at this stage it is only possible to give a general impression that some of them have lived longer than might have been expected."

J. C. McDonald: Before accepting the relation between immunological profile and clinical reaction as one of cause and effect one must consider whether the association might not have been due to selection of cases.

M. Turner-Warwick: The immunoglobulin results reported, especially the preferential increase in serum IgA are similar to our findings. Does secretory IgA refer to saliva or sputum measurements?

*Prof. Webster: The specimens were saliva.

M. Turner-Warwick: We too have found apparent depression of PHA, but in many cases this was related to low lymphocyte counts. When corrected for this, the PHA transformation returned to within the normal range in many cases.

The main differences between your study and our own concern antibodies cytotoxic to lymphocytes. In a separate study (Merchant *et al.*, 1975) we were unable to identify such antibodies in asbestos workers having a range of radiographic changes including pleural and parenchymal shadows. The differences between these two sets of results is likely to be due to technical points which we must now resolve.

J. M. G. Davis: The paper makes a statement to the effect that all asbestos fibres over 5 μm become coated to form asbestos (ferruginous) bodies. This is not in agreement with previous findings. Both in human lungs and lungs from experimental animals it has been reported that only a small minority of fibres ever become coated.

* Prof. Webster: I agree that there are a number of fibres which remain uncoated and in my opinion these fibres are still capable of causing a desquamative alveolitis leading to organization and therefore progression of the degree of fibrosis.

A. G. Heppleston: I support Dr Davis' statement that many of the fibres extracted from human asbestotic lungs are indeed uncoated and may well be pathogenic.

J. Bruch: I wonder whether the immunological changes are caused by the disease or are a sign of disposition to acquire asbestosis. The question is: post or propter?

M. Turner-Warwick: The question about whether immunological changes precede or result from asbestosis is crucial. The problem is difficult because the "beginning" of disease is unknown; it is certainly much earlier than the point at which radiological or clinical manifestations are detected.

The problem can only, I think, be resolved by longitudinal studies and since the progression of lung changes is often and perhaps usually much slower than is sometimes assumed, these studies will have to be prolonged.

P. Cole: The crux of the working hypothesis presented, as I see it, is the assumption that asbestos fibres become antigenic when coated with ferritin protein. The results presented, as an "immunological profile", on patients with pleural or parenchymal disease in no way *directly* support this assumption since no attempt seems to have been made to demonstrate *in vitro* sensitization to asbestos. The results show non-specific depression of delayed hypersensitivity (e.g. reduced PHA response) which may be due to factors entirely unrelated to the asbestos fibre itself, or to interference with the normal course of co-operative events in cell mediated events by the fibre (e.g. diminished macrophage function in the afferent limb of the immune response), but are unlikely to be due to asbestos sensitization itself.

* Prof. Webster: Asbestotic fibrosis in the form of an organized desquamative alveolitis does occur before the immunological profile is altered.

* Written reply.

TOPOGRAPHIC DISTRIBUTION OF ASBESTOS FIBRES IN HUMAN LUNG IN RELATION TO OCCUPATIONAL AND NON-OCCUPATIONAL EXPOSURE

P. SEBASTIEN,* A. FONDIMARE,‡ J. BIGNON,† G. MONCHAUX,*
J. DESBORDES‡ and G. BONNAUD*

Abstract—A topographic study of asbestos fibre content of lung and pleura of diversely exposed cases has been carried out.

For heavily exposed cases with lung fibrosis, this study has stressed the distinctive behaviour of the peripheral lower lobe in the retention of asbestos fibres in the lung. In these areas were found the smallest asbestos concentrations but the largest fibres.

For cases without lung fibrosis, the results clearly demonstrated an accumulation of asbestos fibres, especially of chrysotile type, in peripheral areas. These findings are to be related to the incidence of pleural mesothelioma associated with moderate or low exposure.

The small variation of fibre concentration in the pleural plaques of diversely exposed subjects is pointed out.

INTRODUCTION

The aetiological relationship between the inhalation of asbestos fibres and lung. carcinomas or pleural mesotheliomas is now well established (SELIKOFF *et al.*, 1965; SELIKOFF *et al.*, 1968).

Several epidemiological investigations and environmental measurement studies have indicated that we can find a wide range of asbestos exposures: from environmental to heavy occupational exposures.

Thus, in order to get information about the relationships between type of exposure, diseases and lung residues, it seems interesting to compare the concentrations of asbestos fibres in the different areas of lung parenchyma and in abnormal pleural tissue in subjects diversely exposed to asbestos.

MATERIALS AND METHODS

Selection of cases

This study, involving numerous tedious measurements, has been carried out only on a small number of representative autopsy cases. All the subjects had been living and

* Direction Générale de l'Action Sanitaire et Sociale de Paris.
† Centre Hospitalier Intercommunal de Créteil.
‡ Centre Hospitalier du Havre.

working in the Le Havre area. Occupational inquiries were made by the same team of physicians to establish the duration of asbestos exposure, the number of years from the last exposure and the type of asbestos fibres handled.

Three groups were selected: six asbestos workers with heavy exposure (group I); six subjects who had handled small amounts of asbestos during their professional life (group II); six randomly chosen cases from a series of fifty consecutive autopsies; there was no known asbestos exposure history for these cases (group III).

Pathological study

In all cases, a complete autopsy was carried out, looking carefully for asbestos associated diseases. The degree of lung fibrosis (0 to 4) was evaluated by one of us.

Sampling

After formaldehyde fixation by intratracheal instillation, four blocks of parenchyma were sampled in different sites of the same lung. In case of associated lesions, the less involved lung was chosen. Blocks were sampled according to the following topography:

Central upper lobe (CUL).
Peripheral upper lobe (PUL).
Central lower lobe (CLL).
Peripheral lower lobe (PLL).

When present, parietal pleural plaques, calcified or not, were sampled under the same conditions.

Light microscope study

Samples of a known volume were digested by NaClO. The dissolution product was filtered through a Millipore membrane and examined under 400× magnification using the phase contrast method.

For cases with heavy exposure, the number of coated and uncoated fibres was estimated by a method of randomized examination. It consisted in observing a sufficient number of randomly selected areas in order to obtain the desired accuracy. For that purpose, data from the observation of each field were simultaneously registered by a computer controlling the validity of the sampling by the cumulative means method (SCHROEDER and MUNZEL-PEDRAZZOLI, 1970). The accepted accuracy was 10% of the mean value.

In cases with moderate or no exposure, the whole filter area was examined.

Results were expressed as fibre number per cubic centimetre of fixed lung parenchyma or of pleural tissue.

Electron microscope study

Two electron microscope studies were carried out using different methods:

(i) After chemical "digestion" of a large amount of lung tissue, particulate matter was concentrated by centrifugation. After re-suspension in water, a drop was allowed to dry on a formvar-coated grid. The morphology and diffraction pattern of fibres were obtained after examination under electron microscope Sopelem 75.

(ii) In order to obtain quantitative data, samples were prepared in the following manner: a known volume of lung parenchyma "digested" by NaClO was filtered through a Nuclepore membrane of 0.4 μm pore size. After carbon-coating, small pieces of filter were directly transferred onto electron microscope grids (FRANK *et al.*, 1970).

About 20 squares of 200 mesh grids were examined under a JEOL 100 C electron microscope at a direct magnification of $\times$ 30 000. For each site, several grids were counted and their length and diameter were measured.

RESULTS

Epidemiological and Pathological Data

The data concerning age, sex, duration of exposure, number of years since the last exposure and smoking habits are listed in Table 1. Otherwise, the pathology of the lung is indicated in terms of five grades of fibrosis, and associated diseases are listed as bronchogenic carcinoma (BC), pleural mesothelioma (M), cancer of stomach (SC), cancer of pancreas (PC), breast cancer (Bt C), acute pancreatitis (AP) and laryngeal carcinoma (LC) (see Table 1).

TABLE 1. ASBESTOS EXPOSURE AND DISEASES

	Case	Sex	Age	Years of exposure	Years from last exposure	Smoking habits	Grade of fibrosis	Disease*
Group I	1	M	64	34	4	0	4	BC
	2	M	64	33	3	+	4	BC
	3	F	63	9	10	0	2	BC
	4	F	39	3	20	0	1	M
	5	M	54	6	5	+++	1	BC
	6	M	58	0.5	30	0	0	BC
Group II	7	M	64	10	10	+	0	M
	8	M	68	13	42	++	1	LC
	9	M	53	30	6	0	0	BC
	10	M	54	37	0	++	0	BC
	11	M	64	occas.	?	0	0	BC
	12	M	42	17	0	++	0	M
Group III	13	M	71	0	0	+++	0	BC
	14	M	59	0	0	0	0	BC
	15	F	61	0	0	0	0	Bt C
	16	F	73	0	0	0	0	AP
	17	M	67	0	0	0	0	PC
	18	M	57	0	0	+++	0	SC

* See text for explanation.

Light Microscope Study of Pulmonary and Pleural Asbestos Fibre Content

Lung parenchyma

Pulmonary fibre concentration was expressed as number of fibres per cubic centimetre of lung parenchyma. For groups I, II and III, mean concentrations were, respectively, 2×10^6, 2×10^3 and 2×10^2. Cases of groups I and II showed both coated fibres (CF) and uncoated fibres (UF). For cases of group III, only coated fibres were found under light microscope examination.

For each site in the lung, a local concentration index (LCI) was calculated. LCI is defined as the ratio of the concentration at one site to the mean concentration in the four sites. Values of LCI are listed in Table 2. For cases of group I, LCI mean values were significantly higher in peripheral areas than in central areas. There was no significant difference in upper and lower lobe concentrations. In groups II and III no significant difference occurred in the different site concentrations (peripheral *vs.* central or upper *vs.* lower). For all cases of the three groups, mean value of LCI in the peripheral lower lobe was significantly higher than the mean value of LCI for the three other sites together (1.24 *vs.* 0.92).

Proportions of coated fibres in each site are listed in Table 2. In all but one case of group I, the highest values systematically occurred in the peripheral lower lobe. Examination of mean values for groups I and II showed that proportion of coated fibres was higher in peripheral areas, but these findings had no statistical significance.

In all cases, the average length was significantly higher for coated fibres than for uncoated fibres. Inside the lung, there was no relation between the average length of the fibres and the sampling site. The mean length of CF in groups I, II and III was, respectively, 51, 45 and 37 μm. These values were significantly different.

Pleura. Coated fibres were found in all the samples of pleural plaques (see Table 2). They were shorter than those found in lung parenchyma (average length of 28 μm). Concentrations ranged from 5 to 300 CF per cm^3 of pleural plaque.

Qualitative Findings by Electron Microscopy

Lung parenchyma

In all cases, asbestos fibre content of samples in the peripheral lower lobe (PLL) was studied. The method of sample preparation is described in an earlier section (p. 436(i)).

Asbestos fibres were found in every case of each group. Though this method was not suitable for good quantitative evaluation, it has been estimated that ultramicroscopic fibres readily outnumbered optically visible ones.

Most cases had been exposed to both amphibole and chrysotile fibres. In cases where observations were made a long time after onset of exposure, amphibole fibres were more commonly found than chrysotile. Bundles of chrysotile could be seen, but statistically, ultimate chrysotile fibrils were more numerous.

In most cases, the central fibre of asbestos bodies was of amphibole type.

Pleura. Asbestos fibres were found in all samples of pleural plaques, chrysotile being the variety most commonly found. Most fibres were short ultimate fibrils.

TABLE 2. LIGHT MICROSCOPE STUDY

	Case	Fibre contents of the lung (no. per cm³)	LCI				Proportion of CF (%)				PP	No. of CF per cm³ of PP
			PUL	CUL	PLL	CLL	PUL	CUL	PLL	CLL		
Group I	1	4.3×10^6	1.12	0.68	1.36	0.84	69	50	67	53	+	90
	2	4.1×10^6	1.04	0.80	1.36	0.80	47	48	55	45	+	250
	3	1.5×10^6	1.00	1.12	1.00	0.88	52	29	67	61	+	315
	4	3×10^5	0.76	0.72	1.44	1.12	81	67	84	73	+	180
	5	1×10^5	1.20	0.80	1.28	0.76	25	23	29	20	0	
	6	6.8×10^4	1.04	1.08	1.24	0.64	43	27	44	38	+	25
Mean		2×10^6	1.04	0.84	1.28	0.84	53	41	58	48		126
Group II	7	7×10^3	0.88	0.84	1.48	0.80	89	85	71	73	+	5
	8	4.5×10^3	0.84	1.36	1.24	0.56	79	88	80	80	+	5
	9	1.1×10^3	0.80	0.52	1.56	1.16	78	67	85	77	0	
	10	7.8×10^3	0.72	1.48	0.96	0.84	73	39	67	55	+	0
	11	4.7×10^2	0.64	1.68	0.68	1.00	85	88	77	68	+	—
	12	3.2×10^2	0.68	0.52	1.60	1.16	45	41	48	45	+	20
Mean		2×10^3	0.76	1.08	1.24	0.92	74	68	71	66		
Group III	13	140	0.40	1.36	0.84	1.36					0	
	14	84	1.32	1.44	0.88	0.36					0	
	15	84	1.44	0.36	1.56	0.64		100			0	
	16	65	0.24	1.40	1.52	0.84					0	
	17	55	0.92	0.36	2.28	0.44					+	8
	18	54	0.56	2.40	0.36	0.64					0	
Mean		10^2	0.80	1.24	1.24	0.72						

Quantitative Findings by Electron Microscopy

A quantitative study was carried out in the four lung parenchyma sites, in five cases of group I and five cases of group II. The study is still in progress for cases of group III. For each site, number concentration and fibre size distribution (length and diameter) have been established. The method (p. 437) allowed expression of weight concentration and estimation of the surface of the fibres in the lung.

Results clearly demonstrated that the light microscope method was suitable for CF examination and that the electron microscope was the only practical instrument for assessing the asbestos fibre content of tissues. Indeed, as indicated in Table 3, the mean proportions of optically visible fibres in the whole lung were 10% for cases of group I and less than 1% for cases of group II.

TABLE 3. PROPORTION OF OPTICALLY VISIBLE FIBRES IN DIFFERENT SITES AFTER LIGHT AND ELECTRON MICROSCOPE EXAMINATION (Results expressed in %)

	Case	PUL	CUL	PLL	CLL	Mean value in the lung
Group 1	1	6	9	25	4	11
	2	6	18	37	18	20
	3	6	3	14	7	8
	4	6	4	23	4	9
	5	4	3	7	3	4
Mean		6	7	21	7	10
Group II	7	0.20	0.60	0.70	0.50	0.50
	8	0.04	0.15	0.41	0.20	0.20
	10	0.15	0.50	0.20	0.20	0.26
	11	0.01	0.10	0.01	0.07	0.05
	12	0.01	0.03	0.06	0.09	0.05
Mean		0.08	0.28	0.28	0.21	0.21

The proportion of optically visible fibres according to the different locations in the two groups is also indicated in Table 3. The proportion was higher for cases of group I. In this group, optically visible fibres were significantly more numerous in the peripheral lower lobe (PLL). For cases of group II, the proportion of optically visible fibres was still important in PLL location, but highest values of this proportion did not systematically occur in PLL location as for cases of group I. In group II, lowest proportion of optically visible fibres always occurred in PUL location.

For each sample, concentrations of fibres visible under the electron microscope have been added to concentrations of optically visible fibres and new values of LCI have been calculated (see Table 4). For cases of group I, mean values of LCI were significantly higher in upper lobe. The lowest value was observed in PLL location. In group II no statistically significant difference occurred between upper lobe and lower lobe values,

TABLE 4. VALUES OF LCI BY LIGHT AND ELECTRON MICROSCOPE EXAMINATION

	Case	PUL	CUL	PLL	CLL
Group I	1	1.39	0.63	0.44	1.54
	2	2.32	0.61	0.47	0.61
	3	0.82	2.20	0.35	0.63
	4	0.73	1.22	0.38	1.68
	5	1.33	0.94	0.75	0.98
Mean		1.32	1.12	0.48	1.09
Group II	7	1.74	0.60	0.96	0.69
	8	2.21	1.10	0.35	0.34
	10	0.42	0.26	2.94	0.38
	11	0.42	0.26	2.94	0.38
	12	2.53	0.48	0.63	0.36
Mean		1.59	0.57	1.40	0.43

but results clearly demonstrated an accumulation of asbestos fibres in peripheral areas.

The proportions of chrysotile related to the whole asbestos content of the lung are shown in Table 5, separately for number, surface area and weight of fibres. For chrysotile, the proportion of surface area concentration is higher than the weight concentration because of the specific surface of chrysotile fibres being superior to the

TABLE 5. PERCENTAGE OF CHRYSOTILE OF THE TOTAL ASBESTOS CONTENT IN LUNG PARENCHYMA FOR THE FOUR SITES (N : number; S : surface; W : weight)

	Case	PUL			CUL			PLL			CLL		
		N	S	W	N	S	W	N	S	W	N	S	W
Group I	1	3	1	1	14	7	2	24	3	1	22	6	2
	2	30	12	6	26	13	7	48	19	9	26	9	2
	3	—	—	—	8	2	1	—	—	—	—	—	
	4	53	48	25	69	52	25	80	40	20	54	38	29
	5	7	3	1	1	—	—	2	—	—	—	—	—
Mean		19	13	7	24	15	7	31	12	6	21	11	7
Group II	7	44	16	7	26	17	4	54	21	14	34	11	6
	8	95	67	44	73	46	43	8	35	29	44	12	7
	10	53	15	6	31	7	1	96	77	63	58	68	59
	11	93	97	93	94	84	70	97	95	90	89	79	64
	12	97	99	99	59	66	64	60	40	33	40	63	56
Mean		76	59	50	57	44	37	63	54	46	53	47	38
Mean for Groups I + II		48	36	28	40	29	22	47	33	26	37	29	27

specific surface of amphibole. In most cases of group I, more than 50% of the asbestos fibre surface area in the lung was due to amphibole fibres. When chrysotile was present, it preferentially occurred in PLL location.

All the cases of group II contained chrysotile fibres in their lung. For three cases the proportion of chrysotile was more than 90% and for two cases this proportion was about 50%.

The mean proportions of chrysotile were significantly higher in peripheral than in central areas. Examination of mean values for the two groups confirmed the preferential occurrence of chrysotile in the peripheral area. This difference was more evident when considering number proportion than weight proportion.

Length and diameter distributions of fibres have been established by measuring more than 5000 fibres. All the fibres seen under the electron microscope were less than 0.5 μm in diameter. The proportion of fibres shorter than 5 μm ranged from 70% to 90%.

DISCUSSION

Asbestos Burden in Lung and Pleura

The concentrations measured by light microscopy in subjects of group I and group II are similar to those previously published (ASHCROFT and HEPPLESTON, 1973; FONDIMARE and DESBORDES, 1974). The findings of CF in the lung of all cases of group III agree with previous results (BIGNON *et al.*, 1970). The light microscope study revealed only 10% of the total lung storage in heavily exposed subjects, and even less (0.20%) in the other groups. Results showed that submicroscopic fibres concentration was in the same range for groups I and II ($10^7/cm^3$ for group I and $10^6/cm^3$ for group II), although light microscope examination revealed a more important difference between the two groups ($10^6/cm^3$ for group I and $10^3/cm^3$ for group II). This optical method can be used for a first screening but is unsuitable to study dose–effect relationship in asbestos-related carcinogenesis.

On the other hand, variations between different locations are small compared to the mean concentration of fibres in the lung. Thus, the study of only one block of the peripheral lower lobe, where the proportion of optically visible fibres is highest, is enough for a first screening by light microscopy.

Optical and electron microscope studies of the pleural plaques constantly revealed the presence of coated and uncoated fibres, but with much less variations between the three groups than in lung parenchyma.

These smaller variations might indicate that the number of fibres reaching the pleura is more or less similar whatever the asbestos content in the lung. The fibres encountered in pleura are frequently of chrysotile variety which is very fragmented and short. This preferential localization of asbestos fibres in pleura for a small amount of dust in lungs might explain the occurrence of non-occupational mesothelioma in subjects living in the vicinity of asbestos mines or factories (NEWHOUSE, 1973). Nevertheless, the presence of short fibres in the pleural plaques suggests the pathological effects of these fibres should be further studied in humans (GROSS, 1974; MILLER *et al.*, 1975).

Topographic Variations

Depending on topography, the results for the two groups must be analysed separately.

For cases of group I, results showed a predominance of fibres in the upper lobes; this difference was not observed for cases of group II. Moreover, for cases of group I, the higher proportion of optically visible fibres in lower lobe and especially in PLL indicated a higher concentration of large fibres in these areas.

Several explanations for these findings can be given:

Lung fibrosis was present in all cases of group I, whereas in group II only one patient showed a moderate lung fibrosis. The predominance of fibrosis in lower lobes could influence retention of fibres in these areas.

Zonal clearance varying with lung storage and physical parameters of fibres; it could be expected that aerosol inhaled by patients of group I had a greater concentration of large fibres.

The predominance of dust in the apical parts of the lung has also been found in silicosis and coal-workers' pneumoconiosis (Parkes, 1974). In asbestosis, the predominance of fibrosis in lower lobes might be explained by the larger size of the fibres in these areas.

In group II, results clearly demonstrated an accumulation of asbestos fibres, especially of chrysotile type, in peripheral areas. These findings are to be related to the occurrence of pleural mesothelioma associated with moderate or low asbestos exposure.

Proportion of Chrysotile Fibres

The cases showed various mixtures of amphibole and chrysotile fibres. Although chrysotile was mostly found as ultimate fibrils, bundles of chrysotile were encountered in the different sampling sites. These findings suggest that in spite of the impediment for chrysotile bundles to be inhaled (Timbrell, 1972), such fibres were found in the deep parts of the lung. Bundles of chrysotile were more commonly observed among cases recently exposed to asbestos. Nevertheless, generally, ultimate fibrils readily outnumbered bundles. These findings support rather than contradict the work of Pooley 1972).

Acknowledgement—The technical assistance of Mme Colombel, Mme Naissant, Mlle Moineau and Mr Janson is gratefully acknowledged.

REFERENCES

Ashcroft, T. and Heppleston, A. G. (1973) *J. clin. Path.* **26**, 224–234.

Bignon, J., Goni, J., Bonnaud, G., Jaurand, M. C., Dufour, G. and Pinchon, M. C. (1970) *Envir. Res.* **3**, 430–442.

Fondimare, A. and Desbordes, J. (1974) *Envir. Hlth Perspect.* **9**, 147–148.

Frank, E. R., Spurny, K. R., Sheesley, D. C. and Lodge, J. P. (1970) *J. Microsc. (France)* **9**, 735–740.

Gross, P. (1974) *Archs envir. Hlth* **29**, 115–117.

Miller, A., Langer, A. M., Teirstein, A. S. and Selikoff, I. J. (1975) *New Engl. J. Med.* **292**, 91–93.

NEWHOUSE, M. L. (1973) *Ann. occup. Hyg.* **16,** 97–102.
PARKES, W. R. (Editor) (1974) *Occupational Lung Disorders.* Butterworth, London.
POOLEY, F. D. (1972) *Br. J. ind. Med.* **29,** 146–153.
SCHROEDER, H. E. and MUNZEL-PEDRAZZOLI, S. (1970) *J. Microscopy* **92,** 179–198.
SELIKOFF, I. J., CHURG, J. and HAMMOND, E. C. (1965) *New Engl. J. Med.* **272,** 560–565.
SELIKOFF, I. J., HAMMOND, E. C. and CHURG, J. (1968) *J. Am. med. Ass.* **204,** 106–112.
TIMBRELL, V. (1972) *Assessment of Airborne Particles* (edited by MERCER, T. T., MORROW, P. E., and STÖBER, W.) p. 429. Thomas, Springfield, Ill.

DISCUSSION

J. C. McDONALD: Since the results are based on a small number of subjects, their selection seem important. What do you mean when you state that the autopsy groups were "representative"?

M. SEBASTIEN: Cases were randomly chosen in the same hospital from a series of consecutive autopsies of people with and without asbestos exposure. All the subjects had been living and working in Le Havre, and asbestos exposure inquiries were made by the same team of physicians.

M. JACOBSEN: Was the selection of cases for groups I and II made before or after the autopsies and pathological studies?

M. SEBASTIEN: The selection was made before.

K. ROBOCK: What method did you use to identify the fibre? I think the only satisfactory method is to analyse each single fibre with the electron microscope. I am very doubtful about using the diffraction method in this case.

M. SEBASTIEN: The identification of chrysotile fibres by means of their morphological features and single crystal electron diffraction pattern has been described by many authors to be very reliable, because of the cylindrical lattice of this mineral. With amphibole fibres, it is very easy to get electron diffraction patterns. In this case, because of the very large numbers of reflections, it is quite impossible to distinguish between the different varieties of amphibole, but general features of the pattern are specific of amphibole asbestos.

For this study, more than 5000 fibres have been counted, measured and identified as chrysotile or amphibole by means of their single-crystal electron diffraction pattern.

K. ROBOCK: What is the percentage of asbestos fibres of the total amount of all types of fibres?

M. SEBASTIEN: Cases of groups I and II had occupational or para-occupational exposure and asbestos fibres readily outnumbered non-asbestos ones. For the cases of group III, non-asbestos fibres have been found but not analysed; this problem has been previously investigated by Dr DAVIS and Dr GROSS.

L. LE BOUFFANT: You indicate that there is a difference in the length of the fibres found in the lung and the pleura. Our own observations do not show a significant difference as far as the visceral pleura is concerned; on the contrary, the fibres found in the parietal pleura are on the average much shorter. It would therefore be useful to know if your observations concern the visceral pleura or the parietal pleura.

M. SEBASTIEN: We were talking about the parietal pleural plaques.

M. NAVRATIL: You have shown that only small particles are to be found in pleural plaques. We have proved in our autopsied cases of asbestosis with pleural plaques that only small asbestos bodies can be found in pleural hyalinosis in the parietal pleura; also, we have found isolated ferruginous materials in the collagenous tissue of the plaques. We suggest that this shows that the remains of destroyed asbestos bodies penetrate the fibrous formation of the pleura. What is your opinion?

M. SEBASTIEN: I agree with you, because in cases of group I with lung fibrosis, we have observed a higher concentration of large fibres and coated fibres in subpleural areas and especially in the peripheral lower lobe. As coated fibres remain a long time in these areas, they may break up and ferruginous material reach the pleura.

R. HUNT: Unless all organic structures are removed by low-temperature ashing technique, it is virtually impossible to detect the optical properties of asbestos fibre.

M. SEBASTIEN: I agree with you that we must be very careful in using light microscopy for assessing asbestos fibres in tissues; only trained people can recognize asbestos fibres in light microscopy using their optical properties. Concerning the preparation method, the digestive procedure seems to be very convenient for qualitative and quantitative analysis.

W. SMITHER: You note the common presence of chrysotile fibres in pleural plaques and comment that this is "in spite of the difficult inhalation of chrysotile reported by Timbrell". You also call these "short, ultimate fibrils".

I suggest that not all chrysotile is "curly". There is such a thing as "harsh" chrysotile. Can you comment on the proportion of fine straight harsh chrysotile in the dust cloud originally inhaled by your subjects?

M. SEBASTIEN: For this retrospective study, it was not possible to take air samples to determine the proportion of fine, straight, harsh chrysotile in the dust cloud originally inhaled by the subjects, but such fibres have been found in their lungs.

This study shows that numerous chrysotile fibres—not only ultimate fibrils but also bundles of chrysotile—can penetrate into the deep regions of the lung. We did not observe significant differences. in gravimetric concentration of chrysotile in the different sites of lung parenchyma studied. However, in the peripheral areas the numerical concentration was higher. This might be explained by the fact that chrysotile fibres could have been broken up or longitudinally split in these areas.

V. TIMBRELL: Though it may be difficult for inhaled chrysotile fibres to reach the pleural regions, statistically a small proportion will do so. This type of asbestos can split longitudinally in lung fluids and a fibre 1 μm in diameter may produce as many as a thousand fibrils (number inversely proportional to the square of the diameter). Penetration of a small number of fibrils to the pleura in the first instance can therefore result in a large number of fibres (fibrils) being subsequently recorded in this region.

L. MAGOS: You have found the accumulation of large fibres in the peripheral lower lobe, and also in the subpleural region. This finding is in agreement with that of Dr Morgan (p. 259), who, in animal experiments, found fibrous material mainly in this region after a time delay.

M. SEBASTIEN: Yes, we think that it is a very important point. In every case without lung fibrosis, this topographic study has shown an accumulation of asbestos and especially of chrysotile asbestos in the subpleural areas. By contrast, in cases with severe lung fibrosis, this difference was not found, but a striking fact was the highest percentage (21%) of optically visible fibres in peripheral area of fibrotic lower lobe.

THE BIOLOGICAL EFFECT OF ASBESTOS AND ASBESTOS CEMENT PRODUCTS

K. Robock and W. Klosterkötter

Institut für Hygiene und Arbeitsmedizin des Klinikum der Universität, Essen

Abstract—The importance of the physical characteristics, rather than the chemical composition of fibres, in relation to their alveolar deposition and biological effects is stressed. For alveolar deposition the aerodynamic properties—depending on the fibre diameter—are decisive, whereas in the interaction between macrophages and fibres, fibre length is the decisive factor for cytotoxicity. Probably fibre length could, *inter alia*, be responsible for a pathogenic effect around the lung tissue. The results from measurements of the cytotoxicity of the UICC standard asbestos dusts and pure cement dust are presented and discussed.

INTRODUCTION

Numerous investigations have been carried out by different research institutes into the biological effects of fibrous dusts in lungs (Bogovski *et al.*, 1973; Pelnar, 1974; Pott and Friedrichs, 1972; Reeves *et al.*, 1974; Stanton and Wrench, 1972; Stanton, 1972; Wagner *et al.*, 1974; and others). The results indicate that the cytotoxic, fibrogenic and carcinogenic reactions are based on special characteristics of respirable fibres—probably a mechanical irritation—and not on their chemical composition or their molecular structure (electron structure). Geometric dimensions (diameter and length), elastic properties and insolubility in biological environment are to be understood as the defined characteristics.

In the very extensive inhalation experiment of Wagner *et al.* (1974) with the five U.I.C.C. standard asbestos reference samples, no differences were found between amphibole and serpentine asbestos dusts with regard to their fibrogenic and carcinogenic effects. Reeves *et al.* (1974) as well as Stanton and Wrench (1972) and Stanton (1972) came to the same conclusion. Recent analyses of compensated asbestosis cases between 1968 and 1973 among asbestos mine workers in South Africa by Baunach *et al.* (unpublished) indicate that in the Cape Province where exclusively crocidolite is obtained, only 0.22% of interstitial fibrosis cases have been diagnosed against 0.68% in Transvaal where mainly amosite and chrysotile are obtained. Autopsy diagnoses confirmed the same relationship. All these results disprove the special risk of crocidolite. According to the investigations of Stanton and Wrench (1972), Stanton (1972), Pott and Friedrichs (1972) and Smith (1974), glass fibres, ceramic fibres and fibres of minerals other than asbestos may cause similar pathogenic reactions.

Consequently, the mineral of asbestos cannot of itself be considered as hazardous to health, but generally all single fibres with the above-mentioned characteristics and able to reach the lung alveoli must be presumed hazardous.

Whether fibres are respirable and presumably are deposited in the alveolar area depends on their aerodynamic diameter. This is defined by the geometric diameter of the fibres and their density, and is almost independent of length. This explains why fibres with a length of 100 μm and more have been found in the lung tissue of humans and animals (TIMBRELL *et al.*, 1970) and that, on the other hand, only fibres with a geometric diameter smaller than about 3 μm can reach the alveolar area. Thicker fibres or fibre bundles cannot be inhaled or will be deposited in the mouth/nose area, or in the bronchial area, from which they will be more or less rapidly eliminated. For dusts from asbestos cement products, it is of great importance to take the aerodynamic properties into account. Depending on the type of product and the treatment, we mostly find aggregates consisting of fibres and fibre bundles covered with cement. By selecting certain processing methods, the development of single fibres which can be inhaled into the alveolar area could be reduced and the risk to health be almost excluded.

Finally, after deposition in the alveolar area, the interaction between fibres and macrophages begins. According to our investigations and to those of BECK *et al.* (1971), fibres with lengths smaller than 5 μm become totally incorporated by the macrophages as the spherical equivalent diameter of the macrophages varies between 12 μm and 25 μm. These fibres can be eliminated from the lungs through the macrophages. The results of investigations indicate that these short fibres are neither cytotoxic nor carcinogenic. But if fibres are present which are too long to be totally incorporated by the macrophages, damage of the macrophage membrane will occur. Consequently, the macrophages lose their mobility, elimination from the alveolar area is hindered and the fibres, finally, penetrate the lung tissue. These proceedings in the alveolar area plausibly explain the damaging effect of fibres longer than about 10 μm. In Great Britain this fibre length was initially taken for the lower limit and later—as a factor of safety—reduced by 50% to 5 μm and included in the regulations.

Our own investigations are at present concerned with the cytotoxicity of fibrous dusts, because any penetration of fibres into the lung tissue depends on the interaction of fibres causing damage to macrophages. To what extent additional co-factors, i.e. metal ions or substances adsorbed on the fibre surface, can be a secondary cause of carcinogenic reactions cannot yet be explained.

CYTOTOXICITY OF U.I.C.C. STANDARD ASBESTOS DUSTS

Stereoscan photographs (Fig. 1) of alveolar macrophages after incubation with fibres show how at the point where the fibre departs from the macrophage, the cell membrane places itself around the fibre like a sleeve. According to BECK *et al.* (1971), this incomplete incorporation causes an increased permeability of the cell membrane at the point of exit of the fibre, and thus a chronic stimulus to the cell. A continuous loss of enzymes (LDH) has been biochemically proved (BECK *et al.*, 1971). An increased lactate production is the sign of an energetic compensation of the loss of enzymes (BECK *et al.*, 1971). A lysis of cells follows inevitably.

Figure 2 depicts the depression of the oxygen consumption of alveolar macrophages without and after incubation with the five U.I.C.C. standard asbestos samples. The

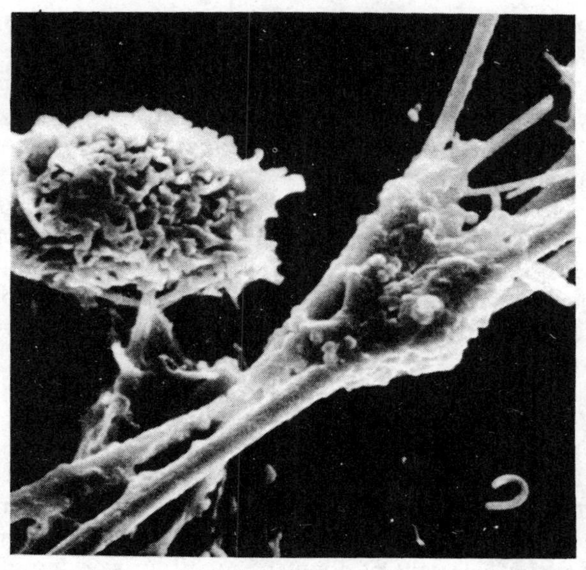

FIG. 1. Stereoscan photograph of alveolar macrophages after incubation with fibres.

polarographic method used in this case is described in another publication (ROBOCK, 1974). The depression of the TTC-reduction activity of the macrophages shows a similar pattern (ROBOCK and KLOSTERKÖTTER, 1971). The two chrysotiles A and B show a much stronger cytotoxic effect (B a little stronger than A) than the three amphibole fibre types. The latter do not differ in their cytotoxic properties. Similar relation-

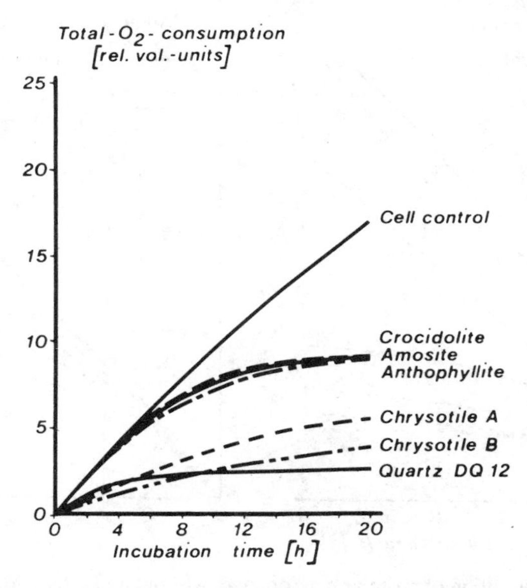

FIG. 2. Oxygen consumption of alveolar macrophages without and after addition of U.I.C.C. standard asbestos dust and quartz DQ 12 as a function of the incubation period.

ships have been found for the fibrogenicity in intratracheal and intraperitoneal tests with rats in our Institute. The results agree with those of the above-mentioned inhalation experiments of WAGNER *et al.* (1974) considering the lower respirability of the two chrysotiles according to TIMBRELL (1972), and the greater leaching from this type of asbestos in the lung. This explains why all five dusts showed the same fibrogenic reaction in these inhalation experiments.

The stronger cytotoxicity of the two chrysotiles can also be explained as follows: in a biological nutrient solution (pH = 7.2) separation of 0.24% magnesium (chrysotile A) and 0.38% magnesium (chrysotile B) after 1 h has been proved. This leads to a shift of the pH value into a range (7.7 and 8.8 respectively) which cannot be endured by the cells and an additional toxic effect is caused. This is not valid for the three amphibole fibre types.

CYTOTOXICITY OF THE DUST OF ASBESTOS CEMENT PRODUCTS

In preparation for animal tests with dusts of different asbestos cement products, first test measurements were made of their cytotoxicity. For this, samples have been collected with a membrane filter unit (EM 100 (Gravikon); Sartorius, Göttingen) with an air speed of 0.8 m/s at a height of about 1.5 m at four working sites (A, B, C, D) at different processing points in an asbestos cement factory. Additional samples were taken in the raw asbestos (E) and cement (F) stores. Samples contained chrysotile only; 7% in asbestos cement dust A, 5% in dust B, 2% in dust C and 5% in dust D. The investigations on free fibres and their lengths and diameter distribution in the samples

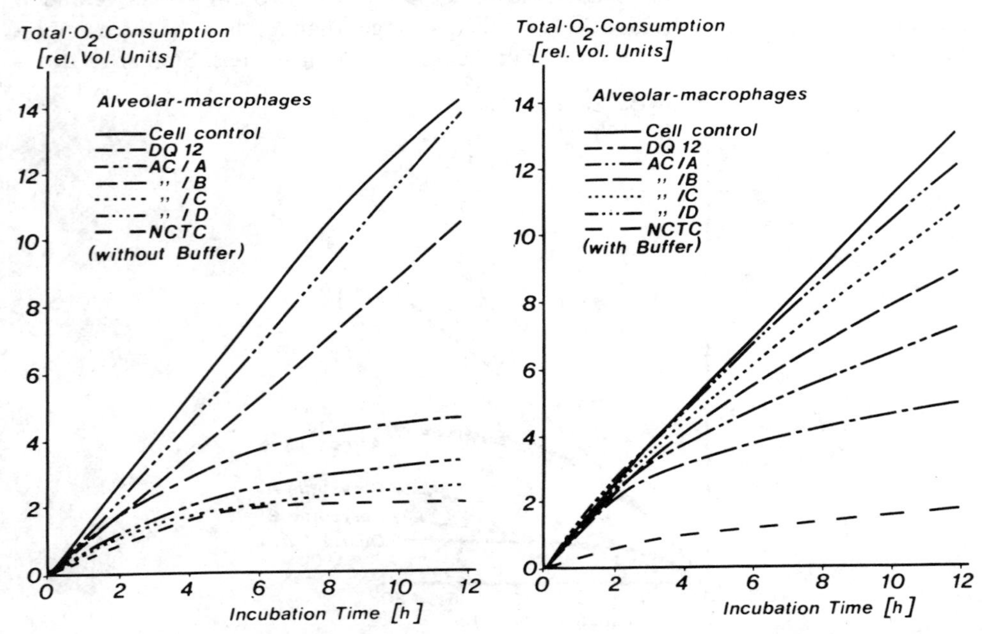

FIG. 3. Oxygen consumption of alveolar macrophages without and after addition of four asbestos cement dusts and quartz DQ 12 as a function of the incubation period (NCTC = normal buffered nutrient solution). (a) Without additional buffer. (b) With additional buffer.

have not yet been completed. The results of the polarographic measurements of the oxygen consumption of alveolar macrophages under the same conditions as the U.I.C.C samples are depicted in Fig. 3a.

A normal buffered nutrient solution (NCTC) was used. One recognizes that under these conditions the samples A and C appear more cytotoxic than the standard quartz DQ 12. Simultaneously, a substantial shift of the pH value in the suspension was seen, i.e. from 6.9 for the basic solution to 10.2 (dust A), 9.66 (dust B), 10.3 (dust C) and 8.7 (dust D). No explanation can as yet be given. Probably the cement plays an essential part, as will be indicated later. By suspension of dust samples in titrisol buffer (pH = 7) we were able to avoid the pH shift. The results (Fig. 3b) show that this additional

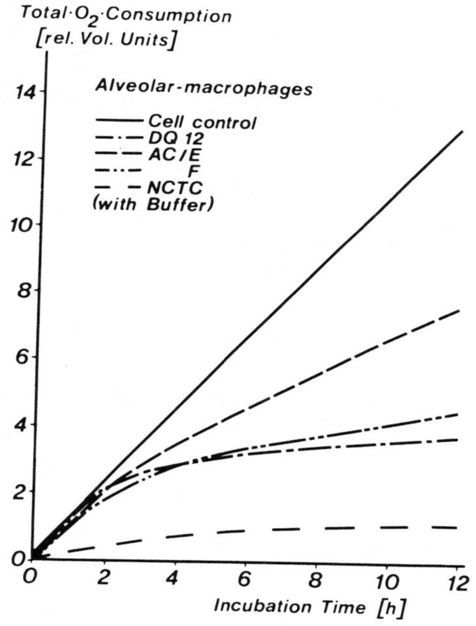

FIG. 4. Oxygen consumption of alveolar macrophages without and after addition of chrysotile (E) and cement (F) as well as quartz DQ 12 as a function of the incubating period (with additional buffer).

buffering strongly affects dust C and also dust A, but not dusts B and D which are of minimal cytotoxicity anyway. The cytotoxic effect of dust A and especially of dust C became much weaker. In order to avoid false interpretations, the cell test, therefore, has to be handled critically. It is obvious that the dust samples react differently in regard to the biological effects. This may be due to the product itself, but also to different treatment, i.e. drilling, sawing, cutting.

Figure 4 depicts the results with the basic asbestos (chrysotile) and the fine dust of cement. Chrysotile influences the oxygen consumption in the same relation as the U.I.C.C. standard chrysotile to quartz DQ 12. The cement dust appears rather cytotoxic so that this influence has to be also considered in connection with the results of Fig. 3b.

In consequence of these first test results in all cell experimental investigations with asbestos cement dusts, not only the influence of Mg ions (pH value shift) but additionally the influence of cement has to be considered. Results from animal experiments suggest that cement particles probably become rapidly dissolved and thus eliminated. The question is whether the cell experiment can deliver a definitive answer on the toxicity of those asbestos cement dusts. We have to wait for the results of corresponding animal experiments and also for those of further cell experiments.

REFERENCES

BAUNACH, F., WILES, F. J. and SOSKOLNE, C. L. (unpublished) Paper to *XVIII International Congress On Occupational Health, Brighton 1975.*

BECK, E. G., BRUCH, J., FRIEDRICHS, K.-H., HILSCHER, W. and POTT, F. (1971) *Inhaled Particles III* (edited by WALTON, W. H.) vol. I, pp. 477–487. Unwin Bros., Old Woking, Surrey.

BOGOVSKI, P., GILSON, J. C., TIMBRELL, V. and WAGNER, J. C. (Editors) (1973) *Biological Effects of Asbestos.* IARC Scientific Publication no. 8. International Agency for Research on Cancer, Lyon.

PELNAR, P. V. (Editor) (1974) *Fibres for Biological Experiments. Transcript of IOEH Conference, Montreal 1973.* Institute of Occupational and Environmental Health, Montreal.

POTT, F. and FRIEDRICHS, K. H. (1972) *Naturwissenschaften* **59,** 318.

REEVES, A. L., PURO, H. E. and SMITH, R. G. (1974) *Envir. Res.* **8,** 178–202.

ROBOCK, K. (1974) *Beitr. Silikoseforsch.* **26,** 112–262.

ROBOCK, K. and KLOSTERKÖTTER, W. (1971) *Inhaled Particles III* (edited by WALTON, W. H.) vol. I, pp. 465–474. Unwin Bros., Old Woking, Surrey.

SMITH, W. E. (1974) *Fibres for Biological Experiments. Transcript of IOEH Conference, Montreal 1973* (edited by PELNAR, P. V.) pp. 54–58. Institute of Occupational and Environmental Health, Montreal.

STANTON, M. F. (1972) *J. natn Cancer Inst.* **48,** 633–634.

STANTON, M. F. and WRENCH, C. (1972) *J. natn Cancer Inst.* **48,** 797–821.

TIMBRELL, V. (1972) *Assessment of Airborne Particles* (edited by MERCER, T. T., MORROW, P. E. and STÖBER, W.) pp. 429–441. Thomas, Springfield, Ill.

TIMBRELL, V., POOLEY, F. and WAGNER, J. C. (1970) *Pneumoconiosis. Proceedings of the International Conference, Johannesburg 1969* (edited by SHAPIRO, H. A.) pp. 65–70. Oxford University Press, Cape Town.

WAGNER, J. C., BERRY, G., SKIDMORE, J. W. and TIMBRELL, V. (1974) *Br. J. Cancer* **29,** 252–269.

DISCUSSION

I. P. GORMLEY: Your data suggest that cement dust alone is more cytotoxic than some asbestos cement dusts collected in the same factory. Would you comment on this?

Dr ROBOCK: At the moment I cannot say any more, but on the other side, in the animal experiments we seem to find very fast clearance of cement particles and no fibrogenic effects. The acute cytotoxicity of the cement particles is perhaps due to a pH shift *in vitro* and may have no connection with specific fibrogenic effects in animals or human beings.

A. MORGAN: In the introduction to this paper it is implied that the U.I.C.C. standard reference samples of asbestos have similar fibrogenic and carcinogenic properties. The work of STANTON and WRENCH (1972) and of WAGNER *et al.* (1974) is quoted in support. With regard to the former, the data they give on fibrogenic activities are only qualitative in nature. Although Wagner *et al.* found that asbestosis was induced by all the U.I.C.C. samples, the amount of chrysotile found in the lungs of rats at the end of exposure was very much less than that in rats exposed to the amphiboles. This could be due either to a smaller alveolar deposition of chrysotile or to its much more rapid clearance from the lung. In either case it would appear that a much smaller dose of chrysotile has resulted in a similar degree of fibrosis to that produced by a large amount of amphiboles. Until more satisfactory data are available it cannot be assumed that the U.I.C.C. samples have similar fibrogenicity, and what information there is, indicates that chrysotile and particularly chrysotile B are more active in this respect.

Dr ROBOCK: I was astonished in former times about the greater cytotoxicity of the chrysotiles. Wagner *et al.* are the first to give an explanation for this. I am observing this very much higher cytotoxicity of the chrysotiles against amphiboles. Therefore, one can explain the same effect in animal experiments in connection with a lower mass concentration of the chrysotiles found in the lung tissue. We started with all these problems and it is too early to say anything more at the moment.

G. BOULEY: What method did you use to measure the amount of O_2 used by the alveolar macrophages *in vitro*?

Dr ROBOCK: We developed a new device for measuring the oxygen consumption by using a Clark electrode. This polarographic method was first described by Munder *et al.* in Münster at the International Pneumoconiosis Symposium in 1967.

J. FERIN: What was the cell/particle ratio in your experiments? If this was not standardized, do you not feel that the number and size distribution of the particles may affect your results?

Dr ROBOCK: We used a standardized method, i.e. the same mass concentration of the U.I.C.C. dusts and the same number of macrophages in the size range between 11 and 25 microns measured each day with the Coulter Counter Equipment. The dust/cell ratio was 4.8 mg dust and 9×10^6 cells for each experiment, but I cannot say anything about the particle number.

J. C. WAGNER: Why did you wish to repeat our experiments if you accept the results?

Dr ROBOCK: I accept your results completely because they are in agreement with mine and there is no necessity to repeat the experiments. In further experiments one should look for more details—deposition probability, solubility and fibre number.

V. TIMBRELL: Our observation of as much fibrosis in rats' lungs containing chrysotile asbestos as in those with a much larger weight of amphibole may be a consequence of fibrogenicity being related to fibre number or surface area rather than to the mass. In future experiments it will be desirable to estimate fibre number and surface area to determine whether (possibly as a result of chrysotile fibres splitting in lung fluids) the chrysotile compares with the amphibole in terms of one of these parameters.

Dr ROBOCK: I agree with you and I explained my opinion in my paper, hoping I would not have to interpret it. By your own theory chrysotile has a lower possibility of reaching the alveolar area and, too, we can assume a higher leaching in the lung tissue. This in conjunction with the higher cytotoxicity for the U.I.C.C. chrysotiles than for the amphiboles may cause the same asbestosis effect and all the other biological effects.

L. LE BOUFFANT: We have been studying this dissociation of chrysotile fibres in the lung after intratracheal injection in rats. The chrysotile consisted of 20-μm fibres prepared on a microtome. After 2 weeks, the animals were sacrificed and the lung content examined by electron microscope. We found a very marked dissociation of the bundles of fibres, much greater than when ultra-sound treatment was used.

THE INFLUENCE OF VARYING LENGTHS OF GLASS AND ASBESTOS FIBRES ON TISSUE RESPONSE IN GUINEA PIGS

G. W. Wright

Saint Luke's Hospital, Cleveland, Ohio

and

M. Kuschner

State University of New York at Stony Brook, New York

Abstract—Intratracheal injection of samples of naturally occurring and man-made mineral fibres into guinea pigs showed that while long fibre samples produced marked fibrosis, short fibre specimens produced only a macrophage reaction. In most cases the long fibre samples were administered in smaller doses than the short. The samples tested were crocidolite asbestos, a synthetic fluoramphibole and two specimens of glass fibre with different mean diameters.

With all the minerals tested some short fibres, but not long fibres, were transported to the hilar lymph nodes. In some instances the numbers of short fibres found in these nodes appeared to be much higher than would be expected from the percentage of short fibres in the original sample, and it is suggested that this may be due to the breakdown of long fibres within the lung.

There is the growing conviction that the fibrogenic effect of asbestos is size dependent. An increasing number of publications demonstrate the lack or relative lack of fibrotic response to "short" fibres and the dependence of fibrosis on the presence of "long" fibres, short and long being variously defined.

These observations are strongly supportive of the concept that stimulation of connective tissue proliferation is a function of the physical properties of fibres rather than of their chemical characteristics. If this is so, it would seem reasonable to expect that fibrous materials other than asbestos might evoke similar reactions. The availability of a series of fibres of asbestos and of glass carefully characterized as to size prompted us to examine and compare the biological response to different fibre types. The test system employed was intratracheal instillation into halothane anaesthetized guinea pigs of suspensions of fibre in distilled water.

In the complete study 28 different groups of 30 animals each received injections of 3 to 25 mg of fibre administered in 2 to 8 instillations. The number of injections and the amount of each injection was in large part determined by the quantity of material that could be held in suspension and instilled without too much clumping and aggregation.

For the purposes of this brief presentation, we have chosen to demonstrate the contrasting effects of long and short fibres of 4 pairs of materials, 2 forms of asbestos and 2 of glass. In the course of the study, animals were sacrificed at 6 months, 1 year and 2 years. We shall only present the findings at 2 years after the last injection.

The first pair of samples is of crocidolite fibres. The long fibre sample is one in which more than 80% of the fibres are over 10 μm in length while the short sample is one in which more than 99% are less than 5 μm in length (Fig. 1). In both samples 70% of the diameters range from 0.10 to 0.30 μm. The long-fibre group received a total dose of 4 mg and the short-fibre group received 25 mg.

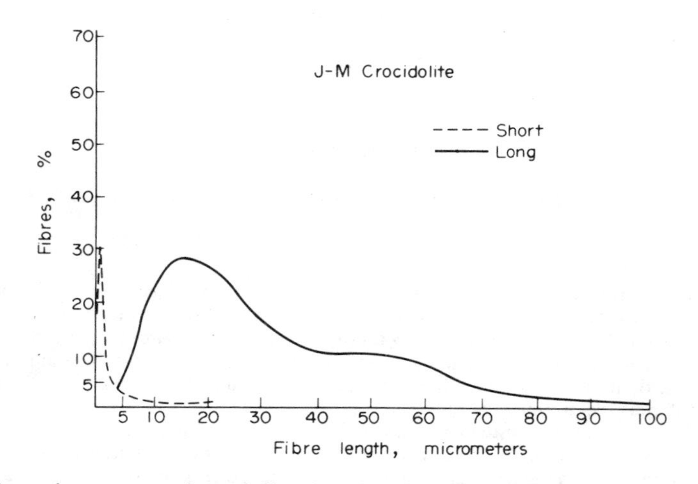

FIG. 1. Schematic representation of fibre lengths of short and long samples of crocidolite.

The long sample produced extensive interstitial fibrosis, most marked in those portions of lung abutting on the terminal bronchioles and involving the respiratory bronchioles and proximal alveoli (Fig. 2a).

In contrast the short sample of crocidolite produced no fibrosis (Fig. 2b).

Higher magnification of the reaction to long fibre reveals an occasional visible fibre in the fibrotic interstitium with asbestos body formation (Fig. 3a).

Some short fibre is retained in the lung within aggregates of macrophages (Fig. 3b).

Within the hilar nodes of the animals exposed to long fibres, there are macrophages containing fibres too small to be resolved (Fig. 4a). None of these are long and thus must represent the result of a "sieving" effect by which the long fibre remains in the lung while the small proportion of fibres which are short are phagocytosed and translocated to the lymph nodes.

It is worthy of note that these short fibres do not lead to fibrosis and in the lymph nodes of animals exposed to short fibres there are many more macrophages with ingested fibre but again without fibrosis (Fig. 4b).

The second set of samples consists of long and short fibres of a synthetic fluoramphibole. Diameters are for the most part less than 1.0 μm although 3.5% of the long fibres are 1 to 2 μm in diameter. The long fibres are such that 16% are longer than

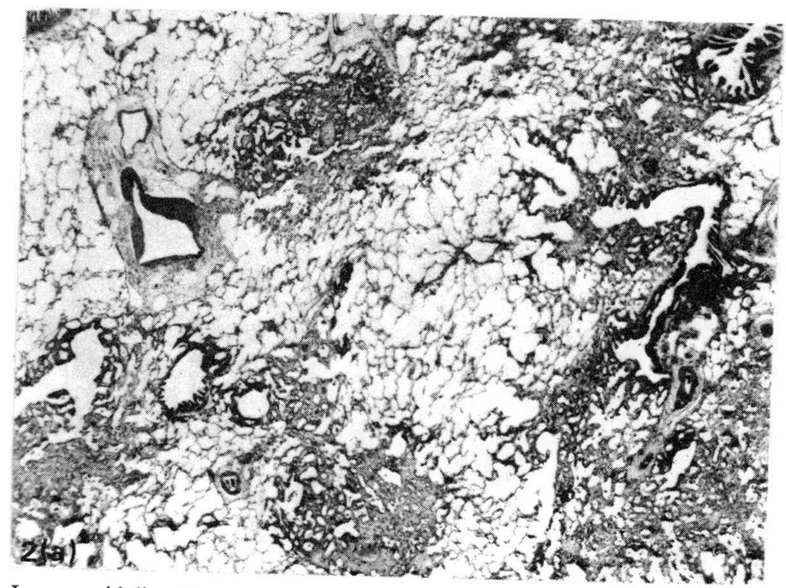

Fig. 2a. Long crocidolite. There are extensive areas of fibrosis abutting on the terminal bronchioles and involving respiratory bronchioles and proximal alveoli (× 10).

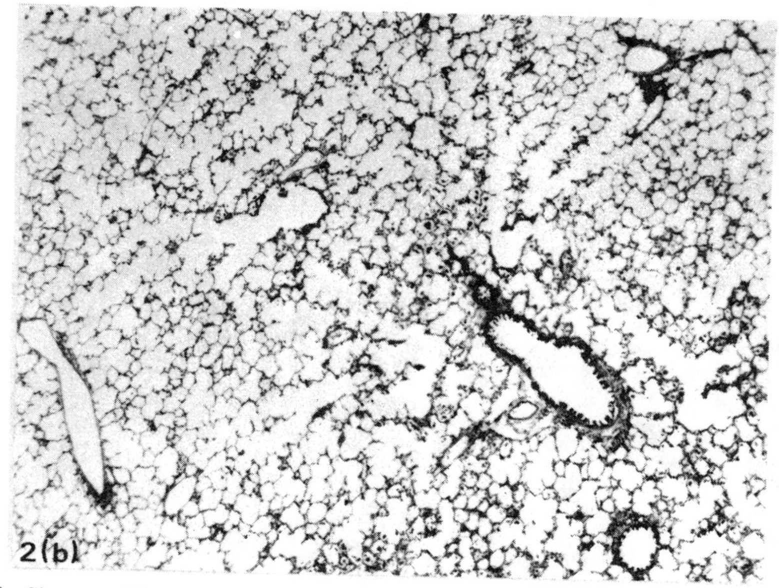

Fig. 2b. Short crocidolite. Fibrosis is absent. Aggregates of macrophages are seen in some alveoli (× 10).

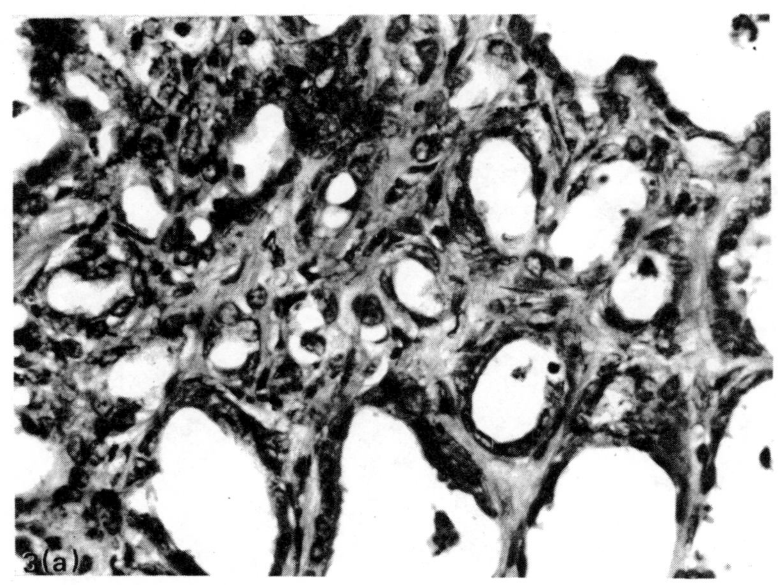

FIG. 3a. Long crocidolite. Dense interstitial fibrosis is seen in the lung. An occasional fibre is visible in the fibrotic interstitium (× 600).

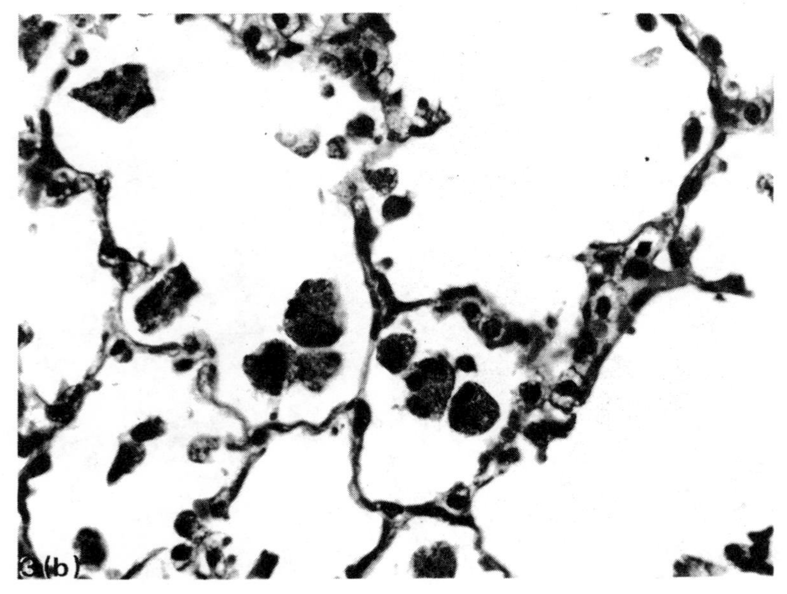

FIG. 3b. Short crocidolite. Short fibres are retained in the lung within macrophages but without fibrosis (× 600).

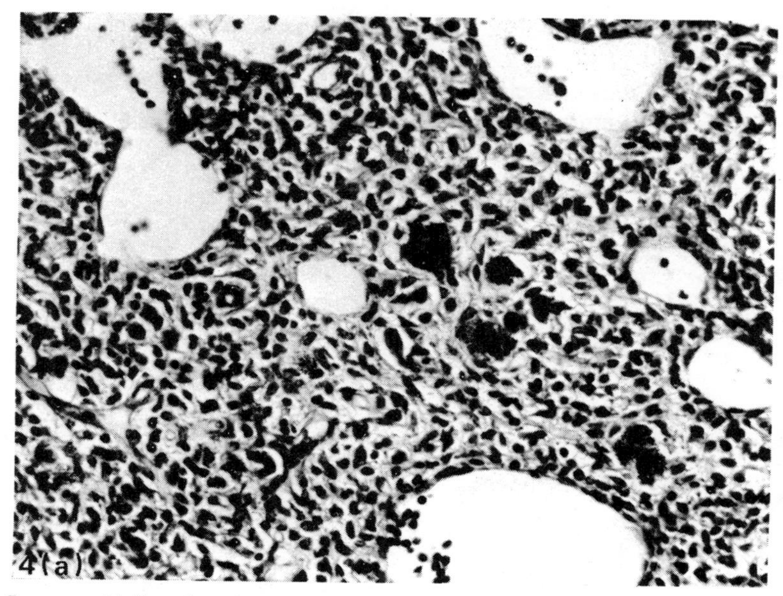

FIG. 4a. Long crocidolite—lymph node. "Sieved" short fibres in macrophages are present within lymph nodes of long-fibre recipients. There is no fibrosis (× 600).

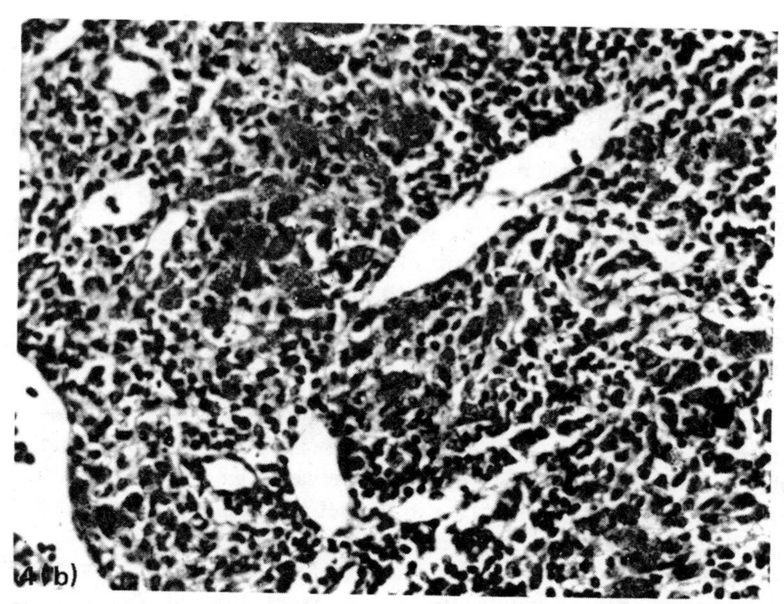

FIG. 4b. Short crocidolite—lymph node. Large numbers of macrophages containing short fibres are seen in the lymph nodes. There is no fibrosis (× 600).

10 μm and 43% are longer than 5 μm. The short-fibre sample consists of more than 99% of fibre less than 5 μm (Fig. 5). Animals exposed to both long and short fibres received a total dose of 12 mg.

The long fibres of this synthetic fluoramphibole again produced striking interstitial fibrosis (Fig. 6a). The short fibres of fluoramphibole left the lung unaltered (Fig. 6b).

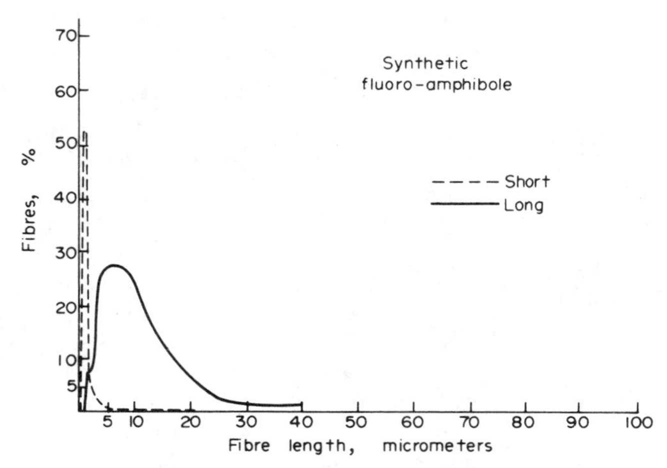

FIG. 5. Schematic representation of fibre lengths of short and long samples of a synthetic fluoramphibole.

In the long-fibre recipients, an occasional asbestos body was observed in association with areas of fibrosis (Fig. 7a). In the short-fibre recipients, an occasional macrophage containing an identifiable fibre was noted (Fig. 7b).

The lymph nodes of the guinea pigs receiving long fibres showed small groups of macrophages containing what must be assumed to be "sieved" smaller fibres (Fig. 8a). The lymph nodes of the short fibre recipients contained large aggregates, indeed sheets, of macrophages but in neither was there fibrosis (Fig. 8b).

Consider the relative effects of a pair of samples of glass fibre of diameters ranging from 0.1 to 1.0 μm. The long fibres are such that 92% are longer than 10 μm while the short-fibre sample contains 93% of fibres which are less than 10 μm in length (Fig. 9). The long-fibre group received a total dose of 12 mg and the short-fibre group received 25 mg.

The long fibre produces a fibrotic lesion which, as in asbestos, involves the area of lung immediately about the terminal bronchiole (Fig. 10a). Although similar in location and character, the quantitative difference between this reaction and that produced by asbestos is striking. The short fibres in this set of samples produce no change other than macrophage aggregation in the alveoli (Fig. 10b).

Occasional fibres can be identified in areas of fibrosis after long-fibre exposure (Fig. 11a). In the short-fibre recipients, the macrophages are stuffed with fibre but unassociated with fibrosis (Fig. 11b).

In the long-fibre recipients the lymph nodes contain large numbers of small fibres in

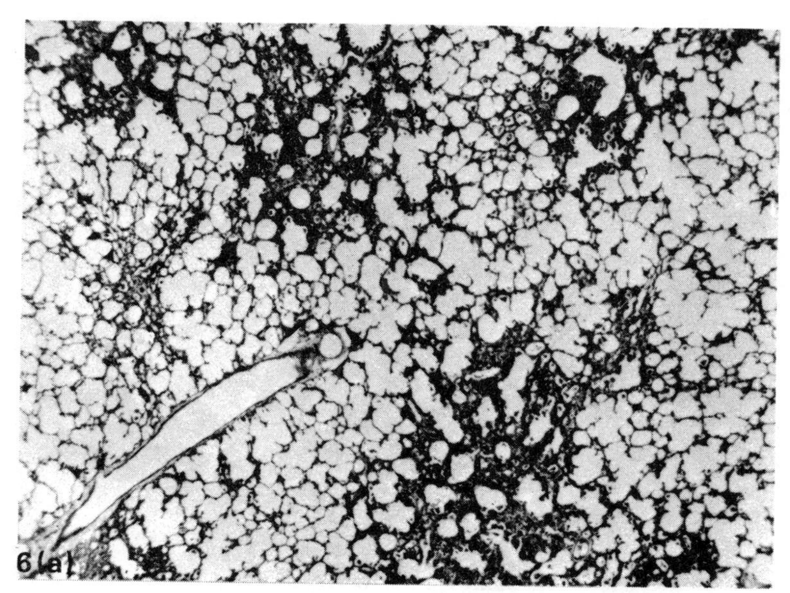

FIG. 6a. Long fluoramphibole. Peribronchiolar fibrosis involves the interstitium about the terminal bronchioles (× 10).

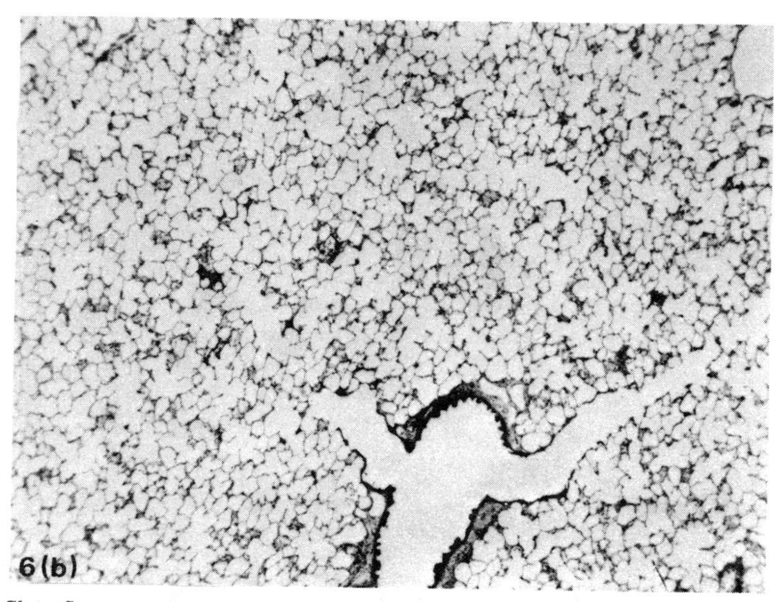

FIG. 6b. Short fluoramphibole. The lung is free of fibrosis. Aggregates of macrophages are present within some alveoli (× 10).

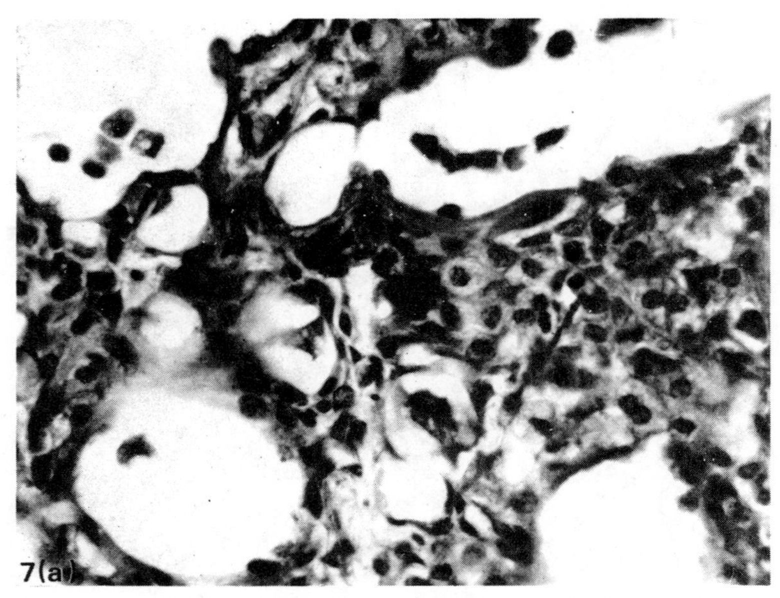

FIG. 7a. Long fluoramphibole. Occasional fibres and "asbestos bodies" are seen in areas of dense interstitial fibrosis (× 600).

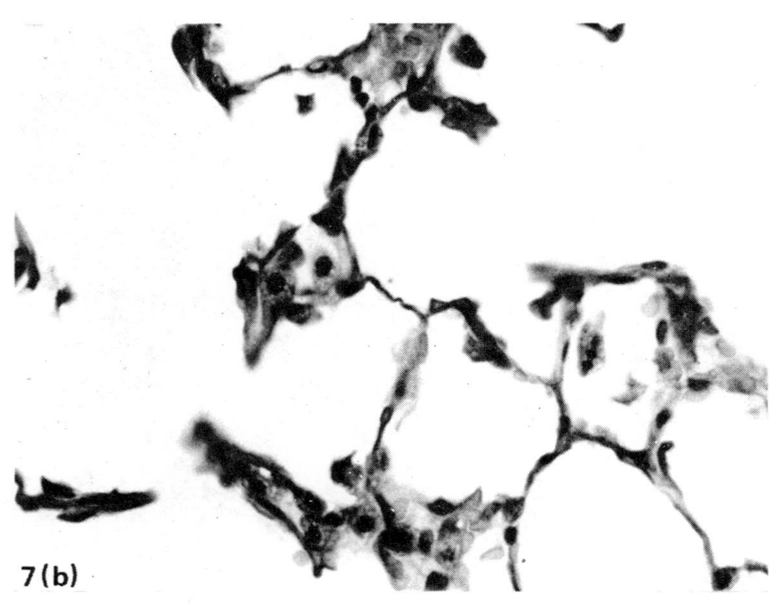

FIG. 7b. Short fluoramphibole. There is no evidence of fibrosis. An occasional fibre or intracellular "asbestos body" is seen within macrophages (× 600).

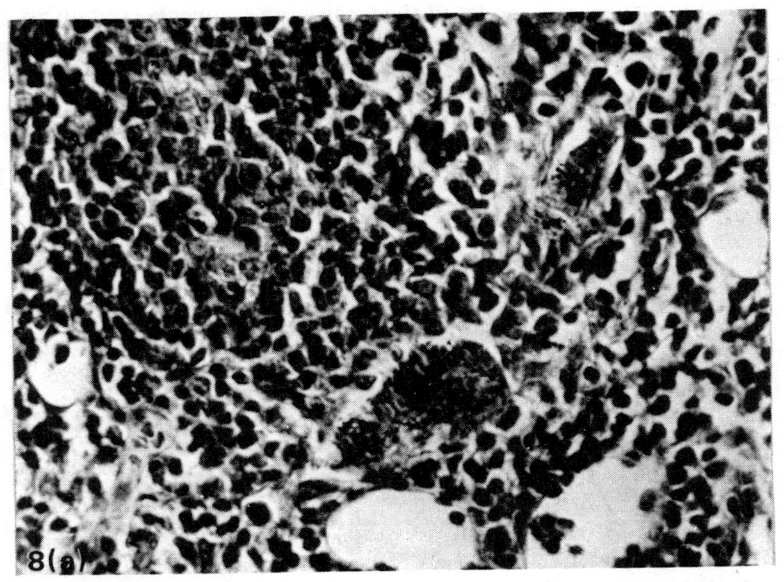

FIG. 8a. Long fluoramphibole—lymph node. "Sieved" shorter fibres are seen within the macrophages of the lymph nodes of long-fibre recipients. There is no fibrosis (× 600).

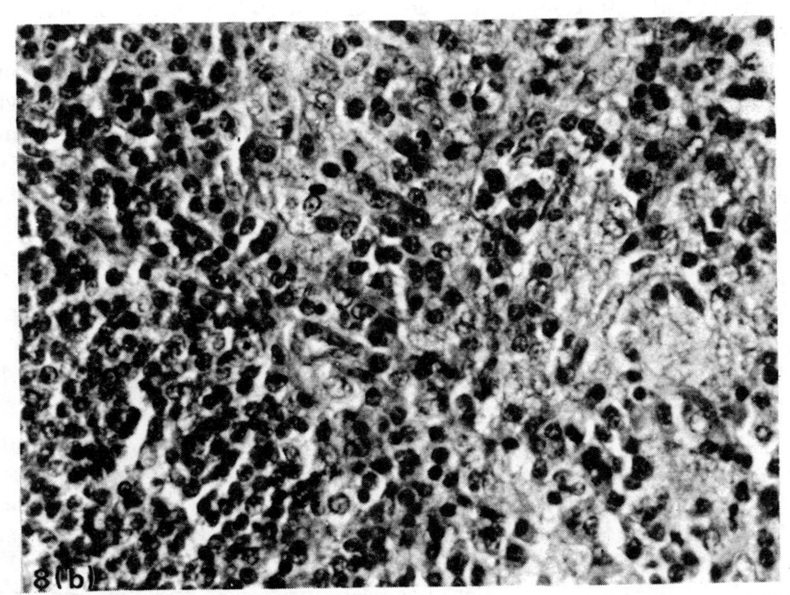

FIG. 8b. Short fluoramphibole—lymph node. Sheets of macrophages are present within the lymph nodes of the short fibre recipients. No fibrogenic reaction is evoked (× 600).

amounts which appear out of proportion to the numbers of small fibres in the original sample (Fig. 12a). The lymph nodes of the small-fibre recipients contain, as one might expect, large numbers of fibre-laden macrophages (Fig. 12b). In neither case is there significant fibrosis.

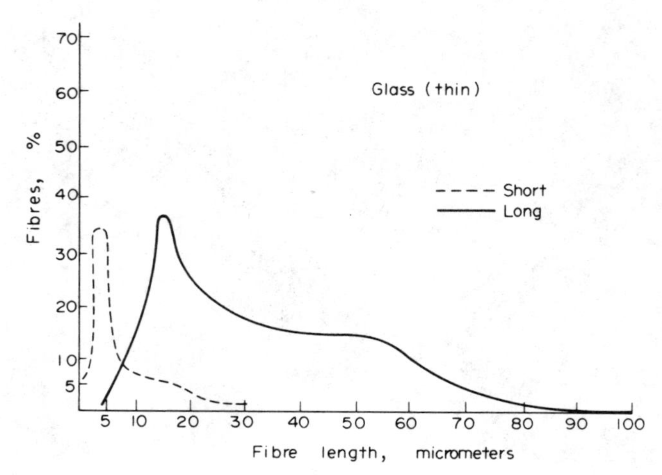

FIG. 9. Schematic representation of fibre lengths of short and long samples of thin glass fibres.

Another pair of samples of very thin glass fibre was used in which mean diameters were less than 0.10 μm. Long fibres were such that 50% were longer than 10 μm and the short fibres were all less than 5 μm in length (Fig 13). Long fibres were administered to a total dose of 12 mg while the total dose of short fibres was 25 mg.

The long fibre again produced a minimal but definite lesion in the same vulnerable area, the zone abutting on the terminal bronchiole (Fig. 14a). The instillation of short fibre did not result in fibrosis of any degree (Fig. 14b).

Fibres of this very fine glass were, of course, not visible in the small but definite areas of cell proliferation and fibrosis found in the long-fibre recipients (Fig. 15a). There was a macrophage reaction in the short fibre recipients (Fig. 15b).

Sheets of macrophages were present in the "long-fibre lymph nodes" (Fig. 16a) and were more marked in the "short-fibre lymph nodes" (Fig. 16b) but fibrosis was not seen in either.

We believe the following conclusions may be drawn from these observations.

Long fibres (longer than 10 μm) of asbestos produce fibrosis. Short fibres (those less than 10 μm) do not produce fibrosis in either lung or lymph nodes. This is confirmatory of a number of investigations of the comparative fibrogenicity of asbestos fibres of various lengths introduced into the lung, the pleural cavity and the peritoneal cavity (VORWALD *et al.*, 1951; TIMBRELL and SKIDMORE, 1973; BURGER and ENGELBRECHT, 1970; HILSCHER, 1970; WEBSTER, 1970; GROSS, 1974; BECK *et al.*, 1971).

Although the fibrogenicity of glass has been questioned, it would appear that long fibres of this material are also fibrogenic. The uncertainty as to its fibrogenicity in past experiments (GROSS *et al.*, 1970) and the marked quantitative difference between its

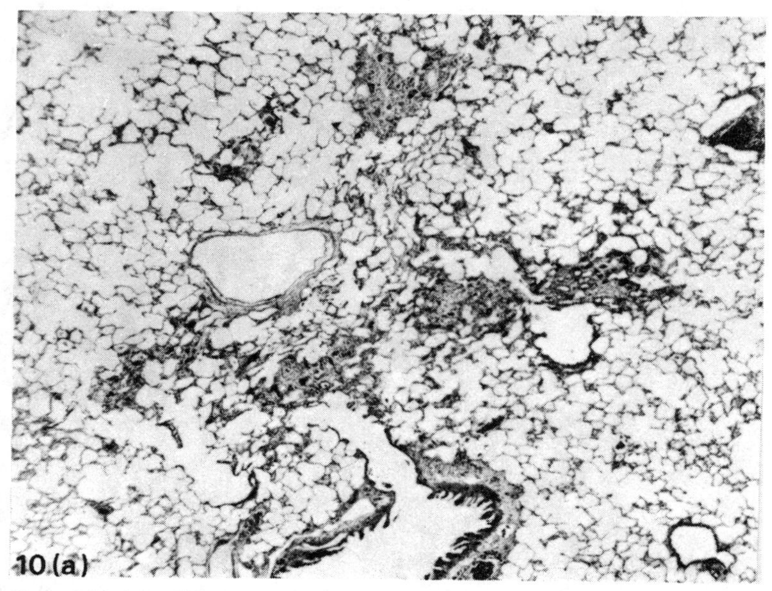

FIG. 10a. Long thin glass. This area represents the zone of most marked fibrotic reaction among all the animals so exposed. The reaction was much less marked in most animals (× 10).

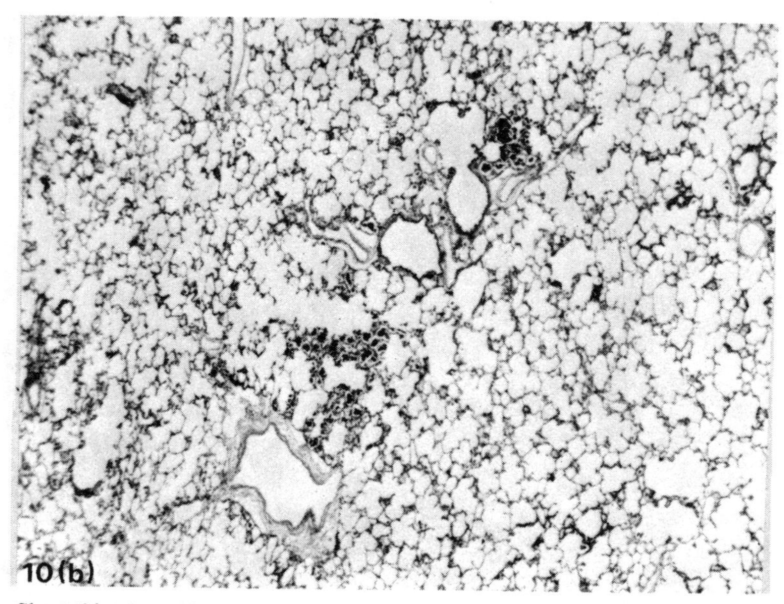

FIG. 10b. Short thin glass. There is no fibrosis. Aggregates of macrophages are seen in groups of alveoli (× 10).

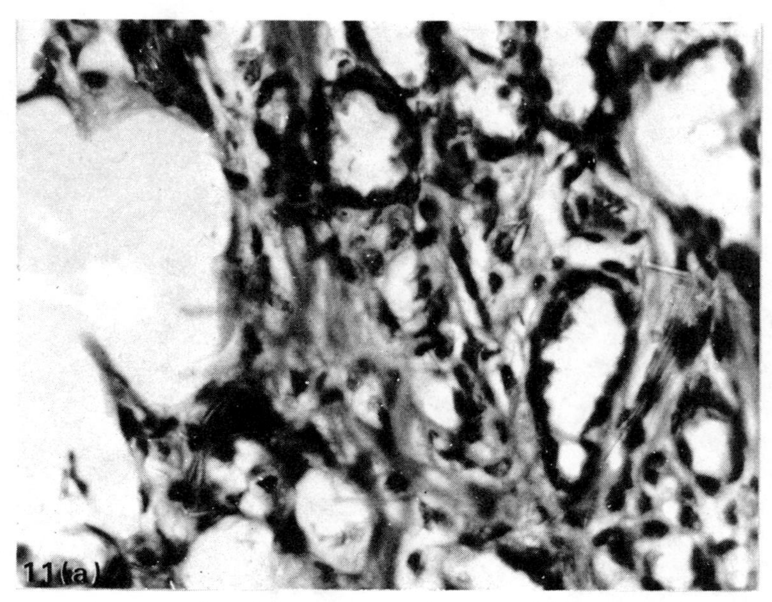

FIG. 11a. Long thin glass. Glass fibres are seen in those interstitial areas which are the site of fibrosis (× 600).

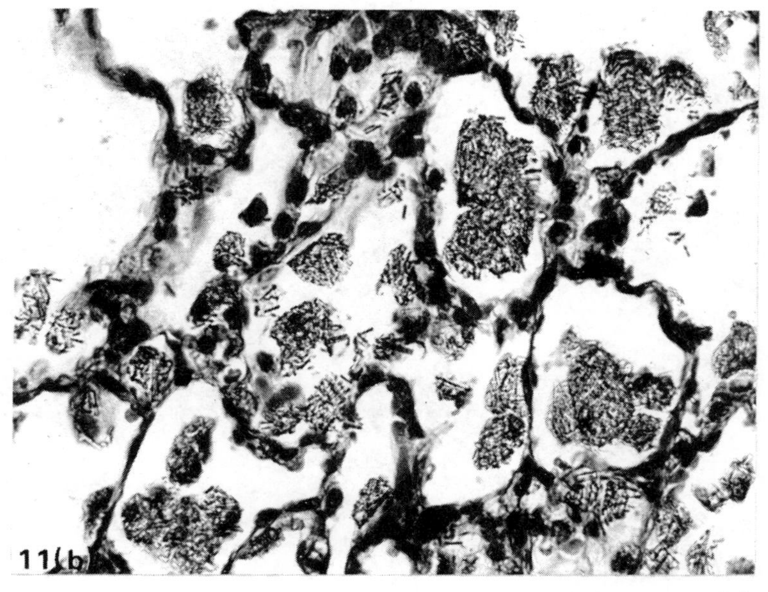

FIG. 11b. Short thin glass. Large numbers of glass fibre are seen within aggregated short fibres within the alveoli. No fibrosis has resulted (× 600).

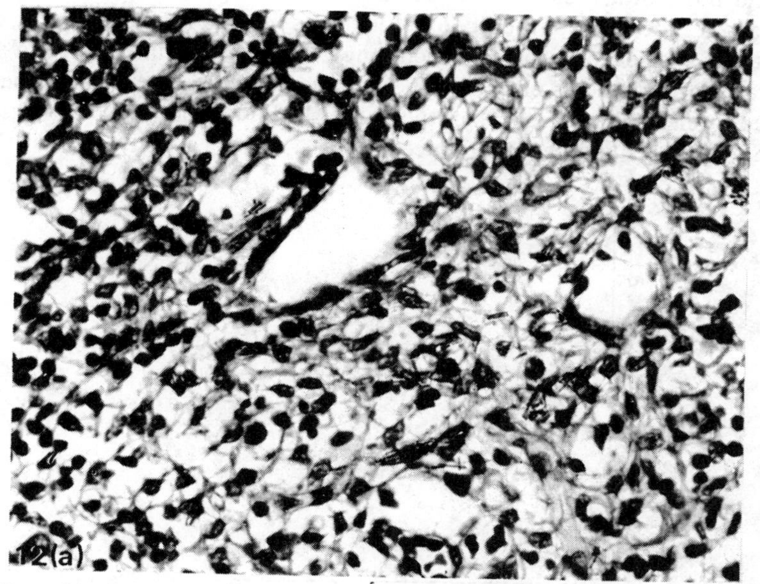

FIG. 12a. Long thin glass—lymph node. A surprisingly large number of short fibres are seen in the lymph nodes of long-fibre recipients. These may be the result of fragmentation of long fibres as well as of the presence of some short fibre in the sample. There is no fibrosis (× 600).

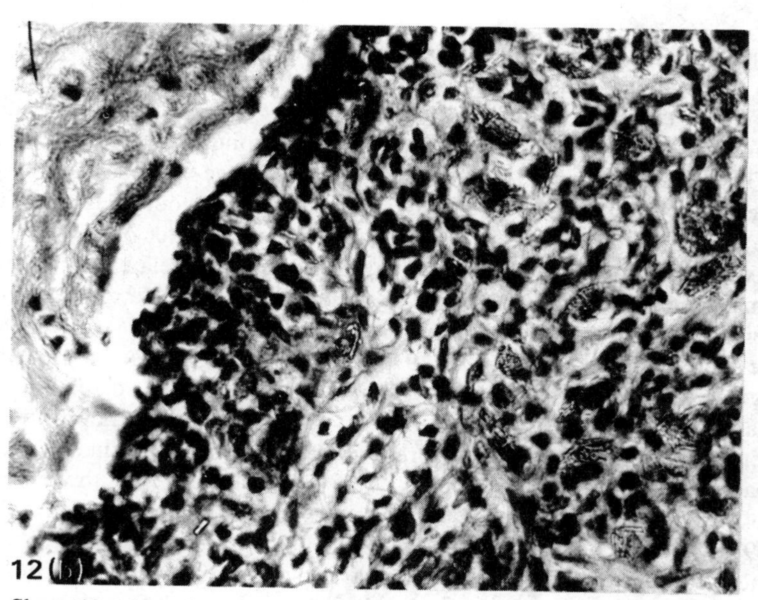

FIG. 12b. Short thin glass—lymph node. Large numbers of fibre-laden macrophages are seen within the lymph nodes. No fibrogenic reaction is evoked (× 600).

effects and those of asbestos in the present series of experiments, we believe to be a consequence of the lesser durability of a long glass fibre as compared to the durability of asbestos. In the experiments in which long glass fibre was introduced, a surprising amount of short fragments of fibres appear in the lymph nodes. This fragmentation is confirmed by electron micrographic studies of ashed lung and lymph nodes of animals in which long fibres had been introduced.

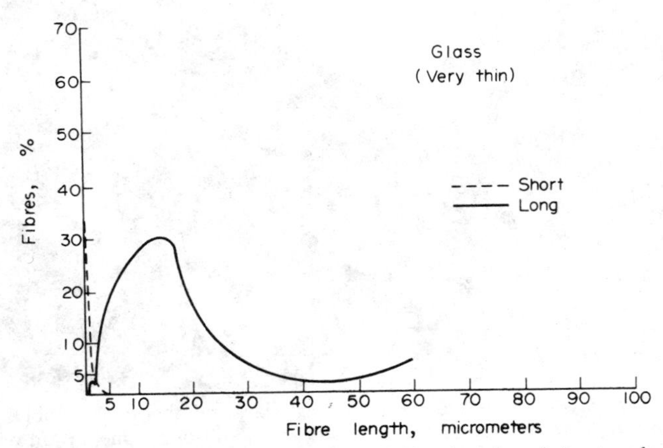

FIG. 13. Schematic representation of fibre lengths of short and long samples of very thin glass fibres.

The mechanism which best explains the similarity of response to a variety of asbestos fibres and to glass is one well worked out for granulocytes (HENSON, 1972) and has been extended to macrophages (BECK *et al.*, 1971; BRUCH, 1974). Cells attempting to engulf long fibres are involved in incomplete or "frustrated" phagocytosis. The process known as exocytosis results in leakage of tissue damaging enzymes from the cell without being specifically toxic to the phagocyte. It is reasonable to presume that tissue damage so produced is the ultimate inciter of fibrosis.

The experiments described and the foregoing discussion relate only to fibrosis. All of this may not, however, be unrelated to tumour induction. Here, too, a specific size dependence of carcinogenicity appears to be emerging (STANTON and WRENCH, 1972; SMITH *et al.*, 1972; MAROUDAS *et al.*, 1973). There is the strong suggestion that the co-carcinogenicity of asbestos with cigarette smoking is the result of the induction of a particularly vulnerable cellular substrate on which the tobacco-derived carcinogen can operate. This substrate is the proliferating peripheral epithelial reaction that accompanies the fibrosis of asbestosis. This may account for the excessive incidence of adenocarcinoma in the lung cancer of asbestotic workers (WHITWELL *et al.*, 1974).

Further, the development of experimental mesothelioma seems to occur *pari passu* with the fibrosis engendered by tumorigenic fibres and argues for a form of malignant transformation not unlike that induced by plastic films, so-called "solid state" carcinogenesis (BRAND, 1975).

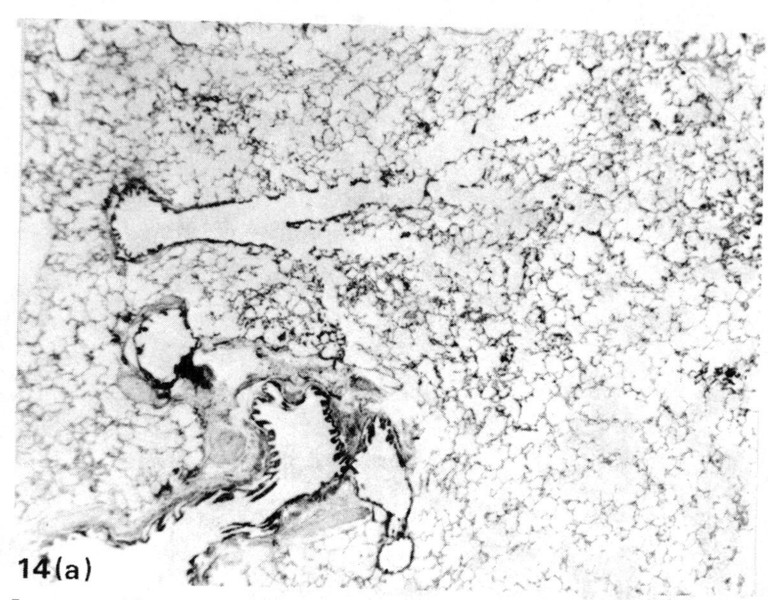

FIG. 14a. Long very thin glass. A mild interstitial fibrosis is noted in the walls of the respiratory bronchioles and adjacent alveoli. Macrophages are also seen within alveoli (× 10).

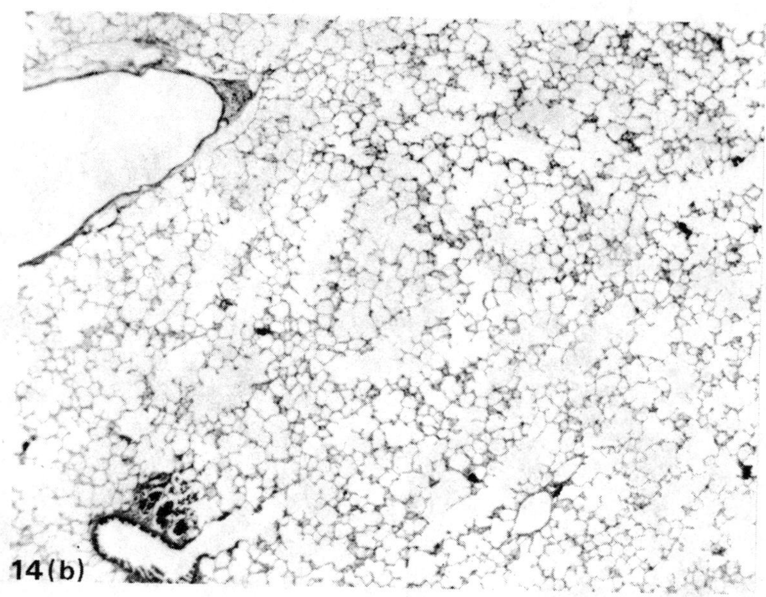

FIG. 14b. Short very thin glass. Except for focal aggregates of intra-alveolar macrophages, the lung is unaltered (× 10).

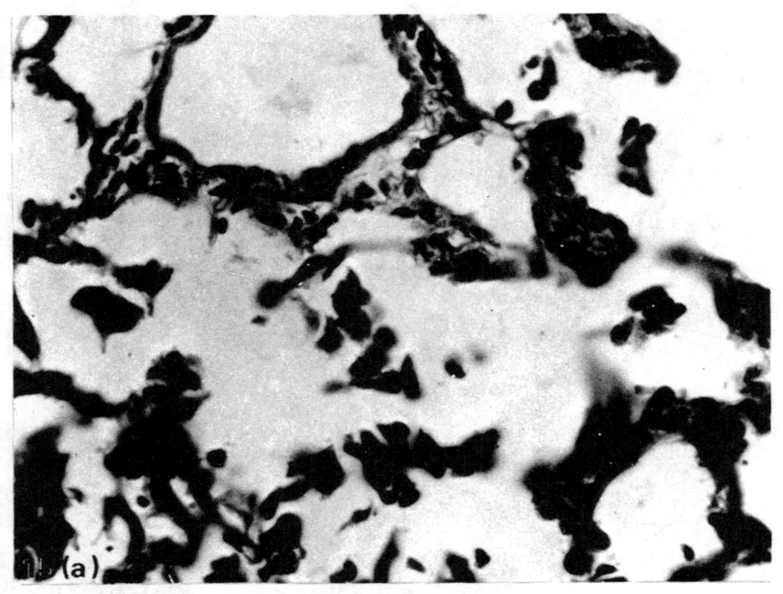

FIG. 15a. Long very thin glass. There is minimal interstitial fibrous thickening together with increased cellularity in alveoli abutting on respiratory bronchioles. Macrophages are also present within air spaces (× 600).

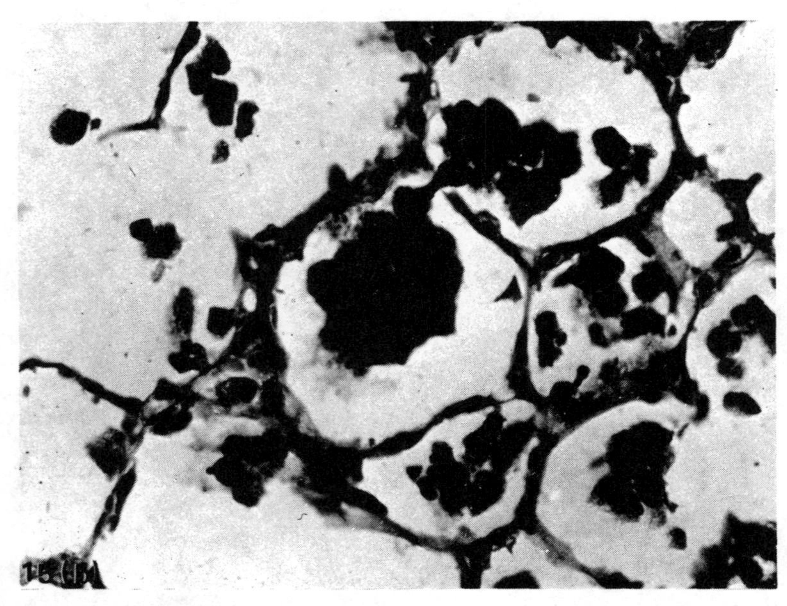

FIG. 15b. Short very thin glass. Aggregates of macrophages are present in focal groups of alveoli. There is no fibrosis (× 600).

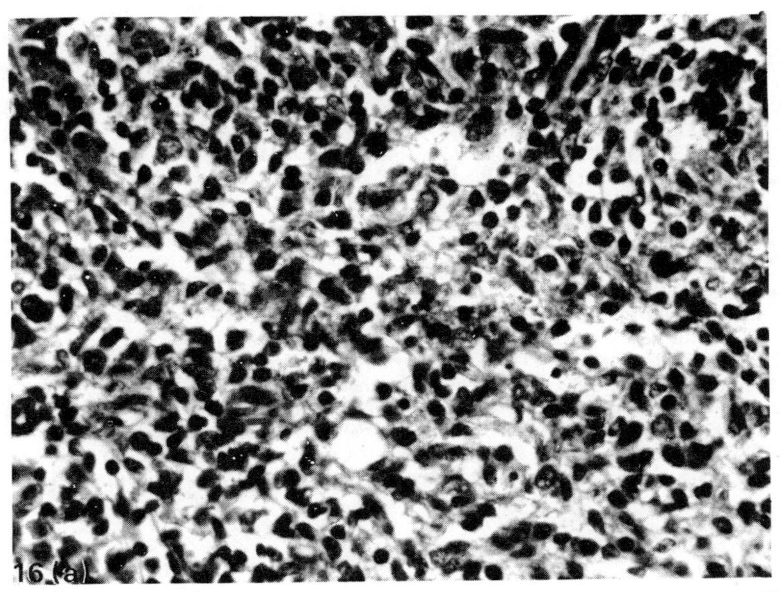

FIG. 16a. Long very thin glass—lymph node. Sheets of macrophages are present within the lymph nodes of the long fibre recipients. There is no fibrosis (× 600).

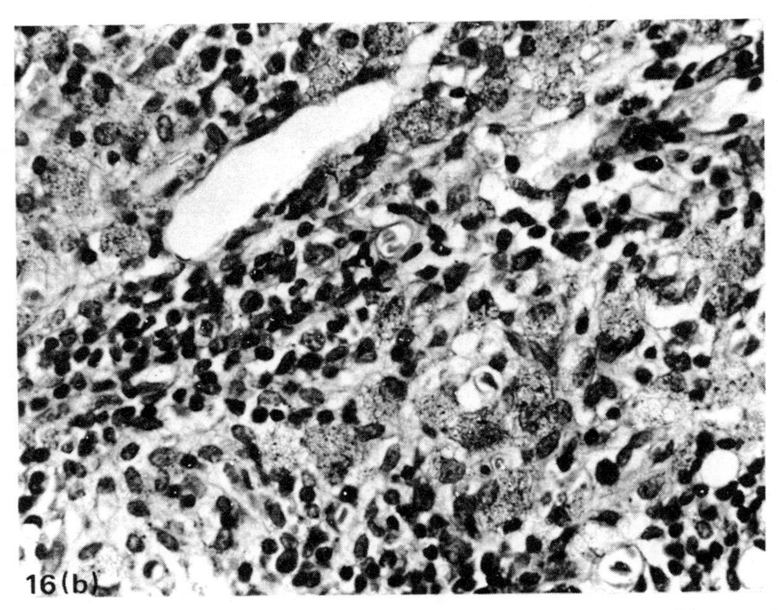

FIG. 16b. Short very thin glass. Large numbers of macrophages are present and have a refractible granular appearance. Individual fibres are not resolvable (× 600).

REFERENCES

BECK, E. G., BRUCH, J., FRIEDRICHS, K.-H., HILSCHER, W. and POTT, F. (1971) *Inhaled Particles III* (edited by WALTON, W. H.) vol. 1, pp. 477–487. Unwin Bros, Old Woking, Surrey.

BRAND, K. G. (1975) *Cancer I* (edited by BECKER, F. F.) pp. 485–511. Plenum, New York.

BRUCH, J. (1974) *Envir. Hlth Perspect.* **9**, 253–254.

BURGER, B. F. and ENGELBRECHT, F. M. (1970) *S. Afr. med. J.* **114**, 1268–1270.

GROSS, P., KASCHAK, M., TOLKER, E. B., BABYAK, M. A. and DE TREVILLE, R. T. P. (1970) *Archs envir. Hlth* **20**, 696–704.

GROSS, P. (1974) *Archs envir. Hlth* **29**, 115–117.

HENSON, M. (1972) *Am. J. Path.* **68**, 593–612.

HILSCHER, W. (1970) *Naturwissenschaften* **57**, 356–557.

MAROUDAS, N. G., O'NEIL, C. H. and STANTON, N. F. (1973) *Lancet* **1**, 807–809.

SMITH, W. E., HUBERT, D. D., and BADOLLET, M. S. (1972) *Am. ind. Hyg. Ass. J.* **33**, A162.

STANTON, M. F. and WRENCH, C. (1972) *J. natn. Cancer Inst.* **48**, 797–821.

TIMBRELL, V. and SKIDMORE, J. W. (1973) in *Internationale Konferenz über die Biologische Wirkungen des Asbestos, Dresden, 1968*, pp. 52–56. Deutsches Zentralinstitut für Arbeitsmedizin, Berlin.

VORWALD, A. V., DURKAN, T. M. and PRATT, P. C. (1951) *A.M.A. Archs ind. Hyg.* **3**, 1–43.

WEBSTER, I. (1970) *Pneumoconiosis: Proceedings of the International Conference, Johannesburg, 1969* (edited by SHAPIRO, H. A.) pp. 117–119. Oxford University Press, Cape Town.

WHITWELL, F., NEWHOUSE, M. L. and BENNETT, DIANE R. (1974) *Br. J. ind. Med.* **31**, 298–303.

DISCUSSION

M. LIPPMANN: For equal masses of fibre instilled in a pair of tests, there would be far greater numbers of the shorter fibres, which would reinforce the conclusion that long fibres are the most important.

Dr KUSCHNER: The masses were not always equal, but when unequal, the short fibre mass was larger. For instance, in the first crocidolite sample, there were 4 mg of long and 25 mg of short fibres, so that you are correct about the number of fibres.

J. C. WAGNER: Why did you not use inhalation experiments rather than intratracheal methods which completely overpower the defence mechanisms of the lung?

Dr KUSCHNER: All animal experiments are unrealistic; one must be quite clear what question one is asking of the experiment. We were not asking about the comparative effects of materials inhaled under natural conditions; but about the differences between the biological effects of series of fibres differing in size which were sure to get into the lung.

G. V. COLES: Were any investigations made of pleural effects after the investigations of fibrogenicity?

Dr KUSCHNER: The pleural reaction was examined with the remainder of the lungs. There was no parietal pleural plaque formation. In animals with a massive fibrosis produced by asbestos there was pleural fibrosis but not mesothelioma. There were no tumours produced in this series of guinea pigs, all of which were sacrificed after 2 years.

R. HUNT: Human studies confirm the fibrogenicity of long asbestos fibres, i.e. 25 μm, as opposed to shorter fibres which are transported away and dealt with by the R. E. system.

Dr KUSCHNER: In an earlier publication, Timbrell and his group made the point that one of the differences between long and short fibres was residence time in the lung. Even if the differing effect these materials have on cell populations is ignored the question of residence time in the lungs must still be considered.

C. J. GÖTHE: The photomicrographs seem to show a considerably larger difference between the histological tissue reactions caused by long-fibred asbestos and long-fibred glass than between the tissue reactions caused by long-fibred and short-fibred glass. How do you explain this difference between asbestos and glass with similar fibre type? Is it due to differences in the physical or chemical properties of your asbestos and glass fibre samples?

Dr KUSCHNER: There was no reaction to the short-fibred glass, but there is, as you say, an extraordinary difference between short- and long-fibred asbestos. This relates to the fact that asbestos is a much more efficient fibrogenic agent and I attribute this in part to its durability. As to the differences between long-fibred asbestos and long-fibred glass, I think that the difference is perhaps based on the fact that glass does not persist in its long-fibred form. If it did, it might be much more like asbestos. A difference can be seen between chrysotile fibrils and other forms of asbestos; possibly because the fibrils are more fragile.

J. BRUCH: Five years ago we tested the fibrogenicity of short and long asbestos fibres and found a strict correlation between the fibre length and the degree of fibrosis. The short fibres were preferentially transported into the lymph nodes. Four months after a single i.p. injection of U.I.C.C. crocidolite and amosite, a relative increase of the longer fibres in the fibrotic lesions compared to the original frequency distribution of the fibre lengths could be observed, the shorter fibres on the other hand predominated in the lymph nodes.

Dr KUSCHNER: Yes, your very clear description of this phenomenon is acknowledged in our paper. I believe that you made the point that the small fibres in the lymph nodes did not produce fibrosis.

F. F. HAHN: Have you made any attempt to quantitate the pulmonary fibrosis, by collagen determinations, or by morphometric or other techniques?

Dr KUSCHNER: No, we did not, but I think it would be very useful. This effect was so remarkable that we presented it without collagen or hydroxy-proline determination.

Dr. J. C. GILSON: Can you give us information about changes in mass and size distribution of fibres within the animals' lungs during the 2 years of observation? You hinted that the glass fibres were being altered.

KUSCHNER: We are just beginning to do that and the concept I advanced was based on an impression derived from the low-temperature ashing of a series of lungs which are now ready to be quantitated. It will be important to do counts at 6 months, 1 year and 2 years after inhalation of fibres of which we have detailed characteristics and see how they compare. Our strong impression, based on the visual observation of electromicroscopy at 1 year and 2 years after inhalation, is that the glass fibres do indeed fragment and that we will have a much larger number at the end of the experiment. We are digesting the lung and the lymph nodes together. It could be useful to make a distinction because a lot of the short fibre that we demonstrated in the total sample may be in nodes even in the animals that received long fibres as a result of fragmentation and carriage to lymph nodes.

L. MAGOS: I would like to suggest that you present the size distribution of fibres in columns and not by continuous lines which give a false impression.

Dr KUSCHNER: We tried it that way. It would have been difficult to superimpose the two. I think the proper way to do it is to plot a cumulative size distribution.

M. CORN: We performed a laboratory study to 'determine changes in lengths and diameters of chrysotile asbestos fibres and glass fibres with milling (ASSUNCAO, J. and CORN, M., *Am. ind. Hyg. Ass. J.*, 1975, **36,** 811–819). We found that the asbestos fibres became shorter and diameters were reduced but, in the case of glass fibres, diameters remained unaltered and lengths of fibres were reduced. If a 3 : 1 aspect ratio is used to define a fibre, then the percentage of fibres relative to total particles (fibres and non-fibres) decreased with milling. Your experiments suggest a similar shortening of glass fibres after deposition in the lung.

Dr KUSCHNER: I should be surprised to see them reduced to particles, but I am reasonably confident that they are being reduced in size.

SESSION 6

Wednesday, 24th September

BIOLOGICAL REACTIONS TO DUST (3)

CHRYSOTILE ASBESTOS: BIOLOGICAL REACTION POTENTIAL

R. J. RICHARDS, P. M. HEXT, RASHMI DESAI, TERESA TETLEY, JENNY HUNT, R. PRESLEY* and K. S. DODGSON

Departments of Biochemistry and Anatomy, University College, Cardiff*

Abstract—Evidence is presented indicating that chrysotile asbestos induces rapid cellular ageing in lung fibroblast cultures. Depending on the dose of asbestos given to these cultures the formation of fibrous collagen is enhanced or suppressed. The reaction of chrysotile at the cellular and molecular level is discussed and is considered to be determined by the organic coating it receives or the manner in which the surface adsorbed material is modified. Studies are included of the ability of chrysotile to adsorb and retain serum proteins, pulmonary surfactant and lysosomal enzymes. Finally, a critical appraisal is given of the theories accounting for chrysotile-induced fibrogenesis particularly related to the lung fibroblast system studied.

INTRODUCTION

Whilst it has been known for many years that chrysotile asbestos is detrimental to health and that it has a role in the induction of lung fibrosis, tumours and possibly emphysema, our knowledge of the cellular response to this material, particularly at the biochemical level, is very slight. It could be argued that this type of situation is common for many diseases and that a better understanding of the chemistry of the cell would help us to alleviate such problems.

Many experimenters have shown that chrysotile is an asbestiform mineral of very high biological activity. It is highly cytotoxic *in vitro* (SAKABE *et al.*, 1971; ALLISON, 1971; BECK *et al.*, 1971; RICHARDS *et al.*, 1974), a powerful haemolytic agent (HARINGTON *et al.*, 1971; DESAI *et al.*, 1975) and it produces a high percentage of tumours in experimental animals (WAGNER *et al.*, 1973; POTT *et al.*, 1974). However, whilst accepting that chrysotile produces fibrosis in man, some investigators dispute its role as an active carcinogenic agent.

At the present time chrysotile accounts for over 90% of the asbestos produced throughout the world and it would therefore seem realistic that studies of asbestos-induced diseases should concentrate on the effects of this material. However, despite its world-wide use and distribution and the fact that it can induce many of the conditions described above, chrysotile is not always favoured for use in many experimental studies. This is probably due to its physical characteristics and instability; fibres can "open out" *in vivo* or in biological media, and elements (particularly Mg^{2+}) can be leached from the surface (MORGAN *et al.*, 1971). Thus there are difficulties for the experimenter in explaining chemical reactions by cells in response to this "altering" fibre. Nevertheless it is probably the very instability of the fibre which indirectly explains its highly potent biological activity. The "physical characteristics" of fibre shape and size must determine the site of chrysotile deposition. However, before the asbestos fibre makes contact with any cell upon deposition in the alveolus it will have been "modified" in a variety of ways, by adsorbed mucus and other bronchial secretions or by a coating of highly charged pulmonary surfactant rich in lipoprotein material. Further modifications will ensue upon reaction with cellular membranes, free enzymes and other biological macromolecules before entry into alveolar cells. Within the cells a complex series of biochemical removal and adsorption reactions may take place on the "dust" surface. Thus in any biological system it is difficult to envisage that chrysotile can ever exist as a completely "naked" magnesium silicate; its biological activity is determined by the organic coating that it receives (see KOGAN, 1970; JONES *et al.*, 1972; MORGAN, 1974) or perhaps more specifically by the ease with which this coating is removed, replaced or modified (DESAI *et al.*, 1975). In addition, the question must be posed as to whether chrysotile (as a result of its potent binding affinity) has the ability to interfere with the action of, or degrade cellular components which are essential to the normal functioning of the cell (HARINGTON, 1973).

The work detailed here shows the results of some initial studies on the biological reaction potential of chrysotile asbestos using simple cellular and acellular test systems. The very simplicity of the *in vitro* systems employed (fibroblast culture, haemolysis experiments, etc.) makes extrapolation to reaction mechanisms in the human lung difficult. Nevertheless, such systems can supply much needed knowledge of the effects of chrysotile asbestos at the molecular level and the results can be applied to animal experiments and finally to studies of human tissue. With this in mind, sections of this paper offer a critical appraisal of some theories related to the biological potential of chrysotile asbestos, particularly those concerned with fibrogenesis. Complete discussion of all the theories relating to dust-induced fibrogenesis are not included as these are adequately covered in recent articles (HARINGTON, 1974; CHVAPIL, 1974).

REACTION OF CHRYSOTILE ASBESTOS WITH LUNG FIBROBLAST CULTURES

The interstitial fibroblast is the architect cell of lung tissue, being responsible for the formation and degradation of collagen (fibrous, pro and tropocollagen) and protein-mucopolysaccharide complexes (proteoglycans, proteoglycosaminoglycans) which form the matrix necessary for the correct conformation of collagen fibres (RICHARDS and WUSTEMAN, 1974b; CHVAPIL, 1974). Thus, in lung fibrosis and probably emphysema the ultimate response to toxins or particulate matter must involve the fibroblast cell. For reasons discussed previously (RICHARDS and JACOBY, 1974) we have considered that the lung fibroblast may be directly affected by dust particles which build up in the interstices of the lung. The results summarized in Table 1 indicate the direct effect of chrysotile asbestos on lung fibroblast cultures where the dust has been added to logarithmically growing cells. Details of dust additions, cell cultures and analyses for cell mat DNA, RNA, protein and hydroxyproline, and the culture fluid for secreted glycosaminoglycans (hyaluronic acid, chondroitin sulphates) have all been described previously (see Table 1). It should be noted that all experiments were carried out in the presence of foetal bovine serum (20%) and Waymouth's medium and consequently the chrysotile asbestos automatically receives an "organic coating" from components in the culture medium (discussed later).

TABLE 1. THE EFFECTS OF CHRYSOTILE ASBESTOS ON LUNG FIBROBLASTS *in vitro*
(L.P. = logarithmic growth phase; S.P. = stationary phase)

A. BIOCHEMICAL STUDIES		
1. Change in glycosaminoglycan release	(L.P. + S.P.)	
2. Alteration in ratio of secreted hyaluronic acid/ chondroitin sulphates	(S.P.)	RICHARDS *et al.*, 1971
3. Increase in cell mat fibrous collagen	(S.P.)	RICHARDS and MORRIS, 1973
4. Little stimulation of DNA		HEXT *et al.* (in preparation)
5. Depression of intracellular activities of lysosomal enzymes	(L.P.)	
6. Stimulation of plasma membrane ecto-ATPase	(late L.P. early S.P.)	
7. Decreased accumulation of amino acids	(late L.P.)	
B. LIGHT MICROSCOPE STUDIES		
1. Some cellular destruction followed by rapid recovery	(L.P.)	
2. Fusion of nucleolar material	(L.P.)	
3. Occurrence of binucleate cells	(L.P.)	RICHARDS and JACOBY, 1974
4. Induction of vacuolization	(L.P.)	
5. Abnormal formation of reticular fibres	(S.P.)	
C. TIME LAPSE PHOTOGRAPHIC STUDIES		
1. Some loss of contact inhibition	(L.P.)	
2. Early shedding of membrane fragments	(L.P.)	Unpublished data
3. Rare mitotic abnormalities	(L.P.)	
4. Uptake of small visible fibres; large fibres not taken up but "heaped" by cell action	(L.P.)	
D. ELECTRONMICROSCOPE STUDIES	(all L.P.)	
1. Early nuclear distortion ($4\frac{1}{2}$ h, after dust addition)		
2. Early alteration of cell surface—loss of "fuzz"-induction of microvilli		RICHARDS *et al.*, 1974
3. Early swelling of endoplasmic cisternae (24 h after dust)		
4. Early induction of pinocytosis		
5. Uptake of fibres (determined by serial sections) some of which are clearly membrane bound but many others appear free in the cytoplasm		

The results (Table 1) have indicated that more cell mat hydroxyproline (a measurement of fibrous collagen) is found in cultures exposed to chrysotile asbestos and that an alteration occurs in the level and ratio of glycosaminoglycans secreted into the culture medium. Chrysotile also has an effect on the cell surface as shown in Table 1

(A6; C1; C2; D2) and it induces early depression of intracellular hydrolytic enzyme activities although the relationship of this phenomenon to the uptake of dust into membrane-bound particles (D5) or the increased pinocytosis (D4) is unclear. It is possible that the membrane and lysosomal alterations as well as pinocytotic enhancement are all secondary changes following the effects of chrysotile on cytoplasmic components (see later) with subsequent alteration in the nucleolus and nuclear material.

Whilst some mitotic divisions are abnormal (one amitosis has been recorded on film) the cells recovering from exposure to chrysotile seem to exhibit normal mitosis. The electron microscopical and biochemical studies have indicated that chrysotile induces an early maturation process in these lung fibroblasts. Nuclear distortion, the appearance of cell surface microvilli, swelling of the endoplasmic cisternae, active pinocytosis, lower accumulation of amino acids and the stimulation of ATPase, all of which are induced within a short time period by chrysotile in logarithmically growing fibroblasts, are all characteristics of stationary phase ("old") normal cells. It was therefore postulated (RICHARDS *et al.*, 1974) that chrysotile speeded up the maturation or "ageing process" in fibroblast cultures and that the end product of this stimulation was an increased level of fibrous collagen (*in vitro* "fibrosis"). However, many questions arising from these studies remain unanswered: what is the original stimulus for this final effect? Are the effects of chrysotile on the cell membrane more important than changes caused by the entry of dust into the cytoplasm? Does the dust always enter the cell in a phagosomal vacuole? Why are lysosomal activities reduced at a time when active pinocytosis is taking place? What effect, if any, is due to the presence of binucleate cells, abnormal divisions and nucleolar abnormalities? In the fibrogenic effect are the collagen/reticulin fibres produced of the correct type? Is more collagen actually synthesized or is less collagen degreaded or does the alteration to the delicate balance of glycosaminoglycans secreted into the medium mean that more fibrous collagen will be laid down from the soluble tropocollagen molecules available (see OBRINK, 1973)?

This final question would seem to be of prime importance and studies using ^{3}H-proline are now in progress to determine the production of soluble and fibrous collagen throughout the culture period and the amount of collagenous material that is degraded in the presence and absence of chrysotile.

Recent studies have indicated that chrysotile can exert a dual effect on fibroblast cultures, i.e. it can cause an increase (*in vitro* "fibrosis") or decrease in the amount of cell mat hydroxyproline after 24 days *in vitro* (Table 2). For the sake of simplicity the first effect will be designated "I.H." and the latter effect "D.H." No complete explanation can be offered for the fact that the same concentration of chrysotile (50 μg/ml of culture medium) can produce two entirely opposite effects in fibroblast cultures. From experimentation it is known that the amount of cellular destruction, the removal of cellular debris and dust and subsequent recovery of the cell population, and/or the state of growth of the culture at the time of dust addition are not singularly responsible for producing the I.H. or D.H. effect. Whilst all of these factors may have a role in the extent of the response, it is considered that the actual mass or number of fibres available to the cell population (and perhaps the number which enter the cells) dictates whether more or less fibrous collagen is present in the chrysotile-treated cultures. Thus

TABLE 2. THE EFFECT OF CHRYSOTILE (50 μg/ml of culture medium) ON CELL MAT COLLAGEN LEVELS IN FIBROBLAST CULTURES

Dust was added during logarithmic growth on day 3 and cultures analysed for cell mat by hydroxyproline on day 24. The results are expressed relative to untreated control cultures taken as =100% and represent studies on ten different strains and twelve different subcultures (total number of treated cultures = 52). The DNA relative to controls (taken as 100%) is shown in brackets alongside each figure for hydroxyproline.

Relative levels of cell mat hydroxyproline in chrysotile-treated fibroblast cultures which gave values HIGHER than those of normal cultures (I.H. effect)			Relative levels of cell mat hydroxyproline in chrysotile-treated fibroblast cultures which gave values LOWER than those of normal cultures (D.H. effect)		
Strain and subculture number			Strain and subculture number		
16/3B	144	(85)	30/7AB	80	(69)
31/4	167	(83)	61/3A	25	(105)
30/4	102	(94)	61/35	37	(151)
40/5	866	(115)	65/2PS	77	(88)
40/6A	276	(107)			
56/F10	222	(84)			
65/4D	110	(94)			
57/7P	285	(140)			
Mean	271	(100)	Mean	55	(103)
Net change	+171%	(0)	Net change	−45%	(+3%)

in the culture system described (where at the point of dust addition there are approximately 1 to 1.5×10^6 logarithmically growing cells) it appears that lower concentrations of chrysotile (25 μg/ml of culture medium) produce the I.H. response whereas very high concentrations (75 μg/ml) produce the D.H. response. Concentrations between these levels can produce either effect although in all the cultures so far examined the fibrotic effect (I.H.) is favoured (>2: 1 at concentrations of 50 μg/ml of culture medium—see Fig. 1). Thus if it were possible to extrapolate to conditions in the lung and if an important effect of the chrysotile was direct action with interstitial fibroblasts in a state of an active repairing process, then it could be argued that only small amounts of this particular dust are necessary to produce a fibrotic response. On the other hand, large deposits or aggregation and continual reaction of small masses of fibres would lead to heavy cellular destruction and finally non-replacement or growth of interstitial tissue.

All the previously described studies have been restricted to strains of cells (derived initially as primary cell lines from rabbit lung) which have been maintained to their 10th passage (subculture) only. It is believed that prolonged subculturing leads to "age" changes in culture (RICHARDS and WUSTEMAN, 1974b) which may in turn induce a modified response to dust fibres as well as alteration in the balance of products. It was decided to study the long-term effects of chrysotile asbestos on a line of lung fibroblast cells and to monitor both the biochemical and morphological response to a

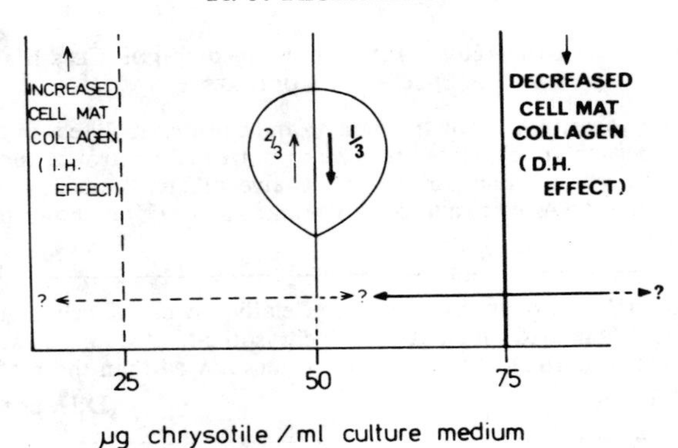

FIG. 1. Suggested response of lung fibroblast cultures to different concentrations (by mass) of chrysotile asbestos.

constant small dose of this dust. Thus a line of cells was isolated and after the first subculture one strain was given a small dose of chrysotile (strain 70/C) in the majority of passages (some subcultures received no dust stimulus, see Fig. 2) and another identical strain was kept as a control (strain 70/N) which received no such stimulus. Subcultures were performed on each cell strain at regular intervals (usually every 6 or 7 days) and dust was added to the chrysotile-treated strain 3 days after each subculture. At intervals, cultures derived from both 70/C and 70/N were set up for biochemical analysis by normal subculturing procedures and test cultures (those from the chrysotile-treated strain) received no further stimulus but were allowed to grow for a 24-day period (medium changes were carried out twice weekly). Control cultures from the normal strain (70/N) were set up in an identical manner and analyses carried out for a variety of parameters (DNA, RNA, protein, hydroxyproline). Changes in the levels of cell mat hydroxyproline (fibrous collagen) produced by cultures from both cell strains

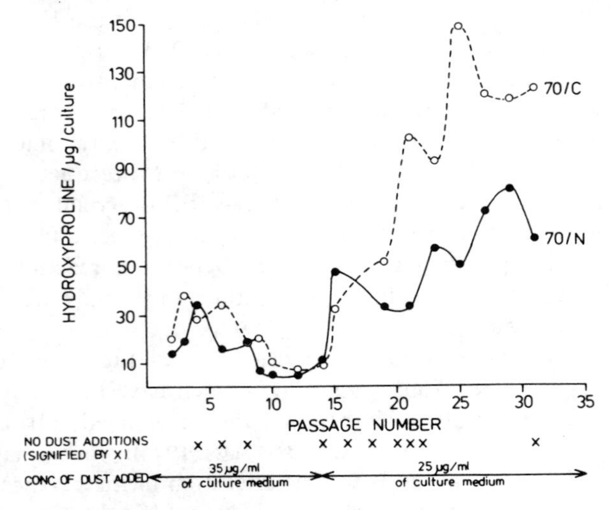

FIG. 2. The long-term effects of chrysotile asbestos on cell mat hydroxyproline levels in lung fibroblast cultures.

in different passages are shown (Fig. 2). It is evident that the chrysotile-treated strain has a higher level of fibrous collagen at most of the passage numbers studied and that this effect is particularly accentuated in test cultures examined after the 19th subculture despite the fact that no dust stimulus was given to the treated strain at the 16th, 18th, 20th, 21st or 22nd passages. Morphological studies have shown that both cell strains are diploid (some tetraploidy is evident although the majority of cells still have 44 chromosomes) although distinct morphological alterations (very large nuclei, increase in nucleoli) were noted at the 11th passage for the treated strain (70/C) and similarly in the control strain (70/N) at the 27th passage. These changes were evident but to a lesser degree for at least 3 or 4 passages on either side of the 11th subculture of 70/C and 27th subculture of 70/N but apart from these times the majority of the cells are of typical fibroblast-like morphology.

A number of interpretations of these data are possible and will be discussed elsewhere (HEXT *et al.*, in preparation). Nevertheless it can again be stated that small quantities of chrysotile asbestos can cause increases in the levels of fibrous collagen in fibroblast cultures and, in addition, removal of the chrysotile stimulus for 3 or 4 passages (hence leaving a small number of cells containing minute amounts of dust—subcultures 20–22, Fig. 2) does not reduce this effect. These data suggest, but still provide no firm proof, that additional collagen is synthesized and laid down by the chrysotile-treated strain. This would seem to be the most logical conclusion when two- to three-fold increases in fibrous collagen occur even when the hydroxyproline levels are expressed relative to cellular DNA. Thus, together with a study of the changes in protein and RNA levels (which are not always related to changes in DNA), the metabolism of collagen in this system would seem to warrant further investigation.

THE BINDING PROPERTIES OF CHRYSOTILE ASBESTOS

As indicated earlier, the binding properties of chrysotile and the subsequent modification of the organic coat may play an important role in the reaction of this dust with cell surfaces and cellular organelles. The positively charged Mg^{2+} ions on the fibre surface, the biochemical potential of trace elements (Cr, Ni, Mn, etc.) in the brucite layer ensures that the reactivity of chrysotile with biological fluids and cell components will be rapid and almost certainly complex (it is envisaged that in such biological fluids as serum, surfactant and interstitial fluid many micro and macromolecular products may adsorb in a multilayer organization on the dust surface). The organic modification of chrysotile dictates its ability to react with cell surfaces. This has been suggested by previous investigators (MCNAB and HARINGTON, 1967; ALLISON, 1971) and recently studied in detail by DESAI *et al.*, 1975. Further results by Desai are shown in Table 3. Serum proteins/polypeptides from the tissue culture medium bind to the chrysotile surface and other studies have shown that the reaction is virtually instantaneous (<30 s). After the reaction, washing of the modified chrysotile with distilled water or hypotonic or isotonic salt solutions removes considerable amounts of proteinaceous (and other?) materials from the surface as shown by the gel electrophoresis patterns and the semi-quantitative estimations of protein remaining on the dust. Thus it might be expected that removal of proteins (the gel electrophoresis studies suggest that particularly the soluble proteins in the 70 000–80 000 molecular weight range, probably albumin and fetuin are removed) from the chrysotile surface would increase the potential of the dust in the haemolytic action. In fact the opposite effect occurs; removal of the soluble proteins reduces the ability of the dust to induce membrane damage (Table 3). This suggests that non-soluble materials (lipids?) bound tightly to the chrysotile surface offer better protection against haemolysis, although the possibility that Mg^{2+} (and other ions) present on the dust surface attach to soluble proteins and may then be removed in the washing procedure, must not be excluded. Nevertheless the former suggestion is attractive and receives support from the fact that rabbit pulmonary surfactant (almost 100% lipoprotein material—79% lipid, 18% protein) completely prevents the chrysotile-induced haemolysis of rabbit erythrocytes when prebound onto the dust surface (DESAI *et al.*, 1975).

In order to obtain good quantitative estimations of materials bound a useful method is that described by MORGAN (1974) who studied the binding of radioactively labelled

TABLE 3. CHANGES IN THE HAEMOLYTIC POTENCY OF CHRYSOTILE BY MODIFICATION OF THE ORGANIC COATING ON THE DUST SURFACE

Haemolysis experiments were performed according to HARINGTON *et al.* (1971) as slightly modified by DESAI *et al.* (1975). In the binding experiments 10 mg of chrysotile was pretreated for 1 h at 37°C in 20% foetal bovine serum + Waymouth's medium and following the desired wash treatments the proteins/polypeptides remaining on the dust surface were removed with sodium dodecyl sulphate and subjected to gel electrophoresis (see FAIRBANKS *et al.*, 1971). A crude estimation of the protein remaining on the surface after each treatment was made by first centrifuging the "dust", removing the organic coat with either 1 M NaOH or 6 N HCl and estimating the total NH_2 groups present with ninhydrin (against standard preparation of leucine) or protein present by the Folin reagent (using bovine serum albumin as a standard).

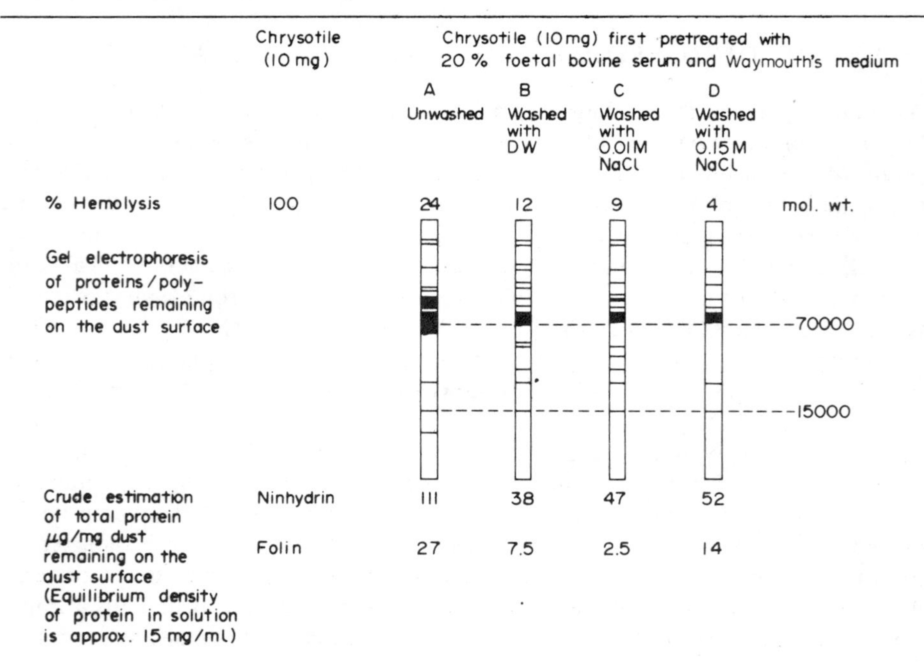

	Chrysotile (10 mg)	Chrysotile (10 mg) first pretreated with 20 % foetal bovine serum and Waymouth's medium				
		A Unwashed	B Washed with DW	C Washed with 0.01 M NaCl	D Washed with 0.15 M NaCl	
% Hemolysis	100	24	12	9	4	mol. wt.
Gel electrophoresis of proteins / polypeptides remaining on the dust surface						70000 15000
Crude estimation of total protein µg/mg dust remaining on the dust surface (Equilibrium density of protein in solution is approx. 15 mg/ml)	Ninhydrin	111	38	47	52	
	Folin	27	7.5	2.5	14	

albumin to dusts. DESAI (data in preparation) has prepared both rabbit serum containing radioactively labelled protein components and labelled pulmonary surfactant for use in binding studies (Table 4). The binding and retention of radioactive serum proteins confirm the findings recorded previously (Fig. 3). It is also evident that chrysotile binds the extracellular lung component, pulmonary surfactant, and that this material is not easily removed from the surface under the conditions of experimentation described (Table 4).

TABLE 4. THE BINDING OF RADIOACTIVELY LABELLED PROTEINS/POLYPEPTIDES FROM RABBIT SERUM AND OF PULMONARY SURFACTANT TO CHRYSOTILE ASBESTOS

To prepare the labelled serum rabbits are given a sterile intravenous injection of ^{3}H-phenyl-lanine in 0.15 M NaCl and sacrificed after 24 h. The blood is drained and allowed to clot and the serum separated at 4°C. Protein estimations and total incorporated radioactivity are recorded following dialysis and the serum sterilized and diluted to the required equilibrium density. Radioactively labelled pulmonary surfactant is prepared by sterile intravenous injection of ^{14}C-palmitate (previously bound to serum albumin in 0.15 M NaCl) into rabbits starved for 24 h. Twenty-four hours after injection the animal is sacrificed by air embolism (nembutal or ether should not be used), the lungs removed intact and pulmonary surfactant prepared, under sterile conditions, by the method of DESAI *et al.* (1975). For full details of the physical properties and biochemical assessment of pulmonary surfactant see HARWOOD *et al.* (1975). Binding studies were performed for 1 h at 37°C. All the washing procedures are carried out in 3 ml of medium for 5 s on a whirlimix, the dust is then spun off and radioactivity counted in both the supernatant and on the amount retained on the dust. Losses due to adsorption on plastic vessels are very slight and insignificant. There is no significant degradation of surfactant (i.e. releasing free ^{14}C-palmitate) over the time course of the experiment.

	(A) Binding and retention of ^{3}H-phenylalanine labelled protein in rabbit serum plus 0.15 M NaCl (Equilibrium density of protein = 5.0 mg/ml)		(B) Binding and retention of labelled pulmonary surfactant in veronal buffered saline (Equilibrium density of surfactant = 1 mg/ml)	
	μg Protein/mg chrysotile	% Retention	μg Surfactant/mg chrysotile	% Retention
Chrysotile asbestos unwashed (2.5 mg)	327		200	
Pretreated dust (2.5 mg) washed once with distilled water	160	49%	186	93%
Pretreated dust (2.5 mg) washed once with 0.15 M NaCl (A) or VBS (B)	160	49%	190	96%

The binding and retention of pulmonary surfactant may be particularly important in studies involving the effect of this dust on alveolar macrophages as presumably these cells live in an environment containing surfactant material and may be responsible for its degradation. A purified preparation of lysosomal enzymes from alveolar macrophages will remove and degrade part of the bound surfactant from the chrysotile surface and experiments are now in progress to study this effect in detail. This type of study is considered important following the work of DAVIES *et al.* (1974) who suggest that when chrysotile enters peritoneal macrophages by phagocytosis it reacts intralysosomally and selectively stimulates the release of hydrolytic enzymes to the cell exterior. These investigators suggest that once hydrolytic enzymes remove the protein coat from the chrysotile then "free" Mg^{2+} groups on the chrysotile surface may interact with lysosomal membrane sialoglycoproteins leading to the formation of membrane protein clusters which is possibly a prerequisite for membrane fusion and exocytosis. It is postulated that the release of lysosomal enzymes may be important in inducing tissue damage seen in chronic inflammation. Some points in these proposals would seem important in future investigations. Once the organic coat (which may not simply be protein) is removed or partially degraded by lysosomal enzymes (either bound to the lysosomal membrane or free in the hydrolytic sap) would not the enzymes or their substrate degradation products then bind onto the "chrysotile" surface? How would this affect the activities of the enzymes? Would released lysosomal enzymes (normally most active in the pH range 3–5 inside the lysosome) produce significant damage in the surrounding tissue matrix (interstitial tissue is considered to be approximately pH 7) unless localized changes in pH occur? WOESSNER (1973) concludes that lysosomal cathepsin D accounts for the digestion of connective tissue protein polysaccharide complexes at pH 5.0 but has no action upon them at pH 7.2. Similarly MORRISON *et al.* (1973) have found that human lysosomal cathepsins B_1 and D have little or no activity in degrading embryonic cartilage proteoglycans at pH 7.0. Nevertheless, as pointed out by DAVIES *et al.* (1974), several agents (including chrysotile) which cause chronic inflammation *in vivo* induce selective release of lysosomal enzymes from peritoneal macrophages *in vitro*. It is clear that whilst precise biochemical conclusions cannot be drawn at the present time this area of research needs further attention.

DESAI (data in preparation) has carried out some studies reacting alveolar macrophage lysosomal preparations with chrysotile asbestos and with dusts pretreated with tissue culture medium (20% foetal bovine serum plus Waymouth's medium) or pulmonary surfactant. The binding affinity of one enzyme, cathepsin D, is shown below (Fig. 3).

Lysosomal enzyme preparations can be maintained for periods of up to 3 weeks at 35°C in isotonic saline or 0.25 M sucrose, buffered at pH 5. The loss of activity is gradual and differs with different enzymes and is dependent on the pH of the medium. There is total loss of activity in all enzymes studied after 14 days when maintained at pH 7. The presence of tissue culture medium is beneficial in retaining enzyme activity although sheep surfactant has no such effect. Chrysotile did not degrade any of the enzymes studied (RNAase, cathepsin D or acid phosphatase) but was found to adsorb the enzymes onto its surface, less binding occurring to dust pretreated with and incubated with tissue culture medium and sheep pulmonary surfactant (Fig. 3).

SPECULATION ON THE MECHANISM OF ACTION OF CHRYSOTILE ON LUNG FIBROBLASTS IN VITRO

The coating of chrysotile asbestos by a range of biological complexes modifies the dust surface prior to any contact with cells in tissue culture (or possibly *in vivo* in the

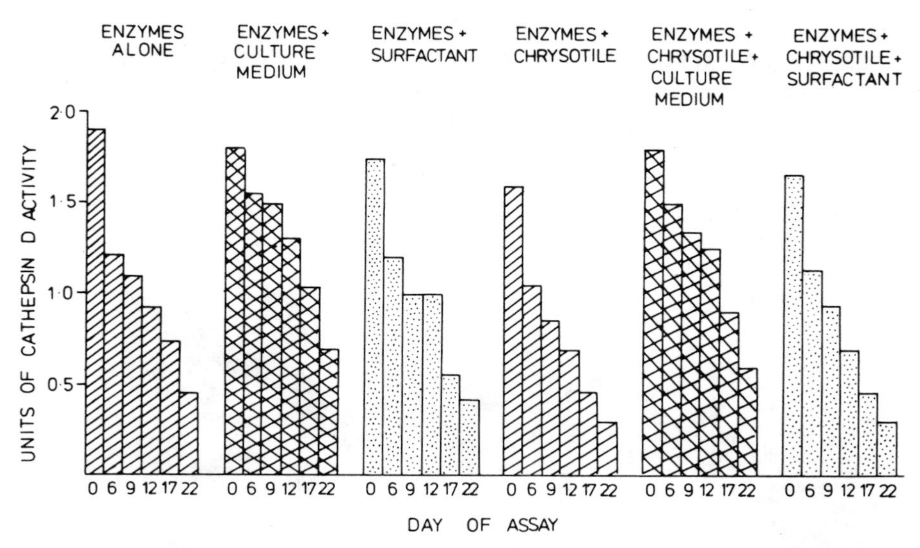

FIG. 3. The ability of chrysotile to bind lysosomal cathepsin D at pH 5 and 35°C. Sheep alveolar macrophages are obtained by standardized lung lavage techniques; the cells are homogenized and a biased lysosomal fraction is obtained by ultracentrifugation in 0.25 M sucrose (EDTA should not be included because of its chelating effect on chrysotile—see HARINGTON *et al.*, 1971). The lysomes are disrupted ultrasonically and sterilized by passage through a 0.45 millipore filter. The enzyme preparations with and without chrysotile are then maintained at 35°C in 0.15 M NaCl buffered either at pH 5 (acetate) or pH 7 (phosphate), the sample being shaken continuously under sterile conditions. Samples were removed at varying time intervals and assayed directly (for total enzyme activity) or first centrifuged and the enzyme activity remaining in the supernatant assessed (for a measure of enzyme activity on the dust). Control assays were performed in all experiments. Cathepsin D was assayed as described previously (RICHARDS and WUSTEMAN, 1974a).

lung). This coating may assist in the phagocytosis or passage of "dust" through the cell surface, particularly for the fibroblast cell which would not "recognize" the material as "foreign". When chrysotile enters fibroblast cells by normal phagocytosis (in a membrane bound phagosomal vacuole) then fusion with primary or secondary lysosomes would result in reactions in the secondary lysosomes including the degradation of some of the organic coat and the possible "opening out" of the dust fibres exposing free Mg^{2+} groups which could then bind but not degrade lysosomal enzymes. In addition, as suggested by DAVIES *et al.* (1974), impairment to the structure of the lysosomal membrane may occur with subsequent exocytosis of hydrolytic enzymes. In chrysotile-exposed fibroblast cultures it is difficult to explain how enzyme release determines whether or not higher or lower levels of fibrous collagen are deposited, unless such hydrolytic enzymes as cathepsin B_1 and D can alter the matrix proteoglycan complexes and thus control the deposition of collagen (OBRINK, 1973). Changes in the levels of proteoglycan secreted into the culture medium by fibroblasts exposed to chrysotile do occur (RICHARDS and MORRIS, 1973) although studies on the cellular levels and the secretion of cathepsin D by such cells are very complex and, as yet, are not fully understood.

It is possible that these events occur following and/or parallel to other pathological reactions in the chrysotile-treated fibroblast cultures. Logarithmically growing fibroblasts have highly active undulating membranes and electron microscopical studies suggest that during this stage of growth some areas of the cell surface are not delineated by a typical plasma membrane but have regions of "fuzz" with associated groups of microfilaments and polyribosomes. This "fuzz" which may consist of mucopolysaccharide/glycoprotein complexes, traps the chrysotile fibres some of which subsequently pass through this layer (and apparently directly) into the cell cytoplasm as non-membrane bound particles (Fig. 4). If these observations are not artefacts due to

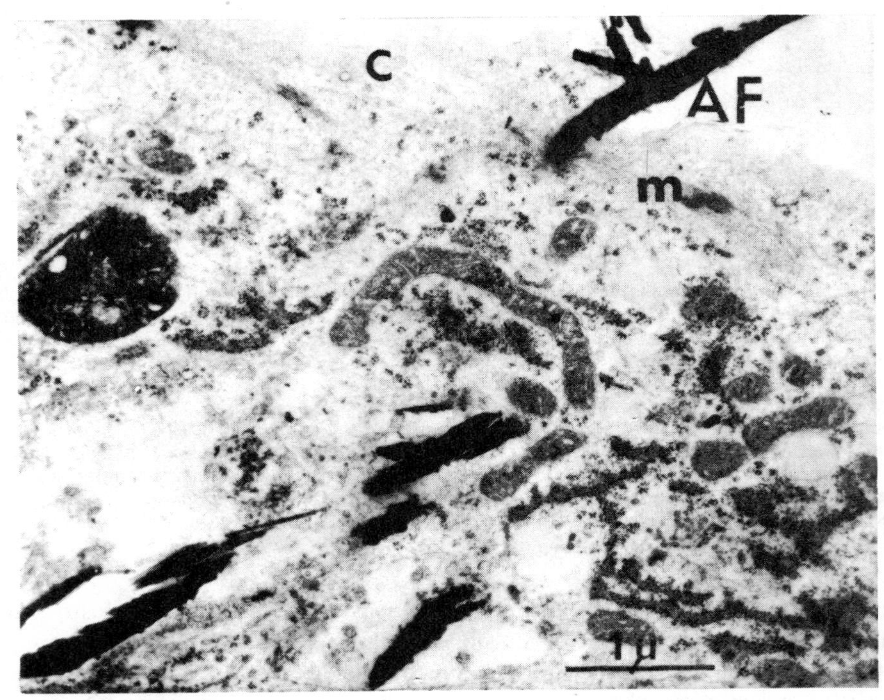

FIG. 4. Electron micrograph of a portion of a logarithmically growing fibroblast cell exposed to chrysotile asbestos. c = cell surface; m = microfilaments; AF = asbestos fibres.

limitations in the electron microscopical techniques employed then chrysotile fibres lie "free" in the cytoplasm of the cell apart from their coating of adsorbed material. Partial loss of this coat as a result of attack by cell sap enzymes or the "opening out" of the fibre to expose highly reactive Mg^{2+} and other positively charged ions would mean that other macromolecules in the cytoplasm could be adsorbed and possibly affected. One such macromolecule could be RNA in which case it is possible to propose a series of events leading to fibrogenesis. The binding of RNA to the chrysotile could lead to cytosol depletion of RNA followed by nuclear stimulation, increased RNA synthesis and hence protein or proteoglycan synthesis. This effect, coupled with lysosomal impairment (i.e. the system may become "clogged" due to the presence of dust and unable to degrade excess protein or proteoglycan), could lead to fibrogenesis.

Certainly, considerable changes in the metabolism of RNA occur in chrysotile-treated fibroblast cultures. In the majority of experiments where a "fibrogenic" (I.H.) reaction occurs correspondingly high levels of RNA are found in the chrysotile-treated cultures, particularly in the long-term studies (Fig. 2). Morphological studies indicate very early changes in the fibroblast nucleolar material soon after the addition of chrysotile and lysosomal RNAase is considerably depressed in all chrysotile-treated cultures. Whilst chrysotile binds RNA preliminary studies suggest that it does not degrade this material. There are apparently no studies in the literature describing the effect of chrysotile on the synthesis and degradation of RNA by cellular systems although HARINGTON (1973) reports some unpublished work by Hawtrey and Bester in which different types of asbestos have been tried as templates for RNA synthesis. In the fibroblast cultures described it would seem to be particularly important to determine whether or not changes in RNA metabolism occurred prior to, parallel with, or as a consequence of, alterations in the lysosomal apparatus.

Thus, in summary, these preliminary findings help to define partially the biological reaction potential of chrysotile at least in simple *in vitro* systems. It would seem to be of importance to establish the primary biochemical lesion induced in fibroblast cultures as a result of exposure to chrysotile thus leading to cellular ageing and excess accumulation of fibrous collagen. Some of the alterations produced in fibroblast cultures by chrysotile are secondary in nature (particularly those associated with changes in plasma membrane structure, amino acid accumulation, pinocytosis) but the primary effect of this fibrous dust is still open to question. The significance of these *in vitro* studies to the reaction of the lung to inhaled chrysotile asbestos is, as yet, unknown although they form the basis of a collaborative study with the M.R.C. Pneumoconiosis Unit, Llandough Hospital, S. Wales, which is designed to determine the sequence of biochemical and morphological changes in lung tissue leading to chrysotile-induced fibrosis. Some of the findings, particularly related to pulmonary surfactant production, are reported in this Symposium (McDERMOTT *et al.*, p. 415).

Acknowledgements—We are grateful to the M.R.C. for financial support; to Mr W. Edwards for excellent technical assistance and to many members of the Biochemistry Department, University College, Cardiff, for their helpful suggestions.

REFERENCES

ALLISON, A. C. (1971) *Inhaled Particles III* (edited by WALTON, W. H.), vol. I, pp. 437–445. Unwin Bros., Old Woking, Surrey.

BECK, E. G., HOLT, P. F. and NASRALLAH, E. T. (1971) *Br. J. ind. Med.* **28,** 179–185.

CHVAPIL, M. (1974) *Envir. Hlth Perspect.* **9,** 283–294.

DAVIES, P., ALLISON, A. C., ACKERMAN, J., BUTTERFIELD, A. and WILLIAMS, S. (1974) *Nature, Lond.* **251,** 423–425.

DESAI, R., HEXT, P. and RICHARDS, R. J. (1975) *Life Sci.* **16,** 1931–1938.

FAIRBANKS, G., STECK, T. L. and WALLACH, D. F. H. (1971) *Biochem.* **10,** 2606–2617.

HARINGTON, J. S. (1973) *Biological Effects of Asbestos. Proceedings of a Working Conference, Lyon 1972* (edited by BOGOVSKI, P., GILSON, J. C., TIMBRELL, V. and WAGNER, J. C.) pp. 304–311. I.A.R.C. Scientific Publication no. 8. International Agency for Research in Cancer, Lyon.

HARINGTON, J. S. (1974) *Envir. Hlth Perspec.* **9,** 271–279.
HARINGTON, J. S., MILLER, K. and MACNAB, G. (1971) *Envir. Res.* **4,** 95–117.
HARWOOD, J., DESAI, R., HEXT, P., TETLEY, T. and RICHARDS, R. (1975) *Biochem. J.* **151,** 707–714.
JONES, B. M., EDWARDS, J. H. and WAGNER, J. C. (1972) *Br. J. ind. Med.* **29,** 287–292.
KOGAN, F. M. (1970) *Proceedings of the Federal Symposium of the U.S.S.R., Sverdlovsk*, 1968 (edited by VELICHKOVSKII, B. T.) pp. 16–34. Inst. Gig. Tr. Profzabol, Sverdlovsk, U.S.S.R.
MACNAB, G. and HARINGTON, J. S. (1967) *Nature, Lond.* **214,** 522–523.
MORGAN, A. (1974) *Envir. Res.* **7,** 330–341.
MORGAN, A., HOLMES, A. and GOLD, C. (1971) *Envir. Res.* **4,** 558–570.
MORRISON, R. I. G., BARRETT, A. J., DINGLE, J. T. and PRIOR, D. (1973) *Biochim. Biophys. Acta* **302,** 411–419.
OBRINK, B. (1973) *Eur. J. Biochem.* **33,** 387–400.
POTT, F., HUTH, F. and FRIEDRICHS, K. H. (1974) *Envir. Hlth Perspect.* **9,** 313–315.
RICHARDS, R. J. and JACOBY, F. (1974) *Tissue Culture in Medical Research. Proceedings of the Symposium, Cardiff, Wales 1973* (edited by JACOBY, F.) pp. 328–335. Heinemann, London.
RICHARDS, R. J. and MORRIS, T. G. (1973) *Life Sci.* **12,** 441–451.
RICHARDS, R. J. and WUSTEMAN, F. S. (1974a) *Life Sci.* **14,** 355–364.
RICHARDS, R. J. and WUSTEMAN, F. S. (1974b) *Tissue Culture in Medical Research. Proceedings of the Symposium, Cardiff, Wales 1973* (edited by JACOBY, F.) pp. 91–99. Heinemann, London.
RICHARDS, R. J., HEXT, P. M., BLUNDELL, G., HENDERSON, W. J. and VOLCANI, B. E. (1974) *Br. J. exp. Path.* **55,** 275–281.
RICHARDS, R. J., WUSTEMAN, F. S. and DODGSON, K. S. (1971) *Life Sci.* **10,** 1149–1159.
SAKABE, H., KOSHI, K. and HAYASHI, H. (1971) *Inhaled Particles III* (edited by WALTON, W. H.) vol. I, pp. 423–435, Unwin Bros., Old Woking, Surrey.
WAGNER, J. C., BERRY, G. and TIMBRELL, V. (1973) *Br. J. Cancer* **28,** 173–185.
WOESSNER, J. F. (1973) *Fed. Proc.* **32,** 1485–1488.

DISCUSSION

V. Timbrell: Is there a limit to the diameter of a fibre capable of entering the cell through the "fuzz"?

Dr Richards: I'm not sure about a limit to the diameter but certainly fibres above a certain length do not enter these cells (20 μm is the largest we've seen inside the cells). If you study the fibroblasts by time-lapse cinematography the longer fibres tend to be "heaped" into masses by cellular action. Presumably there must be some limit to the diameter of a fibre which might prevent its ingestion but I cannot guess what this would be.

K. Robock: (i) Your hypothesis about the action of asbestos fibres inside the fibroblasts requires a pathogenic reaction to short fibres. This is not in agreement with current knowledge that short fibres (shorter than about 10 μm) are not cytotoxic, fibrogenic or carcinogenic. Can you give an explanation for this disagreement?

(ii) Do you know the lysosomal hypothesis of A. C. Allison (*Inhaled Particles III*, 1970, vol. I, p. 437. Unwin Bros., Old Woking) about the mechanism of SiO_2 particles? It seems that this hypothesis applies to a number of unspecific reactions, arthritis for instance, and cannot explain specific SiO_2 or asbestos effects. Is this any different from your hypothesis?

Dr Richards: (i) We used U.I.C.C. Rhodesian chrysotile in our experiments with fibroblasts and so both "long" and "short" fibres were present. Nevertheless we assume that the asbestos fibres which can actually enter the fibroblasts (20 μm seems to be the length limit) are the ones which initiate our *in vitro* fibrogenesis. This is not to say that larger fibres (>20 μm) are not cytotoxic but we would question whether cytotoxicity and fibrogenicity are linked. I find it hard to believe that short fibres (<10 μm) are not cytotoxic, fibrogenic or carcinogenic although I would agree that fibres greater than 10 μm would be more difficult to clear from the lung.

(ii) We have discussed the lysosomal theory as related to the effects of asbestos in some detail in our manuscript. I think that the hypothesis we are suggesting is very different.

J. Bruch: (i) There is little evidence that fibroblasts are directly involved in the phagocytic process *in vivo*. Most of the asbestos inhaled can be detected in alveolar macrophages and to a less extent in type I pneumocytes. Did you test the effect of chrysotile on fibroblasts cultivated together with alveolar macrophages?

(ii) Do you think the lysosomal concept could be applied to the fibroblast system? Can you give any hint as to the size of the digestive apparatus in the fibroblast in comparison to the alveolar macrophages?

(iii) Did you use dust controls, i.e. (a) inert dusts with round particles and (b) other asbestos dust such as amphibole asbestos?

Dr Richards: (i) I agree that there is practically no evidence (however, see Davis overleaf) to suggest that fibroblasts are involved in the phagocytic process *in vivo* possibly because few studies have been directed towards the role of the fibroblast in dust-induced diseases despite the fact it must play an important part in fibrogenesis. We would be the first to point out that the theories we have proposed are taken from results of *in vitro* experiments and therefore we will have to demonstrate that similar events can occur *in vivo*. I think it is generally accepted that one of the primary responses to inhaled dust is by the macrophage cells. We also believe that at certain periods of their lifetime fibroblasts are also potential target cells for dust. We have not tested the effects of chrysotile-treated macrophages on fibroblast cells although we found previously that sufficient numbers of macrophages without any dust pretreatment could stimulate a fibrogenic response in fibroblast cultures (Richards and Wusteman, 1974, *Life Sciences* **14**, 355).

(ii) The lysosomal concept could be applied to the fibroblast system and presumably to other cells which have a lysosomal complement and exhibit normal phagocytosis but I think that many questions must be posed as to the significance of the lysosomal concept in the fibrotic (not cytotoxic or carcinogenic) reaction. We have discussed some of these in the manuscript. There are less lysosomes in the fibroblast cell than, for example, the alveolar macrophage (morphologically speaking). However, the lysosomal enzyme contents may be quite different; for example fibroblast cells show a higher specific activity of cathepsin D than alveolar macrophages although the former cells have lower RNAase and acid phosphatase activities than alveolar macrophages. The enzyme complement of fibroblasts also change with age *in vitro*.

(iii) Very preliminary studies with titanium dioxide, diamond dust and polystyrene particles at equivalent concentrations to the studies conducted with chrysotile have little effect in inducing fibrogenesis (after 24 days *in vitro*). Amosite, anthophyllite and crocidolite (U.I.C.C. samples) are all fibrogenic in our system.

S. Holmes: In your introduction you referred to the possibility of asbestos-induced disease in the general public due to the small amounts present in the atmosphere, liquids, food and drugs. Have you any evidence of this? The most authoritative statement on this question was made at Lyon in 1972 (*Ann. occup. Hyg.* 1973, **16,** 12) when it was said that, so far as is known, there is no risk.

Dr RICHARDS: Thank you Dr Holmes. If anything is considered misleading in the manuscript it will be withdrawn from the published text.

I. P. GORMLEY: You state that "cells recovering from exposure to chrysotile seem to exhibit perfectly normal mitosis". Have you looked at the chromosomes and, if so, are they normal or are there aberrations present?

Dr RICHARDS: Yes, we did. In our long-term studies (see text) where chrysotile was given repeatably to fibroblasts, chromosome counts were performed. With few exceptions the chromosome number stays the same—at 44 in this particular case. Normal mitoses were recorded on film in cells recovering from chrysotile and in one instance only an amitotic division was seen. We do not know if any form of chromosome damage occurs in these cells after exposure to asbestos but it would certainly seem important to find this out.

J. M. G. DAVIS: Some years ago we reported that electron microscope studies of rat lungs after asbestos inhalation did show asbestos fibres in some fibroblasts. I suggest it is most important to determine the relative importance of fibres taken up by macrophages and those taken up by fibroblasts in the stimulation of collagen production.

Dr RICHARDS: I think that we are suggesting the same thing.

A. G. HEPPLESTON: Your cell diagrams referred to "fibroblasts" but suggested to me that the cells taking up chrysotile were macrophages. I wonder if your cultures were a mixture of macrophages and fibroblasts and whether a macrophage factor may be involved in fibre fibrogenesis.

Dr RICHARDS: That is a good question. We never do any work with our cultures until we feel the macrophages have been removed. Certainly in obtaining our cell lines by trypsinization from lung tissue we start off with mixed cell cultures. However, alveolar macrophages are quickly removed because they readily float in culture and are readily killed by repeated trypsinization. Thus we wait for three or four subcultures after the primary isolation before beginning experiments. I think that the diagrams look like "macrophages" because the normally stellate fibroblast cells take on a similar morphology (light microscope studies) to macrophage following treatment with chrysotile. However, from biochemical and electron microscope data the cells that we are growing are clearly fibroblast-like. I see no reason why these findings of the effects of chrysotile on fibroblasts are in disagreement with previous findings about the macrophage factor involvement in fibrogenesis. In fact some of our own earlier studies (RICHARDS and WUSTEMAN, 1974, *Life Sciences* **14,** 355) would suggest a relationship between macrophages and fibroblasts, whether or not the former cells have been pretreated with dust.

R. HUNT: Are you aware of the effects on cell growth in cultures where the liquid substrate has been filtered through sterile asbestos filters? It is assumed that selective protein fraction adsorption has taken place. The same form of adsorption will take place by phagocytosed asbestos and so alter the cytochemistry of the host cell. The inter-lattice spaces on the surface of the fibre must also introduce enormous variations in this phenomenon.

Dr RICHARDS: Yes, we feel that the reaction of any dust particle is related to the material it adsorbs or binds onto its surface or perhaps how material once adsorbed is exchanged in the cell. As you point out the variability of this adsorption must be highly complex. It would be nice to know if it (adsorption) was specific for different dust samples. I think that few cell culture workers use asbestos filters for sterilizing culture medium at the present time.

G. V. COLES: From the practical point of view this morning's papers have thrown much light on the question of substituting other materials for asbestos in the form of fibre-reinforced structural materials. Details of composition of suggested substitutes for asbestos boards of various types as produced in the U.S.A. sometimes show a very high proportion—up to 30%—of free quartz in the matrix. Reinforcing materials proposed have been of many types ranging from carbon fibres to fibrous glass or rock wool. The discussions have suggested that mixed exposure to fibrous asbestos and other fibrogenic materials greatly enhances one of the biological effects of asbestos, namely its fibrogenicity; if the fibres of asbestos also exert their property of inducing neoplasia through becoming templates for RNA production either through surface effects or from their morphology, suspicion must arise that mixed exposure with other fibrogenic materials might enhance the production of neoplasia by asbestos fibres. But the work of Stanton and Wrench and others indicates that the danger of neoplasia from fibres may be independent of the fibre composition and thus of surface effects of the material, and associated with morphology only. Then if the fibre used as reinforcement is one which long maintains a morphology in a dangerous size or shape when deposited *in vivo* in alveoli, the importance of eliminating fibrogenic materials such as quartz from the matrix may be important lest we find substitutes in use which are even more dangerous than previously used asbestos-reinforced materials. However, if the long-term contact with tissue *in vivo* degrades the fibre so that it does not remain in a dangerous size or shape then such a material should be that of choice in the development of substitutes for asbestos-based materials. As WRIGHT and KUSCHNER indicate (p. 455) that glass, for example, degrades *in vivo* in this way it might be possible to satisfy the demands of technology for slender fibres as reinforcement in place of asbestos without the tumour-inducing hazards of the latter.

PREDOMINANCE OF HISTOCOMPATIBILITY ANTIGENS W18 AND HL-A1 IN MINERS RESISTANT TO COMPLICATED COALWORKERS' PNEUMOCONIOSIS*

E. R. HEISE, P. C. MAJOR, M. SHARON MENTNECH, E. J. PARRISH, ANDREA L. JORDON and W. K. C. MORGAN

Appalachian Laboratory for Occupational Safety and Health, National Institute for Occupational Safety and Health, Departments of Microbiology and Medicine, West Virginia University Medical Center, Morgantown, WVa

and

Department of Microbiology, Bowman Gray School of Medicine, Winston-Salem, NC, U.S.A.

Abstract—The possibility that an association exists between susceptibility or resistance to coal workers' pneumoconiosis (CWP) and the distribution of blood group and histocompatibility (HL–A) antigens was tested in a sample of Pennsylvania and West Virginia coal miners with a high prevalence of CWP. Unrelated miners, who were matched by geographic region for age and years in mining, were then divided into three groups composed of men with (1) no radiographic evidence of CWP, (2) simple CWP, and (3) complicated CWP (progressive massive fibrosis or PMF). The distribution of twenty-three HL–A antigens was determined by a two-stage lymphocyte microcytotoxicity technique. The frequency for each antigen was calculated for the total sample ($n = 277$) and for each geographic region and disease category.

Blood-group antigen frequencies were compared by disease category and geographic region on participants in the study in an attempt to detect bias due to ethnic stratification. There were no differences noted within disease categories. One region was found where some stratification might be present.

The serum concentrations of complement and three immunoglobulin classes were measured in an effort to assess disturbances of humoral immunity. No apparent clinical significance could be attributed to the differences in mean values which existed between experimental groups.

When examined at the $P = 0.05$ level there was an excess of the W18 histocompatibility antigen in miners who had no evidence of disease but whose histories of coal-dust exposure were comparable to the two disease groups. The frequency of W18 in miners with simple CWP was approximately that expected for a heterogeneous population of Caucasians. The relative risk of complicated CWP was approximately 300% less in miners who possessed antigen W18 than in those lacking this antigen.

These results suggest an association between W18 and resistance to the development of progressive massive fibrosis and that HL–A1 is associated with resistance to the development of both simple and complicated CWP.

* Work supported in part by the Surgical Tissue Typing Fund of Bowman Gray School of Medicine and NIH grant HL 1676901.

INTRODUCTION

Coal workers' peumoconiosis (CWP) exists in two distinct forms—simple and complicated. The former occurs when the quantity of retained coal dust exceeds the clearance capacity of the lung and is recognized by the presence of small opacities in the chest radiograph. Three categories of simple CWP are defined according to the extent and profusion of these opacities. Simple CWP is associated with minimal respiratory impairment (MORGAN *et al.*, 1972). The second form of CWP, progressive massive fibrosis (PMF), usually occurs on a background of categories 2 or 3 simple CWP and is characterized by the development of large fibrotic masses. PMF is an irreversible process that is often associated with respiratory impairment, permanent disability and premature death (LAPP and SEATON, 1971). The proportion of miners with PMF varies from 0.5% in Utah and Colorado to 3% in central Pennsylvania and approximately 14% in the anthracite miners of Eastern Pennsylvania (MORGAN *et al.*, 1973). It has been suggested that undefined host factors are important in the development of complicated CWP. One of the suspected factors may involve immune responsiveness, since an increased frequency of antinuclear antibodies has been noted in patients with CWP, especially in association with PMF (LIPPMANN *et al.*, 1973; SOUTAR *et al.*, 1974). Whether immunological factors play a role in pathogenesis of this disease remains uncertain (MAJOR *et al.*, 1975).

It is now clear that in animals the genetic region which codes for the major histocompatibility antigens also carries genes important for disease susceptibility (GREEN, 1974). These observations have provided the basis for numerous studies in man of the possible association between genes of the HL–A system and disease. Convincing and consistent differences in the frequency of particular HL–A or related genes have been demonstrated in patients with several diseases of obscure aetiology.

The most widely accepted explanation for the established associations involves immune response (Ir) genes, some of which are linked closely to loci which specify serologically defined and lymphocyte activating determinants of the HL–A system. The fact that the majority of coal miners with simple CWP do not develop PMF raises the possibility that genetic factors may be important in the disease. We therefore compared the frequency of HL–A antigens within a population of active and retired miners in the coal fields of Pennsylvania and northern West Virginia. Our objective was to determine whether particular HL–A antigens were associated with susceptibility or resistance to CWP.

SUBJECTS AND METHODS*

The population under study consisted of 277 unrelated coal miners (273 Caucasian, 2 American Negro, and 2 American Indian) selected on a volunteer basis from a population of miners examined in the first and second series of the United States National Coal Study (MORGAN *et al.*, 1973). The subjects were divided into three experimental groups that were closely matched according to geographic region for age in years (mean 56; range 39–68) and years in mining (mean 34; range 1–54).

As such it is impossible to match the sub-groups according to dust exposure in that

* Mention of brand names does not constitute endorsement by the U.S. Public Health Service.

for the most part it can be assumed that miners with simple CWP and PMF are likely to have been exposed to greater amounts of respirable coal dust than have miners with category 0 (ROGAN *et al.*, 1973). None the less, this need not always be so since the development of CWP is also related to the efficiency of lung clearance. For the purposes of this study, it can also be assumed that miners who have worked for many years but who have clear lungs nevertheless have had fairly heavy dust exposure but for reasons as yet not understood have not developed CWP.

Group I consisted of 97 miners (35% of the total) with no radiologic evidence of disease. Group II was composed of 87 (31%) miners with a diagnosis of simple pneumoconiosis. Group III consisted of 93 (34%) miners with PMF. The number of subjects in each experimental group was similar in each of three defined geographic regions in Pennsylvania and West Virginia (Table 1, Fig. 1).

TABLE 1. HISTOCOMPATIBILITY (HL–A) ANTIGENS FREQUENCIES TABULATED ACCORDING TO CWP DISEASE CATEGORY AND GEOGRAPHIC REGIONS

HL–A antigens		Distribution within disease category				Distribution within regions		
		Group I (no disease)	Group II (simple disease)	Group III (complicated disease)	Groups II + III (simple and complicated)	Western region	Central region	Eastern region
	n= (23)	n= (97)	n= (87)	n= (93)	n= (180)	n= (109)	n= (97)	n= (71)
		% no.	% no.	% no.	% no.	% no.	% no.	% no.
LA Locus	1	35.1 (34)	20.7 (18)	21.5 (20)	21.1 (38)	24.8 (27)	28.9 (28)	23.9 (17)
	2	51.6 (50)	54.0 (47)	49.5 (46)	51.7 (93)	55.0 (60)	45.4 (44)	54.9 (39)
	3	19.6 (19)	29.9 (26)	22.6 (21)	21.6 (47)	22.9 (25)	26.8 (26)	21.1 (15)
	9	22.7 (22)	19.5 (17)	27.9 (26)	23.9 (43)	22.9 (25)	19.6 (19)	29.6 (21)
	10	16.5 (16)	13.8 (12)	7.5 (7)	10.6 (19)	13.8 (15)	13.4 (13)	9.9 (7)
	11	12.4 (12)	8.0 (7)	12.9 (12)	10.6 (19)	11.9 (13)	10.3 (10)	11.3 (8)
	W19	5.2 (5)	3.5 (3)	5.4 (5)	4.4 (8)	4.6 (5)	3.1 (3)	7.0 (5)
	W28	4.1 (4)	8.0 (7)	7.5 (7)	7.8 (14)	3.7 (4)	2.1 (2)	16.9 (12)
	W29	7.2 (7)	6.9 (6)	11.8 (11)	9.4 (17)	10.1 (11)	8.2 (8)	7.0 (5)
FOUR Locus	5	12.4 (12)	14.9 (13)	11.8 (11)	13.3 (24)	9.2 (10)	11.3 (11)	21.1 (15)
	7	21.7 (21)	21.8 (19)	24.7 (23)	23.3 (42)	27.5 (30)	15.5 (15)	25.4 (18)
	8	21.7 (21)	18.4 (16)	12.9 (12)	15.5 (28)	16.5 (18)	17.5 (17)	19.7 (14)
	12	19.6 (19)	28.7 (25)	26.9 (25)	27.8 (50)	23.9 (26)	28.9 (28)	21.1 (15)
	13	6.2 (6)	10.3 (9)	4.3 (4)	7.2 (13)	7.3 (8)	6.2 (6)	7.0 (5)
	W5	18.6 (18)	12.6 (11)	20.4 (19)	16.7 (30)	16.3 (21)	17.5 (17)	14.1 (10)
	W10	11.3 (11)	5.7 (5)	7.5 (7)	6.7 (12)	11.0 (12)	6.2 (6)	7.0 (5)
	W14	3.1 (3)	2.3 (2)	5.4 (5)	3.9 (7)	6.4 (7)	2.1 (2)	1.4 (1)
	W15	16.5 (16)	10.3 (9)	16.1 (15)	13.3 (24)	11.9 (13)	14.4 (14)	18.3 (13)
	W16	2.1 (2)	1.1 (1)	3.2 (3)	2.2 (4)	1.8 (2)	2.1 (2)	2.8 (2)
	W17	7.2 (7)	4.6 (4)	7.5 (7)	6.1 (11)	8.3 (9)	6.2 (6)	4.2 (3)
	W18	15.5 (15)	10.3 (9)	4.3 (4)	7.2 (13)	12.8 (14)	5.2 (5)	12.7 (9)
	W22	5.2 (5)	6.9 (6)	7.5 (7)	7.2 (13)	6.4 (7)	4.1 (4)	9.9 (7)
	W27	9.3 (9)	16.1 (14)	12.9 (12)	14.4 (26)	5.5 (6)	20.6 (20)	12.7 (9)

Heparinized peripheral blood specimens for HL–A typing were transported to the laboratory in Terasaki lymphocyte transport bags (Lifemed Corporation, Campton, California) at ambient temperature. Lymphocytes were separated from other blood cells by a standard ficoll-renograffin technique. The HL–A phenotypes were determined by means of a two-stage microcytotoxicity technique (AMOS *et al.*, 1969). About 100 antisera, obtained from local sources, from Dr Amos, and from the National Institutes of Health were used to detect 9 antigens of the LA (A) series and 14 antigens of the FOUR (B) series. At least three antisera were used to define each specificity. Sera of coal miners were screened for lymphocytotoxic antibodies.

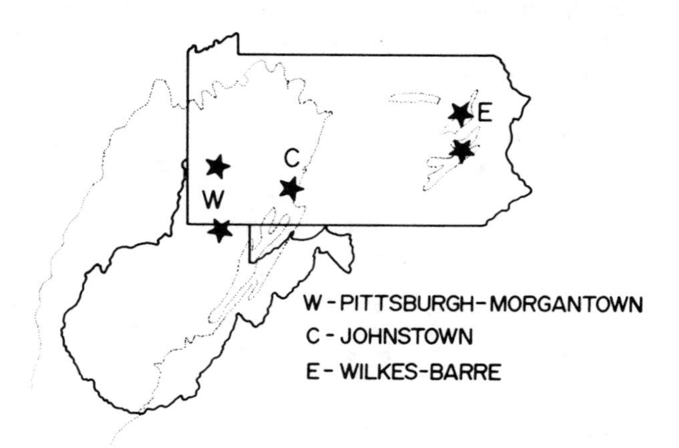

FIG. 1. Geographic regions of Pennsylvania and West Virginia from which coal workers were selected on a volunteer basis for inclusion in the study. The eastern (E) region mines anthracite coal, the central (C) region mines high-ranked bituminous coal and the western (W) region mines lower-ranked bituminous coal.

The ABO, $Rh_o(D)$ and MN blood groups were determined by standard immunohaematological techniques (MILLER *et al.*, 1974). ABO typing results were verified by back-typing with the serum. All $Rh_o(D)$ negative typings were re-examined for the presence of the Du component and all serum specimens were screened for the presence of atypical antibodies with a commercial pooled erythrocyte suspension prepared for that purpose.

Total haemolytic complement levels were determined titrimetrically according to a modification of standard protocol (MAYER, 1961) on serum stored at −70°C prior to assay. CH_{50} units were calculated by probit analysis of the data.

Serum immunoglobulin (IgG, IgA, IgM) concentrations were determined with a microfluoronephelometric autoanalyser (Technicon Corporation, Terrytown, N.Y.) according to the recommended procedure (RITCHIE *et al.*, 1973).

The frequency of a given HL–A antigen or blood group in simple CWP or complicated CWP was compared to its frequency in the CWP free control group using the chi-square test. The frequency of each antigen in the three geographic regions was likewise compared with the chi-square method to test for disturbances of HL–A or blood-group frequencies caused by ethnic stratification.

The relative risk (x) was calculated by the formula:

$$x = \frac{ad}{bc}$$

where a and b are the numbers of affected subjects carrying or lacking a given antigen, respectively, and c and d are the numbers of controls carrying or lacking the antigen, respectively.

RESULTS

The distribution of blood group frequencies by disease category and by geographic region is shown in Table 2. There are no significant differences in the frequency of these antigens when disease categories are compared, indicating that susceptibility or resistance to CWP is not associated with any of these antigens. However, there were differences in the frequencies of blood groups A. M and MN in the central region when compared to the eastern and western regions. The data reflect the different origins of the populations under study.

TABLE 2. BLOOD GROUP FREQUENCIES ENCOUNTERED IN U.S. REFERENCE POPULATION, COMBINED SAMPLE POPULATION, CWP DISEASE GROUPS AND GEOGRAPHIC REGIONS

R.B.C. blood group	Distribution within		Distribution within disease category			Distribution within regions		
	U.S. reference population	Combined sample population	Group I (no disease)	Group II (simple disease)	Group III (complicated disease)	Western region	Central region	Eastern region
		n= (271)	n= (95)	n= (85)	n= (91)	n= (109)	n= (97)	n= (65)
	%	% no.	% no.	% no.	% no.	% no.	% no.	% no.
O	45	40.9 (111)	44.2 (42)	41.2 (35)	37.4 (34)	40.4 (44)	45.4 (44)	35.4 (23)
A	40	38.4 (104)	36.8 (35)	34.1 (29)	44.0 (40)	44.0 (48)	26.8 (26)	46.2 (30)
B	11	13.7 (37)	12.6 (12)	17.7 (15)	11.0 (10)	11.9 (13)	15.5 (15)	13.9 (9)
AB	4	7.0 (19)	6.3 (6)	7.1 (6)	7.7 (7)	3.7 (4)	12.4 (12)	4.6 (3)
Rh_o+	85	80.4 (218)	85.3 (81)	78.8 (67)	76.9 (70)	83.5 (91)	79.4 (77)	77.0 (50)
Rh_o-	15	19.6 (53)	14.7 (14)	21.2 (18)	23.1 (21)	16.5 (18)	20.6 (20)	23.0 (15)
M	28	29.2 (79)	31.6 (30)	30.6 (26)	25.3 (23)	22.0 (24)	43.3 (42)	20.0 (13)
N	22	18.1 (49)	16.8 (16)	16.5 (14)	20.9 (19)	21.1 (23)	16.5 (16)	15.4 (10)
MN	50	52.8 (143)	51.6 (49)	52.9 (45)	53.9 (49)	56.9 (62)	40.2 (39)	64.6 (42)

One source of bias in studies of association between HL–A antigens and disease results from ethnic differences between the disease and control samples, since the frequencies of certain HL–A antigens vary between different population groups. In the current study this source of bias was minimized by having equivalent numbers in the control and disease groups from each geographic area. It was of interest, nevertheless, to compare HL–A antigen frequencies in the total miner population with another study involving normal Caucasians. In Fig. 2, the HL–A frequencies observed in the current study are compared with those reported by ALBERT *et al.* (1972) for a population of mixed Caucasians. The HL–A frequencies between the two studies were comparable except for lower frequencies of W19, W14, W15 and W16 in the miners observed. These differences are attributed, at least in part, to a lack of sera to consistently detect the W30, W31 and W19.6 specificities of the W19 complex and relatively weak antisera for W14, W15 and W16.

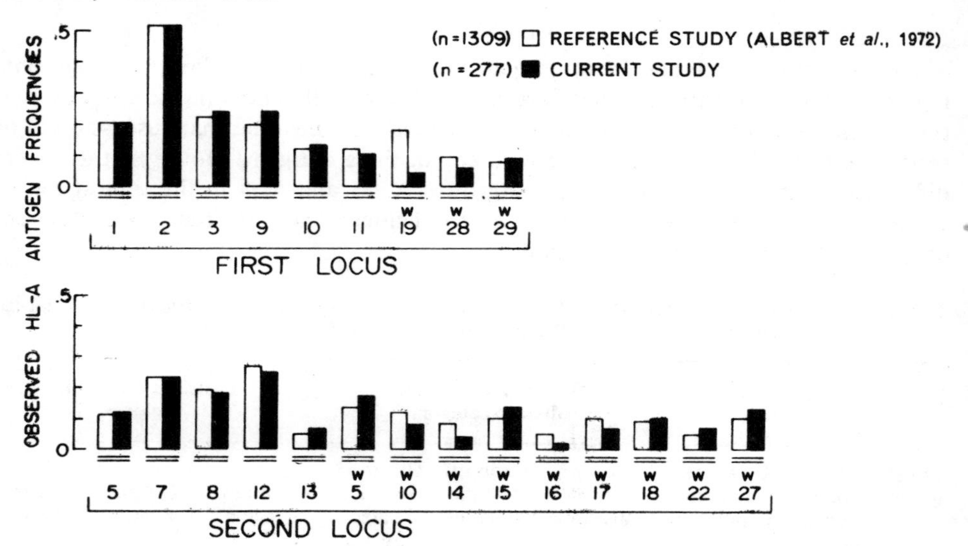

FIG. 2. Comparison of HL–A frequencies observed in the current study of coal workers' pneumoconiosis with those frequencies reported in a reference population of mixed Caucasians.

The distribution of HL–A antigen frequencies is shown in Table 1. HL–A1 was significantly more frequent in the group without evidence of CWP than in the group with simple CWP (Fisher's exact probability = 0.022) or the group with complicated CWP (Fisher's exact probability = 0.027). The frequency of HL–A1 in both CWP groups is equal to the observed frequency of this antigen in a heterogeneous Caucasian population (ALBERT *et al.*, 1972). Antigen W18 occurred significantly (Fisher's exact probability = 0.008) more frequently among miners with no radiographic evidence of disease than in those with PMF. The frequency of W18 in the group with simple CWP is essentially equal to the expected frequency for Caucasians (ALBERT *et al.*, 1972).

When the distribution of HL–A antigens was examined for regional balance, it was found that significant disparities for the W28 specificity existed within the eastern region when it was compared to both the central and western areas. An additional imbalance was evident between the central and western sectors with regard to the W27 antigen. Whether these differences are due to serological, statistical, ethnic bias, or a combination of factors has not been determined.

In order to better compare the association between HL–A antigens and susceptibility/resistance to disease, it is frequently useful to determine the relative risk factor (WOOLF, 1955). The relative risk indicates how many times more frequently the disease occurs in individuals carrying the antigen than in those lacking it. Accordingly, an increased frequency of an antigen in the disease group gives a risk factor above unity and indicates a positive association. Conversely, decreased frequencies in the disease group yield a relative risk factor of less than 1 (negative association). The relative risk factors calculated for the present study are shown in Fig. 3. The data indicate a

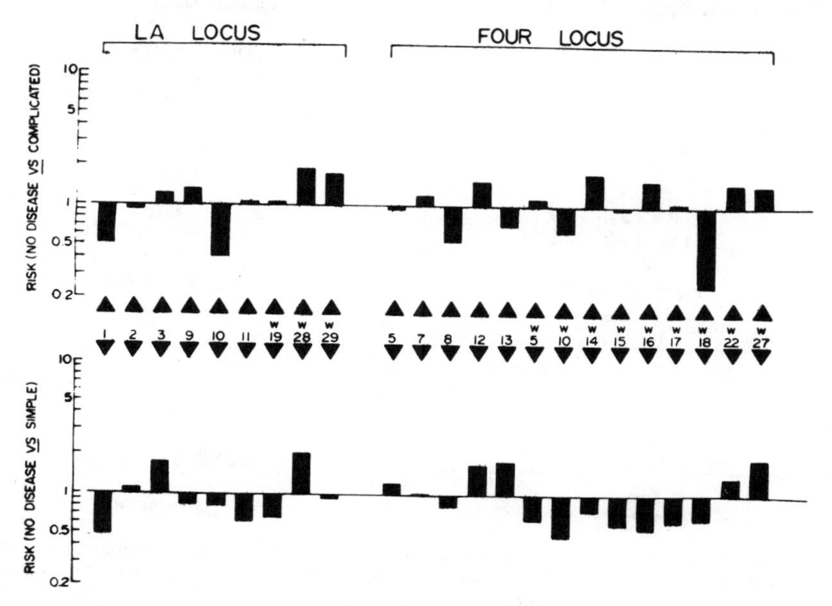

FIG. 3. Relative disease risk factors for twenty-three tested histocompatibility antigens in a population of unrelated coal miners. Relative risk for both simple and complicated CWP is expressed in reference to miners showing no radiographic evidence of CWP.

moderately strong negative association between antigen W18 and PMF (relative risk 0.25). Thus, miners carrying this antigen were about 300% less likely to develop complicated CWP than those who lacked the antigen. A weaker negative association was obtained for HL–A1 and both forms of CWP (relative risk = 0.51 and 0.48 for simple CWP and PMF respectively).

Serum haemolytic complement concentrations were determined in 250 of the miners participating in the study. The results expressed in CH_{50} units/ml are shown in Fig. 4. When the CH_{50} values were compared between disease categories, the mean complement concentrations were equivalent: 101, 98 and 103 CH_{50} units for the group without CWP, simple CWP and complicated CWP, respectively. The mean values between geographic regions were 95, 112 and 93 CH_{50} units in miners from western, central and eastern areas, respectively.

Likewise, there was no apparent clinical significance to the differences in the serum concentrations of IgG, IgA or IgM when compared by disease group but the mean values in the eastern region (177 mg/100 ml) and western region (186 mg/100 ml) were somewhat greater than in the central region (96 mg/100 ml) (Table 3). Cytotoxic antibodies were observed in only 1 of 217 sera.

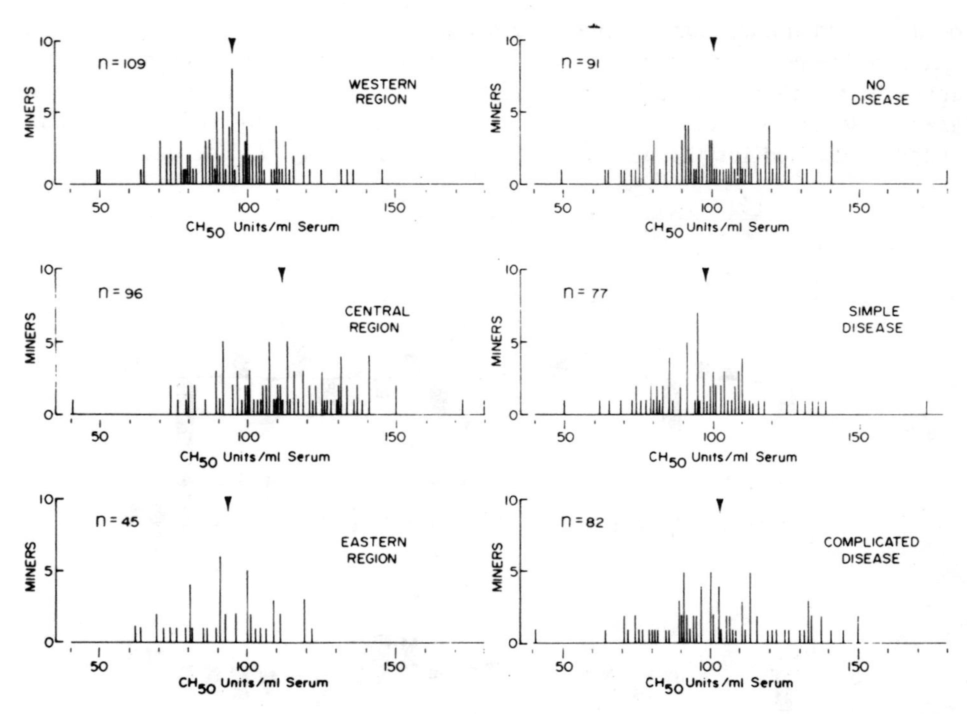

FIG. 4. Distribution of serum haemolytic complement concentrations within the various geographic mining regions and within each experimental disease group. Mean (m) values are indicated by the solid arrows.

TABLE 3. SERUM IMMUNOGLOBULIN LEVELS ENCOUNTERED WITHIN COMBINED SAMPLE POPULATION, CWP DISEASE GROUPS AND GEOGRAPHIC REGIONS

Serum immuno-globulin fraction		Distribution within disease category				Distribution within regions		
		Combined sample population	Group I (no disease)	Group II (simple disease)	Group III (complicated disease)	Western region	Central region	Eastern region
IgG	n	275	97	86	92	109	97	69
	m±s*	1172±267	1120±235	1195±294	1206±267	1242±283	1112±234	1146±263
IgA	n	271	95	85	91	108	95	68
	m±s	259±145	222±127	277±148	281±155	277±155	272±144	211±120
IgM	n	269	95	84	90	106	96	67
	m±s	152±106	150±97	156±112	149±110	186±114	96±59	177±115

* m±s = mean ± s.d. (mg/100 ml).

DISCUSSION

The significant observation in this study was the increased frequency of the HL–A1 and W18 antigens in miners without radiographic evidence of pneumoconiosis. The differences were significant at the 5% probability level, but not when multiplied by the number of antigens tested as recommended by SVEJGAARD *et al.* (1974). Since this latter method is conservative, it is entirely possible that the increased frequencies of HL–A1 and W18 are real and not due to chance. With twenty-three tests (one for each antigen surveyed) this conservative approach amounts to performing each test at the $\alpha = 0.002$ level instead of $\alpha = 0.05$, and thus true differences might be overlooked. However, HL–A1 and W18 were found significant and had values of $\alpha = 0.04$. If the tests were independent and there were no differences for any of the twenty-three antigens, then using the binomial probability function, one finds that the probability of finding at least one test with $\alpha \leqslant 0.04$ out of twenty-three would be about 0.61, and the probability of finding at least two tests with $\alpha \leqslant 0.04$ would be about 0.23. Thus we acknowledge the possibility that our findings could be due to chance, but because of the probing nature of this study, one might reserve judgements on these two antigens until a future study involving only HL–A1 and W18 is undertaken as suggested by SVEJGAARD *et al.* (1974).

It was also found that neither of these antigens were abnormally distributed within the three geographic regions. Thus, if these differences are real, no reason was found to attribute the differences to geographic location.

Approximately a dozen diseases show consistent and significant associations with HL–A antigens (SVEJGAARD *et al.*, 1975). In essentially all previously established associations with disease, there is an increased frequency of one or more antigens as compared to controls. An increased frequency in a disease group indicates that the alleles confer susceptibility to disease. We interpret the increased frequency of the HL–A1 and W18 alleles in the miner group without evidence of CWP as indicating resistance to development of pneumoconiosis. It should be noted that with the possible exception of W18 in the complicated CWP group, the antigen frequencies are essentially those expected for normal Caucasians. Thus, it is the group without disease which appears to be different. For this reason, larger numbers of subjects in the CWP groups would be needed relative to the control group. The data from simple and complicated CWP can be pooled since they do not differ significantly. When the relative risks are calculated on this basis the relative risk factor for HL–A1 is 0.50 and for W18 is 0.43. Expressed differently this indicates that the risk of CWP is 100% and 133% less in miners who carry HL–A1 or W18. This magnitude of relative "resistance" to CWP is approximately the same as the increased susceptibility for insulin-dependent diabetes associated with HL–A8 (SVEJGAARD *et al.*, 1975). By comparison, the classical association between blood group 0 and duodenal ulcer confers a relative risk of 1.33 (an ncreased risk of 33%) for blood group 0 individuals compared to non-0 individuals iVOGEL and HELMBOLD, 1972).

The question as to whether resistance to CWP is dominant or recessive could be approached if the HL–A antigens themselves were responsible for the association in which case it could be determined whether the relative resistance is the same for heterozygotes as for homozygotes. However, if the HL–A antigens are merely passive markers for associated disease-resistance genes then the situation is more complicated. If the reasonable assumption is made that the unknown alleles at the LA and FOUR loci are infrequent, then there is little error in regarding individuals carrying only one antigen of the LA and FOUR series as homozygotes. In this regard, there was not an increased number of two or three antigen phenotypes in the CWP free group of miners as compared to the CWP groups. This may suggest that resistance is a dominant character.

Most of the established HL–A associations with disease involve antigens of the FOUR (B), C or D loci. The accepted explanation is that the associations between FOUR antigens and disease involve immune response (Ir) genes rather than HL–A antigens themselves. This explanation assumes that certain FOUR-locus genes and Ir genes are in linkage disequilibrium. Since the antigens implicated in the present study (HL–A1 and W18) belong to the LA and FOUR series, respectively, the evidence neither supports nor detracts from the Ir gene explanation. However, the strongest association is with W18, a second locus antigen. The hypothetical Ir gene involved in resistance to CWP could be involved with the way in which coal dust is handled by the body.

The question as to whether the apparent association between resistance to CWP is due to a particular haplotype (HL–A1, W18) cannot be answered since family studies have not been carried out.

Recently, MERCHANT *et al.* (1975) reported a significant increase in the frequency of antigen W27 in a group of asbestos workers with definite or suspected asbestosis. An association between W27 and severe asbestosis was also suggested. Despite some similarity between CWP and asbestosis these initial HL–A studies are not in agreement in regard to which, if any, HL–A antigens are definitely associated with pneumoconiosis.

ACKNOWLEDGEMENTS

The authors take this opportunity to acknowledge the technical and administrative assistance of Dr R. Paul Fairman, Dr Mabel Stevenson, Mr John D. Stewart, Ms Nancy J. McGinnis, Mr Gordon L. Stalnaker, Mr. Michael E. Moore, Mrs Carol A. Hando, Mr Jeffrey L. Poling, Ms Martha Lake and Ms Lin Smith. We also thank Mrs Mary Jo. Powell and Mrs Rotha Hall for their typing the manuscript, and Mr Larry F. Boyce and Mr Robert B. Reger and their staffs for computer and statistical support of the project.

A special acknowledgment is extended to all those coal workers from Pennsylvania and West Virginia who donated their time and effort in order to make this study possible.

REFERENCES

ALBERT, E. D., MICKEY, M. R. and TERASAKI, P. I. (1972) *Histocompatibility Testing 1972. Report of an International Workshop and Conference organized by Colloque de l'Institut National de la Santé et de la Recherche Medicale, Evian, France, 1972* (edited by DAUSSET, J. and COLOMBANI, J.) pp. 233–240. Munksgaard, Copenhagen.

AMOS, D. B., BASHIR, H., BOYLE, W., MACQUEEN, M. and TIILIKAINEN, A. (1969) *Transplantation* **7,** 220–223.

GREEN, I. (1974) *Immunogenetics* **1,** 4–21.

LAPP, N. L. and SEATON, A. (1971) *Pulmonary Reactions to Coal Dust* (edited by KEY, M. M., KERR, L. E. and BUNDY, M.) pp. 153–177. Academic Press, New York.

LIPPMANN, M., ECKERT, H. L., HAHON, N. and MORGAN, W. K. C. (1973) *Ann. int. Med.* **79**, 807–811.

MAJOR, P. C., HEISE, E. R., MENTNECH, M. S., PARRISH, E. J., JORDON, A. L. and MORGAN, W. K. C. (1975) *Am. Rev. resp. Dis.* **111**, 917–918.

MAYER, M. M. (1961) *Experimental Immunochemistry* (by KABAT, E. A. and MAYER, M. M.) pp. 133–240. Thomas, Springfield, Ill.

MERCHANT, J. A., KLOUDA, P. T., SOUTAR, C. A., PARKES, W. R., LAWLER, S. D. and TURNER-WARWICK, M. (1975) *Br. med. J.* **1**, 189–191.

MILLER, W. V. *et al.* (1974) *Technical Methods and Procedures of the American Association of Blood Banks*, 6th edn. Am. Ass. Blood Banks, Washington, D.C.

MORGAN, W. K. C., LAPP, N. L. and SEATON, A. (1972) *J. occup. Med.* **14**, 839–844.

MORGAN, W. K. C., BURGESS, D. B., JACOBSON, G., O'BRIEN, R. J., PENDERGRASS, E. P., REGER, R. B., and SHOUB, E. P. (1973) *Archs. envir. Hlth* **27**, 221–226.

RITCHIE, R. F., ALPER, C. A., GRAVES, J., PEARSON, N. and LARSON, C. (1973) *Am. J. clin. Path.* **59**, 151–159.

ROGAN, J. M., ATTFIELD, M. D., JACOBSEN, M., RAE, S., WALKER, D. D. and WALTON, W. H. (1973) *Br. J. ind. Med.* **30**, 217–226.

SOUTAR, C. A., TURNER-WARWICK, M. and PARKES, W. R. (1974) *Br. med. J.* **3**, 145–147.

SVEJGAARD, A., JERSILD, C., STAUB NIELSEN, L. and BODMER, W. F. (1974) *Tissue Antigens* **4**, 95–105.

SVEJGAARD, A., PLATZ, P., RYDER, L. P., STAUB NIELSEN, L. and THOMSEN, M. (1975) *Transplantn Rev.* **22**, 3–43.

VOGEL, J. and HELMBOLD, W. (1972) *Humangenetik* (edited by BECKER, P. E.) Vol. 1, p. 129. Thieme, Stuttgart.

WOOLF, B. (1955) *Ann. hum. Genet.* **19**, 251–253.

DISCUSSION

R. THOMAS: Have you looked at rosette formation in T cells in these exposed cases?

Dr MAJOR: No, we have not. The collection and processing of blood specimens taken from within the eastern parts of Pennsylvania was encumbered logistically and from a technical standpoint we had the minimum number of cells required for HL-A typing. Western Pennsylvania was less of a problem making re-collection of blood for rosette testing a possibility, yet this would exclude the high-risk anthracite areas so I am not sure this would be worthwhile. We have tentative plans to continue this study in the western United States in areas of low incidence of CWP. Perhaps T cell rosette formations could be addressed as a part of this proposed work which could provide information on the status of the delayed response in exposed cases.

D. LIDDELL: (i) One interpretation of the "relative risks" for HL–A1 and W18 is that there was a shortfall of these types of antigen in complicated CWP. However, the frequencies of these types were high in "normal" cases, i.e. where no disease was found. Is there an explanation?

(ii) If the frequencies of ALBERT *et al.* (1972) are to be expected in your selection (*not* population) of miners, should they not arise without disease? Surely not averaged over your complete selection? Are the observed differences in the non-diseased real or artefactual?

Dr MAJOR: (i) I attempted to explain that we felt that the "higher" frequency level for the W18 antigen which was observed in the "no disease" group could possibly be related to an innate constitutional ability by this group to resist the development of disease when exposed to a compromising dust burden. We found that the frequency of this antigen in the "simple" disease category reflected almost exactly those frequencies observed in the general population and in our overall combined population, which makes interpretation difficult. The frequency for the W18 antigen which occurred in the "complicated" category (approximately one-half the normal value) could indicate that the diminished presence of this antigen must be linked to a susceptible posture for the development of progressive massive fibrosis.

(ii) We had no idea before our data were analyzed that our "no disease" or control group would not be characterized by the expected HL-A frequencies reported by ALBERT, *et al.* (1972) unless ethnic statifications were demonstrated within the population studied. The "no disease" group was standardized with the other disease groups by age and longevity of employment and were therefore assumed to have been exposed to comparable dust burdens. I really cannot comment beyond this particular point.

G. BERRY: Presumably there was no *a priori* interest in the W18 antigen as compared with the other twenty-two antigens, it was simply that W18 gave the most significant difference between the three groups? If the fact that W18 was the *most* significant of twenty-three possibilities were taken into account when carrying out the significance test, would differences between the groups still be significant for this antigen?

Dr MAJOR: We have examined 23 antigens and perhaps we should have divided our 0.05 probability level by that number before proclaiming our rejection of the null hypothesis (at least that has been suggested). Such a procedure would technically preclude in multiple testing the recognition of frequency differences which occur by chance alone. However, if we adopted this more conservative approach, we might well be missing differences that are actually there and so we decided to adopt a less conservative procedure in a preliminary study and lay ourselves open to the possibility of error in order to avoid excluding any possible differences at this time.

L. MAGOS: Your conclusions are based on a static study which shows that, in groups of workers with pneumoconiosis, two antigens were less frequent than in miners without pneumoconiosis. However, a definite answer can be obtained only by a dynamic study which starts when the individual enters the mine for the first time. Supposing that the presence of the two antigens HL–A and W18 predisposed the miners to bronchitis, those who had these antigens might have left the mine before the development of CWP. In this case without the suggested relationship the frequency of HL–A and W18 must be lower in the group of workers with pneumoconiosis than in the control group.

Dr MAJOR: That is true in this situation if the HL–A antigens mentioned rendered miners more susceptible to bronchitis and as a result they elected to change their job to one where there was no dust at all (within or without the industry). As a result, one might indeed expect to observe smaller numbers of miners with these antigens in the group of progressive pneumoconiosis. However, this supposition does not explain the higher than expected frequencies of these antigens in the "no disease" category which is an observation in this report.

M. LIPPMANN: Do you have any data on exposure levels to support the assumption that the three groups had equivalent dust exposures? Years of mining are, at best, a very rough index of cumulative dust exposure. Furthermore, even with the same exposures, variations in pulmonary deposition and clearance could easily account for large differences in dust retention even when exposures are similar.

Thus, factors not considered in this study may well have much greater influences on the development of simple CWP or PMF.

Dr Major: The clinical and technical information for this study was taken from our data base of miners examined in the first and second round of the U.S. National Coal Study. Participation of miners was on a volunteer basis which was the best we could achieve.

Dr Morgan: Regarding coal dust exposure levels it is extraordinarily difficult, if not impossible, to select two groups of miners, one with PMF and the other with no pneumoconiosis, both of which have had comparable dust exposures.

M. Lippmann: I do not agree with that.

Dr Morgan: Are you implying that miners with normal films have had the same dust exposure as men with categories 2 and 3 simple CWP. In general this would seem unlikely.

M. Lippmann: I would agree that there is a statistical association and that you are correct if that is all you are inferring, but in view of the variability in deposition and clearance for the same aerosol, there certainly could be an order of magnitude difference in dust retention in these miners and that is a different factor from the one I raised earlier as to whether the dust level was ten times higher for instance in one mine than another.

Dr Morgan: We know from short term studies done by the U.S. bureau of Mines that dust levels were ten times higher in certain mines than in others; but I am beginning to see what you are suggesting—namely, individual susceptibility. This is a most difficult matter to deal with. There were no long term dust measurements made in the U.S. prior to 1969 and, therefore, it would be quite impossible to devise a study in which the groups were matched for dust exposure. Finally, I think it needs to be borne in mind that dust exposure, however much, will not affect one's tissue type.

D. C. F. Muir: I cannot agree with Dr Morgan that years of underground exposure is an adequate measure of dust exposure.

I would like to ask Dr Major whether there was any evidence of consanguinity between members of the sub-groups in the population.

Dr Major: We excluded all siblings and other relatives of miners participating in the study.

J. A. Dick: As the prevalence of PMF varies from coalfield to coalfield, can you explain why the levels of W18 should also vary? And is it possible that PMF causes the absence of W18?

Dr Major: I would not concur that PMF causes the absence of W18 as I am under the impression that the W18 antigen should be with one from womb to tomb. Why does the prevalence of PMF vary from coalfield to coalfield? I do not know but I would suggest that this consideration should not influence our data as we circumvented this problem by selecting miners on a volunteer basis from all coalfields studied according to their diagnosed disease category, that is all regions of study and disease category, were balanced by equal numbers of individuals.

J. S. McLintock: There certainly are differences in the prevalence of PMF in different coalfields in Great Britain (and also in the U.S.A.), but when we looked at the attack rates of PMF and standardised for prevalence in each coalfield (see *Inhaled Particles III*, p. 933), we found the attack rate to be very close in almost all coalfields.

M. D. Attfield: In the light of the statistical significance of your findings, will you be studying a further group of men to see if the two associations still remain significant?

Dr Major: We have tentative plans to continue this study in southern West Virginia which will extend our work from Pennsylvania and northern West Virginia. We also wish to look at this same problem in miners from areas of low prevalence in the western United States such as in Utah and Colorado. As far as expanding our numbers of participants to any great extent we are limited by logistic and technical problems such as dealing with the wide dispersion of miner's residences in the hill and mountain areas and the transport of specimens from the field to the laboratory.

A CELL KINETIC STUDY OF THE ALVEOLAR WALL FOLLOWING DUST DEPOSITION

J. BRIGHTWELL and A. G. HEPPLESTON

Department of Pathology, University of Newcastle upon Tyne, England

Abstract—The stathmokinetic technique was used to study quantitatively the proliferative response of cells comprising the alveolar wall of inbred mice which had inhaled coal or quartz. The exposures occupied 4 weeks and the observations continued over an extended period thereafter.

Control observations suggested that mitotic inhibition was induced solely by residence in the exposure chamber, since cessation of exposure was quickly followed by a temporary rise of proliferative activity. This feature was not apparent when dust was inhaled, though with comparable exposure to both coal and quartz there was an elevation in mitotic incidence of alveolar wall cells in dust-free areas of lung at a later interval. In dust-laden areas the rise was less in evidence, a situation that persisted throughout the post-exposure survival. The difference in mitotic incidence between dust-free and dust-containing areas was more evident after coal than after quartz inhalation, whilst in higher concentration a quartz aerosol induced a continued depression of mitotic activity.

The proliferative response seen in the alveolar walls of control and dusted mice is most likely to be contributed by the interstitial precursors of alveolar macrophages, cells which are recognized to be marrow derived. The changes observed in mitotic incidence are interpreted in terms of demand for alveolar macrophages according to the nature of the dust and the intensity of the exposure.

IT IS now established that the precursors of mononuclear phagocytic cells originate in the bone marrow and are conveyed as monocytes by the blood stream to distant sites where they may emerge to become tissue macrophages, the evidence having been summarized by VAN FURTH *et al.* (1972). Both in the normal state and during sterile acute inflammation, promonocytes or monocytes lose their capacity to proliferate, their cell kinetic parameters being no different from normal 24 h after arrival in the peritoneal cavity (VAN FURTH *et al.*, 1973), though in infective or chronic inflammatory states tissue macrophages may undergo local multiplication (NORTH, 1969; SPECTOR and RYAN, 1970). That pulmonary macrophages also originate from marrow derived precursors has been demonstrated by means of radiation chimeras with chromosome, enzyme or antigen cell markers (PINKETT *et al.*, 1966; VIROLAINEN, 1968; BRUNSTETTER *et al.*, 1971; GODLESKI and BRAIN, 1972). Furthermore, evidence from tritiated thymidine labelling of irradiated animals and of mouse lung explants suggests that, after migration from the circulation into the lung interstitium, monocytes undergo one or more mitotic divisions before entering the alveolar spaces as mature pulmonary macrophages (BOWDEN *et al.*, 1969; BOWDEN and ADAMSON, 1972).

The rate at which inhaled particles are cleared from the lung in the early post-exposure phase is evidently related to the quantity of material deposited. LABELLE and BRIEGER

(1959) found that injected uranium dioxide was cleared faster from rat lung in the presence of 1.5 mg of carbon as compared with 5 μg. The clearance of inhaled silica in rats was also increased by prior inhalation of small quantities (*ca.* 30 μg) of titanium dioxide (FERIN *et al.*, 1965). A similar effect on the clearance of uranium particles was detected when they were given by intratracheal injection along with carbon or aluminium hydrate (LABELLE and BRIEGER, 1960). Parenteral administration of trypan blue (FÉRIN *et al.*, 1965) or inhalation of polyvinylpyridine-*N*-oxide (PVPNO) (SCHLIPKÖTER and BROCKHAUS, 1970) also augmented the elimination of inhaled quartz, probably by mobilizing or preserving alveolar macrophages.

The rate of clearance of injected particles rose in parallel with the number of phagocytes present in lung sections (LABELLE and BRIEGER, 1959). The frequency of "alveolar cells", including alveolar macrophages, increased in relation to fixed cells of the alveolar region following silica inhalation, whilst a small transitory increase was evident after inhalation of "innocuous" dust (STRECKER, 1967). Lung lavage has also been employed to gauge the size of the macrophage pool in various rodents after dust deposition, though the technique is subject to error and unless controlled its quantitative results must be treated with reserve (BRAIN, 1971). It nevertheless appears that brief inhalation of carbon (LABELLE and BRIEGER, 1960) or quartz (RASCHE and ULMER, 1967) soon results in an elevation of the number of macrophages recovered from the lung. A similar rise followed intratracheal injection of carbon, coal, iron oxide or chrysotile (BRAIN, 1971), as well as PVPNO treatment alone (administered intravenously) or in conjunction with dust (both by inhalation) (RASCHE, 1971).

The accumulation of macrophages in the lung as a consequence of dust deposition may reflect local proliferation or systemic recruitment or both. In the present investigation we have attempted to quantify proliferation of alveolar wall cells following inhalation exposure to coal or quartz in low concentration for prolonged periods rather than the short ones characterizing previous studies. In this way the kinetic response to a larger dust burden was elicited. Because the native mitotic incidence of adult mouse lung parenchyma is relatively low, the stathmokinetic technique has been employed. To minimize natural variations in the proliferative activity of alveolar wall cells an inbred strain of mouse was used.

MATERIALS AND METHODS

Inbred, male mice of the A_2G strain were used, the age at death being between 6 and 9 months. Animals were allowed food and water *ad libitum.* Dust inhalation was carried out in chambers based on WRIGHT's (1957) design, the animals being exposed 20 h per day, 5 days per week for a total of 400 h, i.e. over a period of 4 weeks. Samples of respirable dust were taken using a gravimetric thermal precipitator linked to an elutriator with 100% cut off at 7 μm.

Each mouse received an intraperitoneal injection of Colcemid (Ciba) at a dose of 20 μg per g body weight 4 h before being killed by cervical dislocation. The lungs were excised and immersed in ice-cold hypotonic saline for 20 min and then fixed in Carnoy's fluid for 24 h. Sections of the left lung were cut at 5 μm and stained by the periodic acid-Schiff/haematoxylin method. The proportion of arrested metaphases (mitotic incidence or MI) was calculated by scrutiny of approximately 8000 cells; because dust deposited in the lungs tends to form localized alveolar accumulations separate counts were made in areas containing dust and in areas devoid of dust for each animal. To identify areas of lung containing silica, sections adjacent to those stained were incinerated at 560°C for 2 h, washed in concentrated HCl and then viewed by reflected light. In counting alveolar wall cells, circulating leucocytes, endothelium and alveolar macrophages were excluded as far as possible.

Some animals had a comparatively high MI in the dust-free areas of lung and this feature was generally reflected in a high value for dust-containing areas of the same lung. Expression of the MI of dust-containing areas as a percentage of that in dust-free areas gives what may be termed the depression index, which minimizes inter-animal variations.

Each datum point in the Figures represents the mean of at least four animals. Statistical significances were determined by Student's t-test.

RESULTS

Mock Exposure

Mock exposure was carried out in a working inhalation chamber whose dust reservoir was empty. Such an exposure lasted 400 h and was carried out concurrently with the Frances coal and silica II inhalations (see below). The MI at 12 days after exposure is significantly higher ($P < 0.05$) than at 1, 30 or 53 days (Fig. 1).

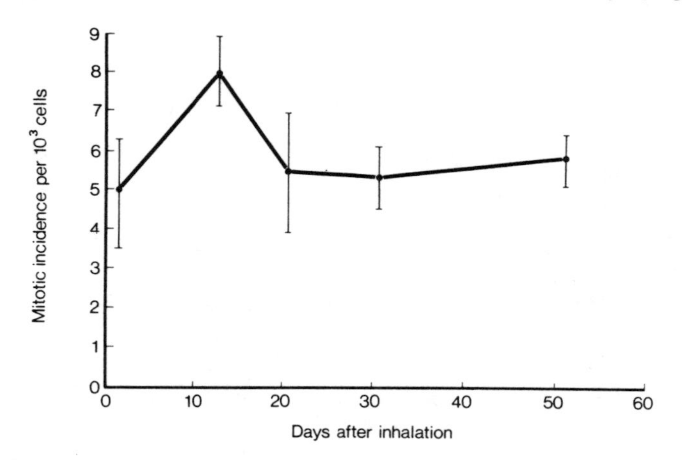

FIG. 1. Mitotic incidence of alveolar wall cells after mock exposure.

A group of ten unexposed stock mice served as further controls for the Wattstown coal and silica I experiments.

Coal Inhalation

Airborne dust from two coal mines, Wattstown, S. Wales (steam coal *ca.* 92% carbon dmmf, NCB rank code 201b/202; Fig. 2), and Frances, Scotland (bituminous coal

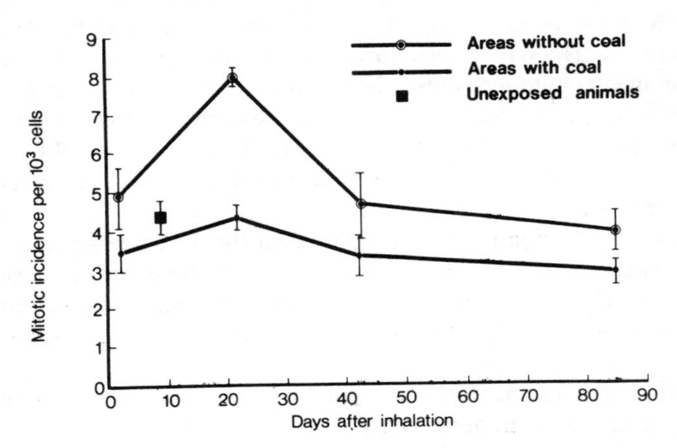

FIG. 2. Mitotic incidence of alveolar wall cells after inhalation of Wattstown coal, 13 mg/m³.

ca. 82% carbon dmmf, NCB rank code 901/902; Fig. 3), was used. The concentrations of respirable dust in the chambers were 13 and 22 mg/m³ respectively.

The MI in dust-free areas is higher than that in dust-containing areas at all time intervals and significantly higher 20 days after inhaling Wattstown coal dust ($P < 0.001$) and at 30 and 53 days after inhaling Frances dust ($P < 0.01$). At these intervals the MI in dust-free areas is also higher than the MI in mock exposed animals (Fig. 1).

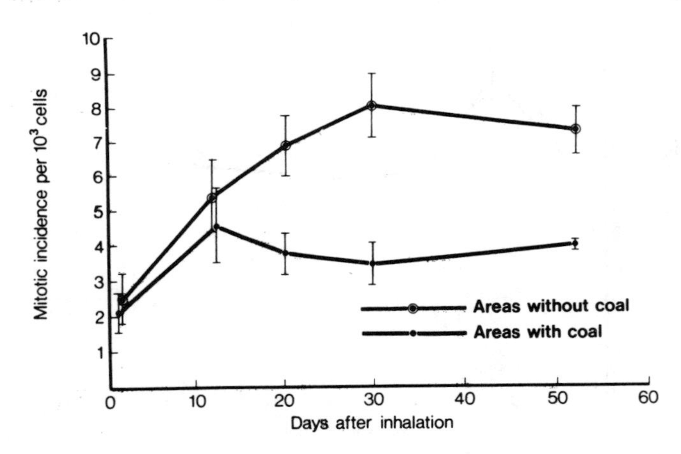

FIG. 3. Mitotic incidence of alveolar wall cells after inhalation of Frances coal, 22 mg/m³.

No rise in MI corresponding to that seen at 12 days in mock exposed animals was evident following Frances inhalation. The initial value for dust-free lung in the Wattstown experiment was similar to the MI of the unexposed controls (Fig. 2).

The depression indices (Fig. 4) give a measure of the difference in MI between dust-containing and dust-free areas. This difference, as shown by the error bars, does not as a rule vary greatly between animals in any one group.

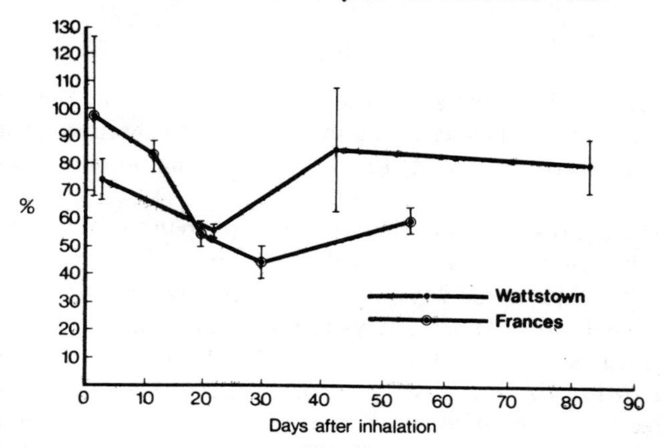

FIG. 4. Depression indices of alveolar wall cells after coal inhalation (MI of dust-containing as per cent of MI in dust-free areas).

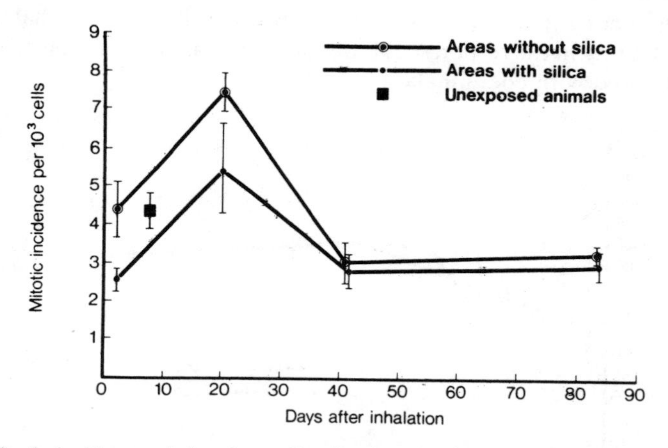

FIG. 5. Mitotic incidence of alveolar wall cells after silica inhalation (experiment I), 12 mg/m³.

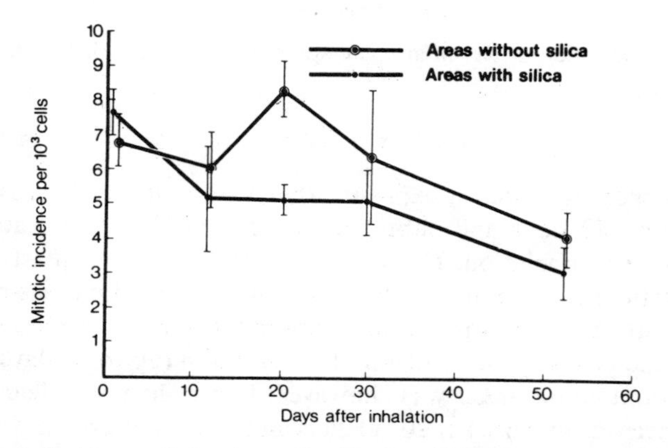

FIG. 6. Mitotic incidence of alveolar wall cells after silica inhalation (experiment II), 28 mg/m³.

Silica Inhalation

Dörentrup quartz with a particle size of 1–3 μm was used. The respirable dust concentration in the chambers was 12 mg/m^3 in the first experiment (silica I; Fig. 5) and 28 mg/m^3 in the second (silica II; Fig. 6) where a lung burden averaging 0.98 mg was achieved.

The MI in dust-free areas is higher than that in corresponding dust-containing areas at all time intervals except day 1 in the silica II experiment. However, this difference is only significant ($P < 0.02$) at 20 days in the silica II experiment (Fig. 6). The MI of mock-exposed animals (Fig. 1) at 53 days is higher than that in both dust-free and dust-containing areas at 41 and 83 days in the silica I and at 53 days in the silica II experiments. The MI of the unexposed controls in silica I is likewise higher than that of either dust-free or dust-containing areas at the two later times, though similar to the initial value for dust-free lung (Fig. 5). The rise in MI seen at 12 days in mock-exposed animals was not reflected in the silica II experiment.

The depression indices (Fig. 7) show that the difference in MI between dust-free and dust-containing areas is generally less than that which follows coal inhalation. There is also more variability in the response of individual animals within each group exposed to silica as compared with coal inhalation.

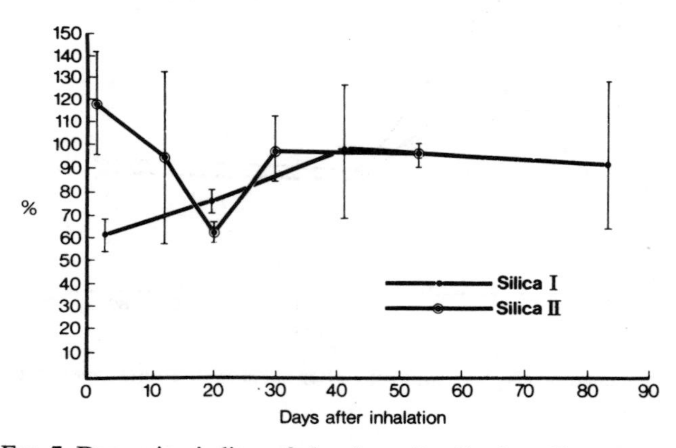

FIG. 7. Depression indices of alveolar wall cells after silica inhalation.

DISCUSSION

The mitotic incidence after dummy exposure, that is without a dust aerosol, increased significantly at about 12 days and subsided by 20 days, but this feature was not apparent following dust inhalation. However, with both coal and quartz there was a distinct rise in mitotic incidence of alveolar wall cells in dust-free areas of lung 20 to 30 days after exposure. This rise was less apparent in dust-containing areas of the same lung. Throughout the post-exposure period of observation (up to 83 days) the mitotic incidence in dust-containing areas was, however, lower than in adjacent dust-free areas. This difference was maximal at 20–30 days and was more evident following coal than quartz inhalation.

Cell division is inhibited by activity (BULLOUGH and LAURENCE, 1961) probably in consequence of adrenalin liberation by stress. The main control experiment (Fig. 1) raises the possibility that exposure itself may engender such a situation. Soon after mock exposure the MI rises temporarily, a response which could represent an attempt to restore the normal level of activity or of cell population in alveolar walls after a depression. The steady state maintained after the burst of mitotic activity is consonant with such an interpretation.

The metaphase arrest technique suggests that in rats there are two dividing populations of lung cells with renewal times of 9 and 27 days (BERTALANFFY, 1964). Although it is not possible to identify with certainty all cell types in mouse alveolar wall using paraffin sections, labelling with tritiated thymidine also points to the existence of two cell populations with renewal times of about 7 and between 28 and 35 days (SPENCER and SHORTER, 1962; SHORTER *et al.*, 1964; BOWDEN *et al.*, 1968). Pulmonary macrophages washed from the lungs of thymidine-treated mice had a generation time of approximately 7 days, suggesting that these cells represent the more rapidly dividing of the two lung cell populations (BOWDEN *et al.*, 1968).

Following the deposition of dust, it may reasonably be assumed that the majority of the mitotic activity was contributed by maturing pulmonary macrophages, although Type II epithelial cells are also increased after silica accumulation (HEPPLESTON and YOUNG, 1972). Alveolar deposition of dust occurs initially throughout the lung and as more dust arrives it may be expected that the demand for alveolar macrophages rises and is met by proliferation of interstitial macrophage precursors or by recruitment from the circulation. Following cessation of exposure, dust-laden cells slowly form focal accumulations, where the demand for more alveolar macrophages is then concentrated. This demand may well exceed the local capacity to supply, so that alveolar macrophages continue to arrive from areas of parenchyma cleared, or largely so, of dust. As the dust burden of individual alveolar macrophages in the aggregates increases the cells disintegrate, creating a further demand for macrophages, a process which might be anticipated to be more in evidence with the cytotoxic silica dust.

After the inhalation of coal dust there is a higher MI in dust-free as compared with dust-containing areas of parenchyma and these higher levels of activity eventually achieve a more-or-less steady state. To account for these changes it may be suggested that, in the case of a relatively non-toxic dust such as coal, the rate of accumulation of macrophage precursors in the interstitium occurs sufficiently slowly for maturation and cell division to take place and that a major contribution to the macrophage requirement of dust-laden areas is met by proliferation in and surface migration from dust-free areas. The existence of a dust burden obscures the transient and probably compensatory mitotic activity seen soon after mock exposure and the delayed onset of cell division may indicate a temporary phase of rapid emigration in which the interstitial residence time is too short to permit division of immature macrophages. As phagocytic needs are gradually met, time is available for cell division and maturation which, in the absence of a further burden, may ultimately subside to the level obtaining in controls.

STRECKER (1967) used the cytostatic technique to assess cellular proliferation in the lungs of rats which had inhaled 500 μg quartz over a brief period. The mitotic incidence in the alveolar region rose three- to five-fold, achieving a maximum 15 days after exposure and then declining: no such rise followed inhalation of an "innocuous" dust in similar amount, although CASARETT and MILLEY (1964) observed an elevated MI in the alveolar cells of rat lung soon after inhaling 10 μg of labelled iron oxide. The present experiments were concerned with the longer-term cellular response to the deposition of a larger dose of quartz over an extended period of exposure. Being cytotoxic quartz destroys alveolar macrophages much more readily than coal when taken up in similar amount and, remaining for the most part in the lung, thus augments the demand for phagocytes. Assuming deposition to parallel aerosol concentration, it appears that a low dose of quartz elicits a kinetic response comparable to that of Wattstown coal (Figs. 2 and 5) and for which a similar explanation may be offered. A higher dose of quartz, however, alters the response and it then seems that, after a mild initial rise, mitotic activity is depressed in the alveolar walls of dust-free areas. Moreover, in relation to aggregates of quartz dust mitotic activity progressively falls (Fig. 6). These features may be interpreted in terms of silica cytotoxicity which persistently raises demand to a level at which immature cells remain in the interstitium of dust-free or dust-bearing areas for too short a period to exhibit a normal level of proliferation.

It would be difficult to explain the present findings in terms of a response from that population of alveolar cells with a prolonged renewal time, especially as it probably consists of Type II pneumocytes which in our experience are non-phagocytic (HEPPLESTON and YOUNG, 1973). Local proliferation of alveolar wall cells in response to dust accumulation therefore refers essentially to the more rapidly renewing macrophage precursors which are marrow-derived. GODLESKI and BRAIN (1972) in fact found that, following inhalation of iron oxide particles by mouse radiation chimeras, macrophages recovered by lung lavage were increased in number and were marrow-derived. Our cell kinetic findings are readily interpreted on this basis and it might then be expected that the recruitment of monocytes from the circulation would assume a larger role with a cytotoxic dose of silica than with the comparatively innocuous coal dust.

Acknowledgements—This investigation was supported by grants to A. G. H. from the Medical Research Council and the National Radiological Protection Board.

REFERENCES

BERTALANFFY, F. D. (1964) *Int. Rev. Cytol.* **17,** 213–297.
BOWDEN, D. H. and ADAMSON, I. Y. R. (1972) *Am. J. Path.* **68,** 521–536.
BOWDEN, D. H., ADAMSON, I. Y. R., GRANTHAM, W. G. and WYATT, J. P. (1969) *Archs Path.* **88,** 540–546.
BOWDEN, D. H., DAVIES, E. and WYATT, J. P. (1968) *Archs Path.* **86,** 667–670.
BRAIN, J. D. (1971) *Inhaled Particles III* (edited by WALTON, W. H.) vol. I, pp. 209–223. Unwin Bros., Old Woking, Surrey.
BRUNSTETTER, M-A., HARDIE, J. A., SCHIFF, R., LEWIS, J. P. and CROSS, C. E. (1971) *Archs int. Med.* **127,** 1064–1068.
BULLOUGH, W. S. and LAURENCE, E. B. (1961) *Proc. R. Soc.* B, **154,** 540–556.
CASARETT, L. J. and MILLEY, P. S. (1964) *Hlth Phys.* **10,** 1003–1011.
FERIN, J., URBANKOVA, G. and VLCKOVA, A. (1965) *Archs envir. Hlth* **10,** 790–795.
FURTH, R. VAN, COHN, Z. A., HIRSCH, J. G., HUMPHREY, J. H., SPECTOR, W. G. and LANGEVOORT, H. L. (1972) *Bull. Wld Hlth Org.* **46,** 845–852.

FURTH, R. VAN, DIESSELHOFF-DEN DULK, M. M. C. and MATTIE, H. (1973) *J. exp. Med.* **138,** 1314–1330.
GODLESKI, J. J. and BRAIN, J. D. (1972) *J. exp. Med.* **136,** 630–643.
HEPPLESTON, A. G. and YOUNG, A. E. (1972) *J. Path.* **107,** 107–117.
HEPPLESTON, A. G. and YOUNG, A. E. (1973) *J. Path.* **111,** 159–164.
LABELLE, C. W. and BRIEGER, H. (1959) *A.M.A. Archs ind. Hlth* **20,** 100–105.
LABELLE, C. W. and BRIEGER, H. (1960) *Archs envir. Hlth* **1,** 423–427.
NORTH, R. J. (1969) *J. exp. Med* **130,** 315–326.
PINKETT, M. O., COWDREY, C. R. and NOWELL, P. C. (1966) *Am. J. Path.* **48,** 859–867.
RASCHE, B. (1971) *Inhaled Particles III* (edited by WALTON, W. H.) vol. I, pp. 391–400. Unwin Bros., Old Woking, Surrey.
RASCHE, B. and ULMER, W. T. (1967) *Inhaled Particles and Vapours II* (edited by DAVIES, C. N.) pp. 243–249. Pergamon Press, Oxford.
SCHLIPKÖTER, H.-W. and BROCKHAUS, A. (1970) in: *Recherche Fondamentale sur les Pneumoconioses,* pp. 39–48. Collection d'Hygiène et de Médicine du Travail no. 10. C.E.C.A., Luxembourg.
SHORTER, R. G., TITUS, J. L. and DIVERTIE, M. B. (1964) *Dis. Chest* **46,** 138–142.
SPECTOR, W. G. and RYAN, G. B. (1970) *Mononuclear Phagocytes* (edited by FURTH, R. VAN) pp. 219–232. Blackwell, Oxford.
SPENCER, H. and SHORTER, R. G. (1962) *Nature, Lond.* **194,** 880.
STRECKER, F. J. (1967) *Inhaled Particles and Vapours II* (edited by DAVIES, C. N.) pp. 141–152. Pergamon Press, Oxford.
VIROLAINEN, M. (1968) *J. exp. Med.* **127,** 943–951.
WRIGHT, B. M. (1957) *Br. J. ind. Med.* **14,** 219–228.

DISCUSSION

J. BRAIN: Throughout your study, you have assumed that the changes in mitotic indices which you have observed are attributable to macrophage precursors. I would question that assumption. In 5-μm sections it is virtually impossible to distinguish macrophage precursors from dividing Type II cells or endothelial cells. Careful studies utilizing electron microscopy reveal that presumptive macrophage precursors account for a relatively small percentage of the cell turnover in the alveolar wall. Furthermore, increases in cell renewal appear to be a non-specific response to any kind of lung injury. For example, ozone, oxygen or NO_2 injury increases the mitotic indices of cells in alveolar walls. Electron microscopy shows that much of the increase is in Type II cells. Perhaps a similar response is occurring here. Only more careful techniques to identify cells (ultrastructure, histochemistry) can answer this question.

Dr BRIGHTWELL: The identity of the alveolar wall cells arrested in metaphase is discussed in the text, but it should be emphasized that our conclusions are based on comparison of mitotic activity in dust-containing and in dust-free areas of lung from individual animals.

Prof. HEPPLESTON: May I add that ultrastructural observations (HEPPLESTON and YOUNG, 1972, 1973) do not suggest that the presence of carbon leads to an increase of Type II epithelial cells, and though some such increase follows quartz inhalation it is greatly overshadowed by the macrophage response. A similar situation was evident in ultrastructural observations (to be published) on the alveolar parenchyma after the inhalation of radioactive particles. Type II cell proliferation following damage by brief exposure to acute gaseous irritants, such as NO_2 and SO_2, is of a different order and is not comparable to the pulmonary reaction following the gradual accumulation of inhaled dust, a situation in which macrophages are in great demand.

J. FERIN: What is the evidence for your statement that alveolar macrophages move from dust-free areas of the lung into areas with particle accumulation?

Prof. HEPPLESTON: The capacity of macrophages to move or be transported over alveolar surfaces was shown by serial killings of rats after brief dust exposure. Initially the dust was widely dispersed, mostly within phagocytes, over alveolar surfaces throughout the lung. As time passed focal collections of dust-laden cells formed in the alveoli near the apex of the acinus, that is just distal to the terminal bronchiole. There seems no reason to doubt that this represents a normal clearance route for macrophages which is accentuated and often overloaded by dust exposure.

IMMUNOLOGICAL STUDIES OF EXPERIMENTAL COALWORKERS' PNEUMOCONIOSIS*

ROBERT BURRELL, DENNIS K. FLAHERTY and JOSEPH E. SCHREIBER

Department of Microbiology, West Virginia University Medical Center, Morgantown, WV,

and

Allergy Section of the Department of Preventive Medicine, University of Wisconsin School of Medicine, Madison, WI, U.S.A.

Abstract—A comparative immunological and microbiological study of experimental coalworkers' pneumoconiosis (CWP) was made in rats and mice subjected to long-term exposures of coal-mine dust aerosols. Such aerosols were realistically prepared at a concentration equal to the maximal level of respirable dust permitted by Federal standards and animals were exposed for lengths of time equal to human work contact. Among the factors studied were the production of IgA and lung reactive antibody, lung microflora and changes in pulmonary clearance. Additional experiments were concerned with the effects of passively administered lung antibody on the pulmonary clearance.

It was found that both species responded immunologically in a similar manner to humans with CWP in that IgA levels were significantly elevated and lung reactive antibodies were stimulated. Coal-mine dust inhalation had little effect on the pulmonary inactivation of inhaled bacteria, but the concomitant occurrence of passively administered lung reactive antibody seemed to enhance the inactivation.

INTRODUCTION

Many histopathologic studies have been performed on various laboratory animals exposed in different ways to coal dust in attempts to determine the pathogenesis of coal-workers' pneumoconiosis (CWP), but little attention has been given to the immunological and microbiological aspects of such exposure. Moreover, many of these studies, which have been ably reviewed by ZAIDI (1969), are open to serious criticisms. Many employed intratracheal injections of aqueous suspensions of coal dust. KING *et al.* (1958) pointed out that such artificial means of dust administration do not lead to the same kind of tissue reactions seen in spontaneous disease due to dust inhalation.

Another criticism of some early studies concerns the use of the rat, an animal almost always subject to chronic respiratory disease due to *Mycoplasma pulmonis* (LINDSEY *et al.*, 1971) which produces pathogenic effects that often render the experimental results valueless. These effects due to chronic infection are often accentuated by other forms of pulmonary stress.

* Supported in part by National Institute of Occupational Safety and Health Contract EHS–R–71–001.

Additional defects of some of the early work include exposing the animals to exaggerated concentrations of suspended dusts and using powdered coal instead of realistic dust samples obtained from a working mine which would include powdered sand from blasting or motoring operations, other mineral dusts produced as by-products of mining, organic matter other than coal, micro-organisms indigenous to these substrates and other materials. With modern air samplers, it has been possible to collect large quantities of all airborne "coal-mine dust" (CORN *et al.*, 1972) which can then be used more realistically in experimental studies.

The immunological consequences of silicosis, both spontaneous and experimental, are well known (VIGLIANI and PERNIS, 1963; ESBER and BURRELL, 1967; MILLER and ZARKOWER, 1974a). They include the production of lung reactive antibodies and rheumatoid factor, the deposition of globulin in silicotic lesions, depressed B cell function, but enhanced T cell responsiveness, and a decrease in phagocytic ability of alveolar macrophages. The present report describes a series of immunological and microbiological studies on two different species of laboratory animals chronically exposed to realistic respirable levels of coal-mine dust.

MATERIALS AND METHODS

Animals

Outbred Swiss-Webster albino male mice, weighing 20–22 g, were obtained from Carworth Laboratories, New York City, N.Y. Male CFN rats, weighing 150–175 g, were obtained from the same source. Neither species was pathogen free. All animals were housed in the animal room facilities of the Chronic Toxicology Laboratories, NIOSH, Cincinnati, Ohio. Although the experiments with each species were not done concurrently, each species was housed in separate facilities.

Coal-mine Dust

Coal-mine dust was obtained from a mine in Cambria County, Pennsylvania, known to be associated with a fairly high prevalence of coalworkers' pneumoconiosis among its employees. The dust No. 51408 was of respirable size (geometric mean 1.23 μm, 34% < 1 μm, 90% < 2.4 μm diameter) and contained 3.0–4.0% free crystalline SiO_2 and 17.8% ash. The dust was dispersed in chambers containing the animals by means of a Wright dust-feed mechanism at an average concentration approximately equal to the maximum Federal compliance level of 2.0 mg/m^3.

All test animals were exposed to this coal-mine dust 6 h/day, 5 days/week for periods ranging from 3 weeks to 12 months. Control animals were treated similarly except that their chamber had a by-pass so that they were not exposed to the dust.

Immunological Parameters

Mice and rat sera were serologically examined for antibodies to homologous lung connective tissue by the antiglobulin consumption test (HAGADORN and BURRELL,

1968). Mouse IgA was measured by commercially available radial diffusion kits (Meloy Laboratories, Springfield, Va.). Rat splenic lymphocytes were isolated and tested for lymphocytotoxin production upon stimulation with soluble lung connective tissue antigen by previously described methods (CATE and BURRELL, 1974).

Lung antibodies, reactive for only the collagen components of the lung, were prepared against homologous lung connective tissue by immunizing mice in a way to produce ascitic fluid (BURRELL *et al.*, 1974). Ascitic fluids containing at least six units of anti-globulin consumption per 0.2 ml against lung antigen were pooled. Two dozen mice to be treated were passively immunized with three 0.05 ml i.v. injections of this pooled homologous fluid per week for the duration of the experiment. An equal sized group of control mice was similarly injected with non-reactive ascitic fluid.

Microbiological Parameters

Following killing by cervical separation, mouse lungs were lavaged with 0.6 ml sterile saline and this fluid was then cultured aerobically for bacteria, fungi and mycoplasma. Mycoplasma were cultured on media specially formulated for murine strains (KOHN and KIRK, 1969) as certain media formulated for human strains may not support growth of *M. pulmonis*.

Media used for culturing fungi and mycoplasma were held for 6 weeks before calling them negative, while all others were held for 2 weeks.

Methods of Assay

Assay for the bactericidal ability of individual mouse lungs was performed according to the method of GREEN and GOLDSTEIN (1966) using aerosolized, ^{32}P radiolabelled *Staphylococcus epidermidis* as the indicator particle. These bacteria were aerosolized in a specially constructed chamber capable of exposing eight mice in individual restrainers at one time (BURRELL, 1970). Since only the snouts of the animals are exposed to aerosol and the mice may be left in the restrainers after exposure when using this device, error due to entry into the mice of radiolabel from grooming activity of contaminated fur is minimized. Approximately 3.0 ml of the radiolabelled bacterial suspension was aerosolized over a 30-min period using a no. 40 DeVilbiss glass nebulizer driven by a pump at 3 psi.

Half of the animals were removed immediately following this exposure for analysis and the remainder at 2 or 4 h afterwards. The remainder of the assay and the calculations were performed as in the Green–Goldstein method.

RESULTS

CWP in Rats

In the first experiment, 200 rats were divided into a test group of 132 animals that were exposed to the coal-mine dust regimen and the remainder served as the control group. After every 3 months, animals were removed at random from each group for bleeding and killed for pathological examination. All bleedings were tested for the occurrence of lung antibodies. A summary of the serological findings may be found in Table 1. No evidence of lung reactivity appeared until after 9 months of exposure, while such reactivity never did appear in the controls.

TABLE 1. THE DEVELOPMENT OF LUNG REACTIVE ANTIBODIES IN RATS EXPOSED TO COAL-MINE DUST

Category		Length of exposure (months)				
	Pre-exp.	3	6	9	12	16
Treated	0/40*	0/25	0/25	6/24	5/25	6/22
Control	0/20	0/12	0/12	0/12	0/10	0/10
					↑ Exposure terminated	

* Results are expressed as the number positive/number tested. Positive samples were any sera showing two or more units of consumption in the antiglobulin consumption test using lung connective tissue as antigen.

Histological examination of the lungs from the test animals initially revealed indications of chronic inflammatory changes of the bronchi, emphysema which became pronounced after 6 months' exposure, pleural thickening and fibrosis. Except for some perivascular and peribronchiolar accumulations of mononuclear cells, the controls failed to show similar changes. However, after 9 months of the sham treatment, the controls also began to show evidence of chronic bronchitis, focal aggregates of alveolar histiocytes, and early formation of granuloma and fibrosis, characteristics of chronic respiratory disease (LINDSEY *et al.*, 1971). *Mycoplasma pulmonis* was cultured with ease in both the treated and control animals from 9 months on. The number of isolates increased as the animals aged. Often, culture of the lungs from diseased animals failed to develop characteristic mycoplasma, but cultures from the obviously caseated middle ear, the organ most affected by this infection in rats, invariably were positive.

The exposure was terminated after 12 months, but immunological and pathological monitoring continued. Sixteen months after initiation of the experiment, the spleens from 14 treated rats, 4 control rats and 7 new, young rats purchased from the same source were evaluated for the presence of lymphocytes reactive with soluble lung connective tissue antigen by means of lymphocytotoxin assays. None of the lymphocytes cultured from either control group demonstrated antigen induced lymphocytotoxin, but 8 of the 14 spleens from rats exposed to the coal-mine dust contained lymphocytes producing sufficient lymphocytotoxin upon antigen stimulation to cause 20% or more cytopathogenic effects on monolayers of rat embryo fibroblast target cell cultures.

CWP in Mice

Since it was impossible to differentiate between coal-mine dust and mycoplasma-induced pathology in rats, the experiment was repeated using mice as the experimental animal, a species which does not exhibit the extensive pathology due to chronic *Mycoplasma* infection. In this experiment, more attention was paid to the infectious aspects of the disease. The mice were divided into a group of 120 that were exposed to the coal-mine dust regimen and 60 controls that received the sham treatment. Bleedings and pulmonary lavages were performed at monthly intervals. The results of the lung reactive antibody studies are given in Table 2. Although the number of

TABLE 2. THE DEVELOPMENT OF LUNG REACTIVE ANTIBODIES IN MICE EXPOSED TO COAL-MINE DUST

Category		Length of exposure (months)			
	Pre-exp.	3	4	5	6
Treated	0/5*	1/6	1/4	2/8	4/7
Control		0/2	0/2	0/4	1/5

* Results are expressed as the number positive/number tested. Positive samples were any sera showing two or more units of consumption in the antiglobulin consumption test using mouse lung connective tissue as antigen.

samples tested was admittedly small because of the limitations in serum sample size, the same general trend in serologic reactivity seen in the treated rats prevailed. Most of the mouse serum samples were used to measure serum IgA to determine if mice reacted in a manner similar to humans (HAGADORN and BURRELL, 1968).

The results, shown in Fig. 1, show that there occurred an increase in IgA in the

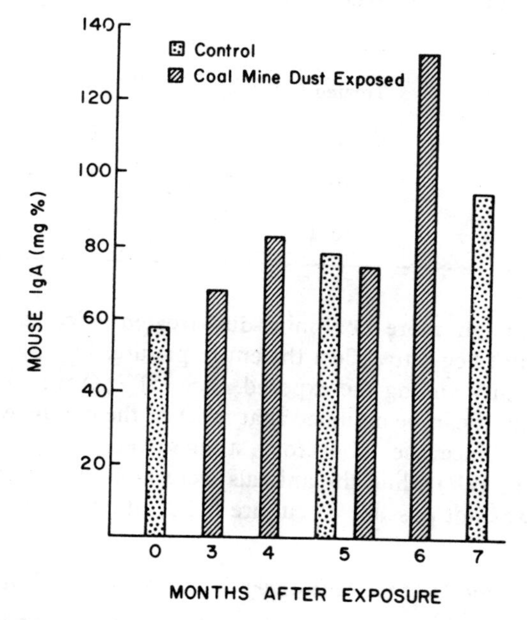

FIG. 1.—Comparison of serum IgA levels between mice exposed to coal-mine dust and sham treated controls.

group exposed for 6 months to the coal-mine dust when compared to the control value even though the latter value was obtained 1 month later.

Lavages from six control and twelve treated mice were cultured at 3, 4, 5 and 6 months after beginning exposure. Of the controls cultured, only one 3-month animal and two each from each of the other sampling periods yielded bacterial growth. *Staphylococcus aureus* was the usual isolate, but there was no pattern among the other isolates. At least three to six mice of each treated sample yielded positive cultures and although there again was no discernible pattern, *Neisseria* spp., alpha haemolytic streptococci, and *Streptomyces* spp. predominated. At no time were fungi or *Mycoplasma* recovered from the pulmonary lavages.

Of greater value was the number of bacterial colonies isolated per 0.1 ml sample of each lavage. Table 3 shows a comparison of the counts of each isolate obtained from

TABLE 3. NUMBER OF MICROORGANISMS PER LUNGS OF COAL-DUST-TREATED MICE COMPARED WITH CONTROLS

Months of exposure	No. of animals cultured	Category	No. of animals showing quantities of bacteria/0.1 ml lavage		
			1–100	10^2–10^3	10^3–10^4
3	12	Treated	2	1	0
	6	Control	0	1	0
4	12	Treated	5	0	1
	6	Control	0	1	0
5	12	Treated	3	3	0
	6	Control	2	0	0
6	12	Treated	4	0	0
	6	Control	1	1	0

the two groups. Although more coal-mine-dust-treated mice yielded quantifiable cultures, the data do not begin to reflect the entire picture. During the last 2 months of exposure, the mortality among the exposed mice (51.7%) was much greater than the controls (8.3%) and it can be assumed that most of the deaths were due to severe pulmonary infections. Since the laboratory studies were being conducted in one location (Morgantown, WV) while the animals were housed and exposed elsewhere (Cincinnati, OH), it was not possible to culture the dead or dying mice.

Effects of Coal-mine Dust on Pulmonary Inactivation of Inhaled Bacteria

A second group of eighty new mice was divided into equal control and test groups for the third experiment. These mice were assayed at 1, 2 and 3 months of exposure for pulmonary inactivation of inhaled, radiolabelled bacteria. A comparison of clearances between treated and control mice tested at each sample period is presented in Table 4.

TABLE 4. EFFECT OF COAL-MINE DUST ON PULMONARY INACTIVATION OF INHALED BACTERIA

Months of treatment	N=	Category	% Bacteria inactivated (4 h after aerosolization)	S.D.*	Average number of bacteria inhaled/mouse
1	10	Treated	98.24	1.23	1.5×10^5
	3	Control	99.09	0.23	1.7×10^5
2	10	Treated	95.56	3.86	2.9×10^4
	5	Control	96.14	2.34	2.6×10^4
3	9	Treated	94.94	3.46	2.9×10^3
	5	Control	96.66	2.85	3.1×10^3

* S.D.—standard deviation.

The percentage of bacteria inactivated 4 h after aerosolization was very uniform, however, no significant differences were seen between the two groups of mice at each sample period. There was a tendency for a greater disparity between control and treated mice as exposure lengthened. The method of assay had the further advantage of allowing the quantity of bacteria inhaled to be measured in each group and such observation indicated that both groups inhaled the same amount of labelled bacteria throughout the exposure period. Although there was a logarithmic decrease in number at each sample period, there was no difference between each group. The decrease noted was due to technical differences in sample preparation.

Effect of Lung Antibody on Pulmonary Inactivation of Inhaled Bacteria

One final experiment was conducted to determine the effect of lung antibody seen in spontaneous CWP on the pulmonary inactivation process. This was accomplished by passively immunizing normal mice with highly reactive lung antibody fluids for 45 days, during which time sample treated and untreated groups of mice were removed for pulmonary inactivation assays. The comparison of percentage inactivation and numbers of bacteria inhaled are shown in Table 5. The results show that after 31 days of passive immunization treatment, the treated mice killed a greater percentage of bacteria than the controls. The difference was about one standard deviation and although the *t*-test for independent samples shows this not to be a significant difference, it was borderline at the 95% confidence level. Of further note was that the control mice inhaled more bacteria throughout the course of the experiment and this difference was statistically significant by the 45th day at the 95% confidence level.

TABSE 5. EFFECT OF LUNG ANTIBODY ON PULMONARY INACTIVATION

Days of treatment	N=	Category	% Bacteria inactivated (2 h after aerosolization)	S.D.[a]	Average number of bacteria inhaled per mouse
17	2	Treated	98.91	N.D.[b]	1.9×10^{3}[c]
	2	Control	98.22	N.D.	2.0×10^{3}[c]
31	5	Treated	94.45	2.87	5.1×10^{4}[d]
	5	Control	90.86	3.99	6.0×10^{4}[d]
45	5	Treated	94.37	2.70	1.0×10^{5}[d]
	5	Control	91.89	3.45	1.3×10^{5}[d]

[a] S.D.—standard deviation.
[b] N.D.—Not done.
[c] Average of counts from four animals.
[d] Average of counts from eight animals.

COMMENT

Although the rat has been a popular laboratory animal for experimental pathologists in the study of silicosis and other pneumoconioses, it has become increasingly clear that it is a poor choice for pulmonary pathology studies because of the almost universal prevalence of chronic *Mycoplasma* infections. Unless investigators employ pathogen-free rats, maintain strict quarantine during the experiments, and carry out a rigid microbiological monitoring programme, their results will be inconclusive. The rat is also a poor choice immunologically since rat IgA exists in such small amounts that it cannot be technically isolated or quantitated readily (BISTANY and TOMASI, 1970). The disadvantages of rats aside, the coal-mine-dust-treated rats did produce lung-reactive antibodies and some evidence of cell-mediated immunity to appropriate antigens that were not found in the controls. In these respects, rats have responded immunologically in a similar manner to coal miners.

The mice proved to be a better immunological and microbiological model of CWP up to a point. They produced lung antibody and exhibited rises in IgA, as do humans, if exposed long enough. However, exposed mice displayed a severe mortality at about the same time these immunological findings became apparent. Since an occasional living mouse sampled at this time exhibited a severe pneumonia, it is assumed that this was responsible for the mortality.

The study was designed primarily to examine the microbiological and immunological aspects of CWP in mice, and although histopathologic studies were not performed on the mice, gross examination of their lungs at time of sacrifice revealed well-developed coal macules on the pleura of most of the exposed mice.

GOLDSTEIN *et al.* (1969) studied the effect of intratracheal injections of aqueous silica suspensions on the pulmonary inactivation of aerosolized bacteria. Although this treatment produced extraordinarily severe silicosis, it failed to alter the bactericidal activity of the lungs. Since the primary defence against inhaled organisms is by alveolar macrophages (GREEN and KASS, 1964) and since it is well known that silica is extremely toxic to such cells (KESSEL *et al.*, 1963), one might have expected a marked decrease in bacterial inactivation. The authors concluded that their results indicated that these defences can incur severe anatomic injury without functional derangement.

In the present experiments, natural exposure to realistic levels of coal-mine dust exhibited surprisingly little effect on bacterial inactivation by the lungs in view of the high mortality seen after 6 months' exposure. Since the inactivation studies only extended for 3 months of exposure, it is quite possible that an indication of functional impairment might have been obtained if such observations could have been made on animals exposed to the coal-mine dust for longer periods. As with humans who must work many years underground before showing evidence of CWP (MORGAN *et al.*, 1973), animals must be subjected to long periods of exposure to coal-mine dust inhalation before developing external evidence of disease.

ZARKOWER and MORGES (1972) have shown that carbon dust alone when administered by inhalation brought about measurable depressions of certain humoral immune responses. The methods used demonstrated almost certainly only IgM responses whereas in CWP the major immunoglobulin class stimulated appears to be IgA (HAGADORN and BURRELL, 1968). In further studies, MILLER and ZARKOWER (1974b) were able to show that carbon dust inhalation enhanced T cell mediated responses systemically, but depressed them in the mediastinal nodes. Additional experiments with silica dust inhalation (MILLER and ZARKOWER, 1974a) concluded with similar results. Thus, although these dusts do not seem to alter *in-vivo* phagocytosis, they conceivably could have an effect on other cells of the afferent limb of the immune response.

Since it is known that patients with CWP produce lung antibodies (BURRELL *et al.*, 1964), especially if their disease is of the complicated types (unpublished observations) and since a variety of data indicates these antibodies to be pathogenic (BURRELL *et al.*, 1974), an experiment was conducted to determine if the presence of these antibodies over an extended period of time had any effect on the bacterial inactivation of the lungs. Although statistical analysis suggested that such antibodies did enhance bacterial inactivation, it was not dramatic. Our methods employed the more easily phagocytized *S. epidermidis*, but had we used the more phagocytic resistant *S. aureus*, the disparity might have been greater. Also, if observations could have been extended beyond 45 days, the difference between treated and control animals might have been even more apparent. Previous studies showed a similar enhancement of clearance of bacteria from the internal circulation (BURRELL *et al.*, 1974).

Perhaps of more importance was the observation that lung antibody-treated mice inhaled significantly smaller amounts of aerosolized bacteria, suggesting that the ventilatory patterns of the treated mice had been changed. Tachypnoea and shallow breathing are associated with fewer bacteria being deposited in more proximal regions of the bronchial tree (G. M. Green, personal communication). It appears that the action of the antibody may have exerted its effects by this mechanism.

Thus, the combined effects of inhaled coal-mine dust and the production and presence of lung antibodies over extended periods of time may lead to anatomic and functional changes in the lung that allow more micro-organisms to be deposited, both from the internal and external environments. Chronic irritation by such micro-organisms might in certain individuals be an important factor in developing complicated types of pneumoconiosis.

As with rats and mice, natural human CWP disease is most likely complicated by infection as well as other environmental stresses. Although it might be argued that there is no human parallel to the *Mycoplasma*-induced chronic respiratory disease, we feel compelled to offer the reminder that rats do not smoke. With individual species differences aside, it is also worth noting that rodents chronically exposed to levels equal to the current American compliance levels of respirable dust concentrations still produce evidence of disease and tissue alteration not seen in aged matched, sham treated controls.

Acknowledgements—The work would have been impossible without the collaboration and advice of William D. Wagner and Edward S. Thompson of the Chronic Toxicology Section, NIOSH, Cincinnati, OH, and the excellent technical assistance of Rosemary Ruff. We would also like to thank Dr G. M. Green of the Vermont Lung Center, Burlington, VT, for reviewing portions of this work.

REFERENCES

BISTANY, T. S. and TOMASI, T. B., Jr. (1970) *Immunochemistry* **7,** 453–460.
BURRELL, R. (1970) *Appl. Microbiol.* **20,** 984–985.
BURRELL, R., WALLACE, J. P. and ANDREWS, C. E. (1964) *Am. Rev. resp. Dis.* **89,** 697–706.
BURRELL, R., FLAHERTY, D. K., DENEE, P. B., ABRAHAM, J. L. and GELDERMAN, A. H. (1974) *Am. Rev. resp. Dis.* **109,** 106–113.
CATE, C. C. and BURRELL, R. (1974) *Am. Rev. resp. Dis.* **109,** 114–123.
CORN, M., STEIN, F., HAMMAD, Y., MANEKSHAW, S., BELL, W. and PENKALA, S. J. (1972) *Ann. N.Y. Acad. Sci.* **200,** 17–30.
ESBER, H. J. and BURRELL, R. (1967) *Envir. Res.* **1,** 171–177.
GREEN, G. M. and GOLDSTEIN, E. (1966) *J. lab. clin. Med.* **68,** 669–677.
GREEN, G. M. and KASS, E. H. (1964) *J. exp. Med.* **119,** 167–176.
GOLDSTEIN, E., GREEN, G. M. and SEAMANS, C. (1969) *J. infect. Dis.* **120,** 210–216.
HAGADORN, J. E. and BURRELL, R. (1968) *Clin. exp. Immunol.* **3,** 263–267.
KESSEL, R. W. I., MONACO, L. and MARCHISIO, M. A. (1963) *Br. J. exp. Path.* **44,** 351–364.
KING, E. J., ZAIDI, S., HARRISON, C. V. and NAGELSCHMIDT, G. (1958) *Br. J. ind. Med.* **15,** 172–177.
KOHN, D. F. and KIRK, B. E. (1969) *Lab. Anim. Care* **19,** 321–330.
LINDSEY, J. R., BAKER, H. J., OVERCASH, R. G., CASSELL, G. H. and HUNT, C. E. (1971) *Am. J. Path.* **64,** 675–716.
MILLER, S. D. and ZARKOWER, A. (1974a) *J. Immunol.* **113,** 1533–1543.
MILLER, S. D. and ZARKOWER, A. (1974b) *Infect. Immun.* **9,** 534–539.
MORGAN, W. K. C., BURGESS, D. B., JACOBSON, C., O'BRIEN, R. J., PENDERGRASS, E. P., REGER, R. B. and SHOUB, E. P. (1973) *Archs envir. Hlth* **27,** 221–226.
VIGLIANI, E. C. and PERNIS, B. (1963) *Adv. Tuberc. Res.* **12,** 230–279.
ZAIDI, S. H (1969) *Experimental Pneumoconiosis*, pp. 64–120, Johns Hopkins Press, Baltimore.
ZARKOWER, A. and MORGES, W. (1972) *Infect. Immun.* **5,** 915–920.

DISCUSSION

H. SMITH: I would agree that the rat is not a suitable animal because of the common occurrence of CRD. Therefore would you suggest a more suitable species?

Dr BURRELL: Dr Weller yesterday presented an excellent paper on work using the monkey. Although it is very expensive for long-term inhalational studies, you can almost do everything on a monkey that you can on a human and were I to have the proper facilities and funds that's what I would use.

J. C. WAGNER: The majority of British pneumoconiosis experiments are done with SPF animals, as a reading of the literature will show.

Dr BURRELL: The papers I have been reading do not say that specific pathogen-free rats were used. In addition, a pathological study recently published shows that even these animals are not free of *Mycoplasma* disease (LAMB, D. *Lab. Animals*, 1975, **9**, 1–8). The mouse does not show the same kinds of lesions according to Lindsey's paper that the rat does and besides, our mice were cultured for *Mycoplasma*. They were always *Mycoplasma* negative.

A. G. HEPPLESTON: How do you justify the use of the term "experimental coalworkers' pneumoconiosis" to compare with either the simple or the complicated form of the human disease in the absence of any histological evidence on the response of your rat and mouse lungs to the presence of coal dust? Subpleural black spots seen by naked eye only in the mice hardly constitute pneumoconiosis. Furthermore, the microbiological and immunological observations are open to serious question since the animals used were not specific pathogen free, and hence bore their own spontaneous microflora in their respiratory tracts to the extent that many had severe pulmonary infection.

Dr BURRELL: Well that's the point I made and why I am here today is to point out to those people who are not familiar with it, what can happen when you do not use specific pathogen-free rats. We did do histological examinations in the rats, but not in the mice. I am an immunologist and I neglected the pathology and, I thought on good grounds, because that was not my main point.

P. COLE: Even reputedly SPF mice and rats cause problems as regards *Mycoplasma* in the respiratory tract. The hamster, however, is remarkably clean with regard to this organism in the respiratory tract.

Dr BURRELL: I don't believe I can measure hamster IgA which was really my reason for using mice.

F. F. HAHN: I would agree that the lung of the Syrian hamster is very clean, but the other organs are not.

J. M. G. DAVIS: Is it really justifiable to use results from SPF animals in studies relating to disease in non-SPF human lungs? I suggest results from both SPF and non-SPF animals should be compared to determine the importance of infections in some human conditions basically caused by dust inhalation.

Dr BURRELL: Of course the scientist tries to separate things into components to find out what the individual contribution is, and that would be the justification for using SPF animals. There are microbiological factors that I didn't consider, for instance, the animals should have been kept at the temperature and humidity of the working mine because these affect the naso-pharyngeal flora, and that is just one more complicated variable. Cigarette smoking is another.

THE ACTIVATION OF PHOSPHOLIPASE A IN MACROPHAGES AFTER THE PHAGOCYTOSIS OF SILICA AND OTHER CYTOTOXIC DUSTS*

P. G. MUNDER and ST. LEBERT

Max-Planck-Institut für Immunbiologie, Freiburg i Br., Fed. Rep. Germany

Abstract—The phospholipid and lipid metabolism of mouse peritoneal macrophages has been studied in the presence of various silicogenic dusts and asbestos particles. These extensive kinetic studies were possible as a reproducible method was developed to determine these major cellular constituents after labelling macrophages with 1-^{14}C-oleic acid. The following results have been obtained so far:

1. Silicogenic dusts activate a phospholipase A in macrophages leading to a concentration and time-dependent degradation of lecithin and cephalin.
2. Using low doses of SiO_2 (<1 mg/10^7 cells) the split-off free fatty acid can still be transesterified into the triglycerides.
3. High doses of silica (>2 mg/10^7 cells) induce also a lipolysis.
4. Silica specifically inhibits a plasma membrane-bound acyltransferase.
5. Asbestos particles induce in long-term cultures a moderate degradation of diacyl-phospholipids with transesterification of 1-^{14}C-oleic acid into the triglycerides.

INTRODUCTION

Since the classical studies of MARKS *et al.* (1956) it is a well-known fact that silicogenic SiO_2 destroys macrophages as measured by the release or inhibition of cellular enzymes or cellular functions (COMOLLI and PERIN, 1963; HARINGTON, 1963; KESSEL *et al.*, 1963; MUNDER and FISCHER, 1965; ALLISON *et al.*, 1966; KLOSTERKÖTTER and ROBOCK, 1967; MODOLELL *et al.*, 1967).

In previous studies on the metabolism of phagocytes during and after the uptake of silicogenic and non-silicogenic dusts we have noted that silica does not only inhibit cellular enzymes but actually activates enzymes of the phospholipid metabolism like phospholipase A_2 (MUNDER *et al.*, 1967; MUNDER *et al.*, 1970). This activation of phospholipase A has been confirmed in a completely different system (GOERKE *et al.*, 1971) and is used to study the presence of phospholipases in cellular membranes which are difficult to determine otherwise (ZAHLER, P., personal communication). The kinetics of this alteration of phospholipid metabolism in macrophages after the uptake of various SiO_2-modifications could, however, only be studied after it was noted that macrophages are rapidly labelled with 1-^{14}C-oleic acid which is incorporated as a rather stable marker in all major phospholipids and lipids. The principal metabolic pathway studied is demonstrated in Fig. 1.

* This work has been supported by a grant no. 6244/00/1/001 of the CEC.

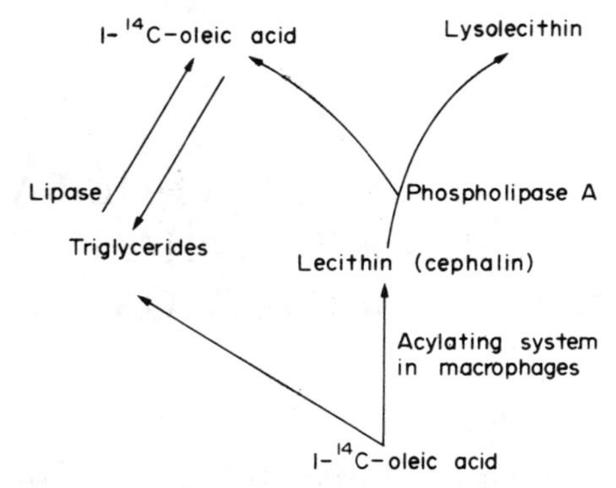

FIG. 1. Investigated pathway of 1-^{14}C-oleic acid.

MATERIAL AND METHODS

SiO_2-modifications, TiO_2 and asbestos particles were obtained from Dr K. Robock, Bergbauforschung GmbH, Essen, Germany.

Triolein: Sigma Company, St. Louis/U.S.A.

1-^{14}C-oleic acid: Radiochemical Centre, Amersham, England.

The cells were cultivated in Eagle's Medium (Dulbecco modification) + streptomycin + penicillin, buffered with (a) mM *N*-2-hydroxyethylpiperazine-*N*-2-ethanesulphonic acid (HEPES), (b) 24 mM $NaHCO_3$.

Macrophages

Mouse peritoneal macrophages were collected and prelabelled with 1-^{14}C-oleic acid as described elsewhere (MUNDER and MODOLELL, 1974). The phospholipids and lipids of the macrophages were extracted and separated by thin-layer silicic acid chromatography as previously described (MUNDER and MODOLELL, 1974; LEBERT, 1975). The separated compounds were scraped off and measured in a scintillation counter.

Tissue Culture

The cultivation of macrophages for longer than 24 h carried out on gas-permeable membranes (MUNDER *et al.*, 1971; JENSEN *et al.*, 1974).

RESULTS

The mean values of the relative distribution of 1-^{14}C-oleic acid incorporated in the various phospholipids and neutral lipids of normal mouse peritoneal macrophages is given in Table 1. After 2 h most of the 1-^{14}C-oleic acid (FFA = free fatty acid) is incorporated into the two diacylphospholipids lecithin (LEC) and cephalin (CEPH) and the neutral lipids (NL). In the absence of serum this labelling pattern will be stable for at least 4 days. If, however, the prelabelled macrophages are incubated with sili-

TABLE 1. RELATIVE DISTRIBUTION OF 1-^{14}C-OLEIC ACID IN PHOSPHOLIPIDS AND LIPIDS IN MOUSE PERITONEAL MACROPHAGES

Time	n		%LL	%SPH	%LEC	%CEPH	%FFA	%NL
10 min	5	x	2.2	3.2	37.9	8.7	26.6	21.4
		s.d.	0.5	1.4	5.7	1.2	2.0	6.4
1 h	5	x	1.9	3.0	54.9	13.5	8.5	18.2
		s.d.	0.4	1.4	6.9	2.3	1.9	6.2
2 h	10	x	1.1	3.6	56.9	15.2	4.4	18.8
		s.d.	0.3	1.2	8.1	3.0	2.0	7.9
24 h	10	x	1.4	3.8	53.3	15.1	5.7	20.2
		s.d.	0.5	1.3	5.5	3.9	2.5	7.6

Cells were prelabelled as described in material and methods.
n = number of experiments. x = arithmetic mean. s.d. = standard deviation.

cogenic or non-silicogenic particles a dose- and time-dependent change in the relative distribution of the radioactivity occurs as shown in Table 2.

TABLE 2. RELATIVE DISTRIBUTION OF 1-^{14}C-OLEIC ACID AFTER PHAGOCYTOSIS OF SiO_2 (DQ)[a]

		% Lecithin			% Free 1-^{14}C-oleic acid		
Time:		1 h	6 h	24 h	1 h	6 h	24 h
Control		62.5	61.7	60.5	5.0	4.8	4.7
DQ 12	1 mg	61.0	51.8	50.3	5.9	10.8	12.2
DQ 12	2 mg	52.4	49.0	43.3	9.1	19.5	27.2
DQ 12	4 mg	51.4	42.6	37.4	14.9	25.9	36.1
F + T[b]		55.3	55.4	56.0	12.3	13.4	14.0

10^7 cells were incubated with the dusts in 4 ml Eagle's Medium at 37°C, pH 7.1.
The remaining percentage of radioactivity is distributed among lysolecithin (LL), sphingomyelin (SPH) and neutral lipids (NL).
[a] DQ 12 = Dörentruper Quarzsand containing 86% quartz.
[b] Cells were frozen and thawed 3 times.

From these results the following conclusion can be drawn:

1. The higher the amount of DQ 12 added the more labelled lecithin is degraded.
2. The degradation of lecithin and accumulation of 1-^{14}C-oleic acid continues after the actual phagocytosis of the quartz and after the actual death of the cells.
3. Destroying the cells by freeze–thawing leads to a slight decrease in labelled lecithin which does not increase during the following hours, demonstrating only a short lasting activity of the liberated phospholipase A as compared to the enzyme in quartz-treated cells.

The change in distribution pattern of the other labelled phospholipid is as follows: cephalin (CEPH) is degraded at the same rate as lecithin. Usually there is only a slight increase in lysolecithin (LL) as the unsaturated 1-^{14}C-oleic acid is incorporated mostly into position 2 of the 1-acyl-3-glycero-phosphorylcholine, the bond of which is split by the phospholipase A_2 (for review see FERBER, 1973).

In all experiments no measurable degradation of sphingomyelin (SPH) has been observed. There are, however, remarkable changes in the labelling of neutral lipids during and after phagocytosis of SiO_2 and other dusts. Table 3 illustrates the observed alterations.

TABLE 3. % 1-^{14}C-OLEIC ACID IN THE TRIGLYCERIDES AFTER PHAGOCYTOSIS OF DQ

		% Triglycerides		
Time:		1 h	6 h	24 h
Control		20.3	20.9	21.4
DQ 12	1 mg	22.1	29.8	30.8
DQ 12	2 mg	22.3	17.1	15.1
DQ 12	4 mg	21.4	17.1	10.4
TiO_2	4 mg	20.8	—	23.9
F + T		16.4	16.7	15.2

Cultivation: see Table 2.

Surprisingly, incubation of 10^7 macrophages with 0.5–1 mg cytotoxic DQ 12 still allows the continuous energy-dependent transfer of 1-^{14}C-oleic acid from the diacyl-phospholipids to the neutral lipids, i.e. triglycerides. Thus, phospholipase A_2 will degrade these phospholipids but the degraded 1-^{14}C-oleic acid does not accumulate as the cells are still able to carry out the energy-dependent transesterification into the triglycerides. This startling phenomenon is even more apparent if the incorporation of 1-^{14}C-oleic acid is measured as shown below (see Table 7). Incubating mouse macrophages (10^7) with 2 mg or more of DQ 12 induces only a short lasting transesterification during the first hour followed by a continuous degradation of triglycerides, i.e. increased lipolytic activity.

On the other hand, destroying macrophages by other means like freeze-thawing induces an immediate lipolytic reaction which then declines. At this point the observed alterations of the lipid metabolism in macrophages can be summarized in 3 stages.

1. Low doses of DQ 12 (<1 mg/10^7 cells) induce a measurable degradation of diacylphospholipid by phospholipase A which, however, is accompanied by a transesterification of the split-off free fatty acids.
2. Doses of 2 mg/10^7 cells clearly enhances the activity of phospholipase A with a marked accumulation of free fatty acids.
3. Beyond that, still higher doses of DQ 12 (4 mg/10^7 cells) induce an increased lipolytic activity in the destroyed cells in addition to the described activation of phospholipase A.

These concentration-dependent changes in the cellular lipid metabolism after the phagocytosis of a highly silicogenic dust can also be observed when other SiO_2-

modifications of different cytotoxicity are used. The mineralogical, chemical and physical characteristics of these dusts as well as their cytotoxicity have been described (KLOSTERKÖTTER and ROBOCK, 1967; BECK *et al.*, 1973; ROBOCK and KLOSTERKÖTTER, 1973; ROBOCK *et al.*, 1973; ROBOCK, 1974).

Table 4 illustrates these three different stages of altered lipid metabolism as induced by different SiO_2 modifications.

TABLE 4. RELATIVE DISTRIBUTION OF 1-^{14}C-OLEIC ACID 24 H AFTER THE PHAGOCYTOSIS OF VARIOUS SiO_2-MODIFICATIONS

Quartz 2 mg	%LEC	%CEPH	%FFA	%NL
Control	48.9	13.9	5.7	26.8
Tridymit TS	45.2	11.6	5.9	33.1
Kristallquarz H	43.7	10.4	6.3	35.7
Sipur 1400	40.2	9.8	7.5	38.1
Bergkristall	37.5	7.0	30.7	20.9
Kristallquarz 3	37.9	7.8	19.6	30.5
DQ	38.9	9.9	28.1	17.6
Tridymit 3a	32.7	10.4	41.9	9.7
Sipur 1500	36.2	7.5	44.5	7.8

Cultivation of cells: 10^7/4 ml, 37°C, pH 7.1, 24 h.

The effect of the SiO_2 modifications used can be grouped into three categories corresponding to the above-mentioned stages: Tridymit TS, Kristallquarz H and Sipur 1400 induced the changes as described in stage 1. Bergkristall and Kristallquarz 3 activates phospholipase A with concomitant accumulation of free fatty acids without lipolysis of triglycerides (stage 2). The highly cytotoxic DQ, Tridymit 3a and Sipur 1500 (see ROBOCK 1974) degrade both phospholipids as well as triglycerides as described (stage 3). None of these three stages can be observed when macrophages have phagocytosed inert dusts like TiO_2 or very low doses of quartz (0.2 mg/10^7 cells).

On the other hand, highly silicogenic SiO_2 like tridymite or DQ 12 quartz can be manipulated in such a way that their strong effect on the lipid metabolism (stage 3) can be changed into stages 2 or 1. In systematic studies the quartz has been modified chemically, physically and by adsorption of organic substances. Treating DQ 12 with hot 1 N H_3PO_4 or 1 N NaOH in a glass beaker changes the effect of 2–4 mg quartz from stage 3 into stage 1. The same is true if DQ 12 is heated up to 800°C.

Finally, covering the surface of DQ 12 with lecithin isolated from the rinsing fluid of the lung has also a very remarkable effect. Even 20 μg lecithin adsorbed on 2–4 mg DQ 12 almost completely inhibits the accumulation of free fatty acids and any lipolytic effect although phospholipase A activity and the energy-dependent transesterification is still clearly demonstrable (stage 1). Several other organic substances like sera, triolein, albumin and globulins have also been used without significant protective effects. This possible protective and modifying effect of lung surfactant might be an important factor in the pathogenicity of a pneumoconiosis.

Similar changes in the quartz-induced alterations of the lipid metabolism of macrophages can be observed when the phagocytosis of silicogenic dusts is impeded as demonstrated in Table 5. It should be pointed out that the lowering of the incubation temperature does not inhibit the adsorption of quartz on the cellular plasma membrane but markedly inhibits the uptake into the cytoplasm.

TABLE 5. RELATIVE DISTRIBUTION OF 1-^{14}C-OLEIC ACID AFTER INCUBATION OF MACROPHAGES WITH DQ 12 AT DIFFERENT TEMPERATURES

Temperature	Quartz	%LEC	%CEPH	%FFA	%NL
37°C	control	64.6	15.1	2.8	12.7
4°C	2 mg DQ	65.0	12.6	2.9	14.7
	4 mg DQ	63.3	11.5	4.6	15.1
18°C	2 mg DQ	54.8	12.9	5.9	21.5
	4 mg DQ	51.9	11.3	12.5	19.8
30°C	2 mg DQ	42.6	8.9	19.8	23.5
	4 mg DQ	38.5	7.3	38.8	10.7
37°C	2 mg DQ	41.5	7.7	28.7	16.6
	4 mg DQ	35.8	6.4	44.8	7.7

Cultivation of cells: 10^7/4 ml pH 7.1, 24 h.

Table 5 clearly demonstrates that activation of phospholipase A and lipases by 4 mg DQ/10^7 cells at 37°C is changed into the stages 2 or 1 if the temperature is lowered to 30°C or 18°C, respectively. At 4°C no changes at all are observed.

Asbestos Particles

Experiments have been carried out and are still under way in which other fibrogenic dust like asbestos or certain coal dusts have been tested for their influence on these different pathways of the lipid metabolism. Table 6 summarizes the results obtained so far with various asbestos dusts.

TABLE 6. RELATIVE DISTRIBUTION OF 1-^{14}C-OLEIC ACID IN MACROPHAGES 4 DAYS AFTER INCUBATION WITH DIFFERENT ASBESTOS[a]

	%LEC	%CEPH	%FFA	%NL
Control	55.7	9.9	6.3	18.8
Crocidolite	48.5	7.1	10.8	18.4
Anthophyllite	38.5	6.1	8.1	35.2
Chrysotile A	38.1	4.4	8.03	40.1
Chrysotile B	43.9	4.7	8.1	34.3
DQ 12	32.9	3.8	27.5	18.5

[a] 2 mg/10^7 cells, pH 7.1, Eagle's medium + 24 mM $NaHCO_3$.

As shown in Table 6 there is a quantitative difference between crocidolite and the other asbestos particles. Asbestos particles lead to a rather low degradation of phospholipids but no accumulation of free fatty acids. The degraded 1-^{14}C-oleic acid is transferred into the triglycerides starting after the first day. The only exception is crocidolite. These changes in the phospholipid metabolism resemble the changes observed either with very low doses of DQ 12 (<1 mg) or with silica of low cytotoxicity (Tables 3 and 4).

Incorporation of 1-^{14}*C-oleic acid in quartz-treated cells*

Recently, we began to study the incorporation of 1-^{14}C-oleic acid into the phospholipids and neutral lipids after the cells had been preincubated with quartz for different lengths of time. The reaction is shown in Fig. 2. As the activation of 1-^{14}C-oleic acid

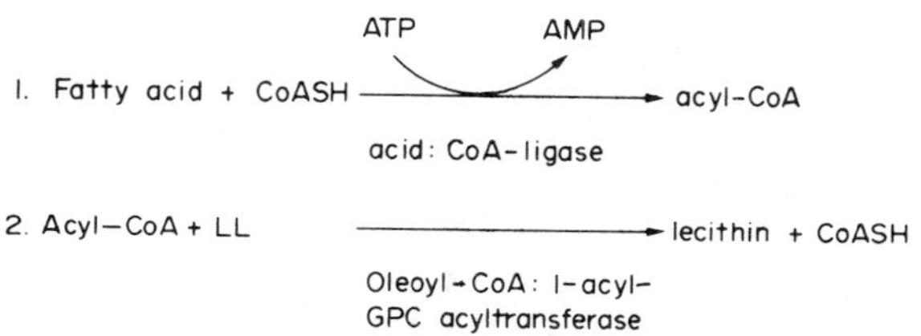

FIG. 2. Incorporation of fatty acid into lecithin.

into oleoyl-CoA is an ATP dependent step carried out in the mitochondria, cytotoxic dust should inhibit this energy-requiring reaction and, therefore, inhibit the incorporation into phospholipids and neutral lipids more or less completely. With rather high concentrations of DQ 12 (2 mg/10^7 cells) this was indeed found. Incubating macrophages with lower concentrations of DQ 12 gave, however, a surprising result as shown in Table 7.

TABLE 7. INCORPORATION OF 1-^{14}C-OLEIC ACID INTO MACROPHAGES AFTER PREINCUBATION WITH DQ 12

Time of preincubation	Quartz	%LEC	%CEPH	%FFA	%NL
	Control	60.4	9.9	8.5	17.5
20 min	0.5 mg DQ	49.4	9.6	14.9	23.3
	1 mg DQ	45.4	8.9	19.4	23.2
	2 mg DQ	40.3	6.4	31.0	19.7
2 h	0.5 mg DQ	45.4	6.1	21.3	24.9
	1 mg DQ	16.4	1.9	47.3	39.5
	2 mg DQ	2.0	1.2	90.0	6.4
24 h	0.1 mg DQ	61.7	11.0	5.5	17.9
	0.5 mg DQ	24.4	4.9	32.7	36.5
	1 mg DQ	9.6	3.5	64.3	21.6
	2 mg DQ	1.8	0.9	94.6	2.4

Twenty minutes after the addition of 2 mg DQ a slight, distinct inhibition of the incorporation is detectable, whereas 0.5 or 1 mg DQ have no effect at this time. The ratio of labelled lecithin to labelled triglycerides is 2 : 1 as in the controls. But after 2 h the patterns are changed completely. 2 mg DQ have completely destroyed the cells, as 90% of the added 1-^{14}C-oleic acid is not incorporated. 1 mg DQ 12/10^7 cells leads, however, to a distinct shift in the labelling pattern of the macrophages. Incorporation into triglycerides is clearly favoured. The ratio phospholipids/triglycerides changes from 2: 1 to more than 1 : 2. This is even more apparent after 24 h. Now 0.5 mg DQ has almost the same effect as 1 mg after 2 h, i.e. markedly favoured incorporation into the triglycerides. 0.1 mg or less DQ 12 has no effect, but different results may be obtained when the cells are incubated longer than 24 h with the dusts.

This surprising finding of a favoured incorporation of 1-^{14}C-oleic acid into the triglycerides instead of the phospholipids after the preincubation with morphologically clearly damaging doses of quartz is difficult to explain.

Moderate doses of cytotoxic DQ 12, high doses of modified DQ 12 or silica of lower cytotoxicity still allow the ATP-dependent conversion of fatty acid into acyl-CoA (see Fig. 2) followed by an almost normal rate of incorporation into the glycerides (Table 7) but an increasing inhibition of the labelling of cellular phospholipids. This means that the acid CoA-ligase is not inhibited under these conditions. As, however, the second step transfer-reaction is carried out by specific transferases one has to assume that silica does inhibit directly or indirectly the plasma-membrane-bound oleoyl-CoA: 1-acyl-glyceryl-phosphorylcholine-acyltransferase. Studies are under way to investigate further this possibly specific interaction of silica with this membrane bound enzyme.

The significance of this observation lies in the fact that silicogenic dust inhibits an enzyme which has apparently an important function in controlling the phospholipid permeability barrier in cellular membranes. This happens before the cells are actually destroyed. This early effect might then be followed by an increasing cellular damage. Whether silica interacts directly with the enzyme or whether it is inhibited by a disturbed phospholipid bilayer in the cell membrane after the adsorption of silica remains an open question.

CONCLUSIONS

Based on the finding that silica interferes with the normal phospholipid metabolism of macrophages at different points, the following hypothesis can be formulated. Low doses of cytotoxic dusts or high doses of dusts with lower cytotoxicity inhibit first the membrane-bound acyl-transferase (see Fig. 2) leading to an increasing disturbance of the permeability barrier of the plasma membrane. This would also explain the permeability changes in non-phagocytic cells like erythrocytes. On the other hand, the phagocytosed silica activates intracellular phospholipase A which, however, is counteracted by the phagocytes, as the free fatty acids are still transferred into the triglycerides. If, however, high doses of silica ($>$2 mg DQ/10^7 cells) are added, enough silica is phagocytosed immediately per single cell preventing any compensatory reaction of the cells. The intracellular silica activates strongly the phospholipase A and lipases leading to a continuous degradation of lecithin, cephalin triglycerides with massive accumulation of free fatty acid and also of lysophosphatides as shown before (MUNDER *et al.*, 1966).

The observed alterations allow one to determine where and to what extent the various silicogenic and other cytotoxic dusts influence the normal phospholipid metabolism. After further different dusts from different coal mines and other sources have been tested in this sensitive system, attempts will be made to correlate the effect on the phospholipid metabolism with their cytotoxic and silicogenic properties, as we believe that the described disturbance is causative for the development of fibrotic tissue reactions. The rate of accumulation of surface active, cytotoxic, free fatty acids and lysophosphatides in the presence of dusts might actually mediate, together with other factors (HEPPLESTON, 1971; ALLISON, 1973), the grade and development of a pneumoconiosis or asbestosis. This suggestion seems reasonable as other substances, known to cause long-lasting formations of granulomatous tissue reactions, disturb the phospholipid metabolism of macrophages in much the same way (MUNDER *et al.*, 1973, MUNDER and MODOLELL, 1974). As to the real mechanism of the interaction of biological substances with SiO_2-modifications on the subcellular level, the extensive work of ROBOCK (1974) has seriously to be considered. It is indeed tempting to speculate whether the relationship between the cytotoxicity of silica and the electron transfer between the semiconductor SiO_2 and the membrane as described by ROBOCK (1968, 1974) can be correlated with the observed activation of phospholipase A or the inhibition of the plasma membrane bound oleoyl-transferase.

Acknowledgement—We gratefully acknowledge the technical assistance of Miss B. Fischer and Mr K. Widmann.

REFERENCES

ALLISON, A. C. (1973) *Biological Effects of Asbestos. Proceedings of a Working Conference, Lyon, 1972* (edited by BOGOVSKI, P., GILSON, J. C., TIMBRELL, V. and WAGNER, J. C.) I.A.R.C. Scientific Publication no. 8. International Agency for Research on Cancer, Lyon.

ALLISON, A. C., HARINGTON, J. S. and BIRBECK, M. (1966) *J. exp. Med.* **124,** 141.

BECK, E. G., ROBOCK, K., GRÜNSPAN, M. and MANOJLOVIC, N. (1973) *Ergebn. Unters. geb. Staub-Silikosebekämpf. Steinkohlenbergbau* **9,** 131–135.

COMOLLI, R. and PERIN, E. (1963) *Proc. Soc. exp. Biol. Med.* **113,** 289.

FERBER, E. (1973) *Biological Membranes* (edited by CHAPMAN, D. and WALLACH, D. F. H.) vol. 2, pp. 221–250. Academic Press, New York.

GOERKE, J., DE GIER, J. and BONSEN, P. P. M. (1971) *Biochim. Biophys. Acta* **248,** 245–253.

HARINGTON, J. S. (1963) *S. Afr. med. J.* **37,** 451.

HEPPLESTON, A. G. (1971) *Inhaled Particles III* (edited by WALTON, W. H.) vol. I, pp. 357–369. Unwin Bros., Old Woking, Surrey.

JENSEN, M. D., WALLACH, D. F. H. and LIN, P. S. (1974) *Exp. Cell Res.* **84,** 271–281.

KESSEL, R. W. I., MONACO, L. and MARCHISIO, M. A. (1963) *Br. J. exp. Path.* **44,** 4.

KLOSTERKÖTTER, W. and ROBOCK, K. (1967) *Ergebn. Unters. geb. Staub- Silikosebekämpf. Steinkohlenbergbau* **6,** 51–54.

LEBERT, S. (1975) *Biochemische Untersuchungen zum Einfluß von SiO_2-Modifikationen auf den Phospholipoidstoffwechsel von Makrophagen.* Thesis, University of Freiburg i. Br.

MARKS, J., MASON, M. A. and NAGELSCHMIDT, G. (1956) *Br. J. ind. Med.* **13,** 187.

MODOLELL, M., MUNDER, P. G. and FISCHER, H. (1967) *Fortschr. Staublungenforsch.* **2,** 179–186.

MUNDER, P. G. and FISCHER, H. (1965) *Beitr. Silikoseforsch. S. Bd. Grundfragen Silikoseforsch.* **6,** 93.

MUNDER, P. G. and MODOLELL, M. (1974) *Rec. Results Cancer Res.* **47,** 244–250.

MUNDER, P. G., FERBER, E., MODOLELL, M. and FISCHER, H. (1967) *Fortschr. Staublungenforsch.* **2,** 129–144.

MUNDER, P. G., MODOLELL, M., FERBER, E. and FISCHER, H. (1966) *Biochem. Zeitschr.* **344,** 310–313.
MUNDER, P. G., MODOLELL, M., FERBER, E. and FISCHER, H. (1970) *Mononuclear Phagocytes* (edited by FURTH, R. VAN) pp. 445–460. Blackwell, Oxford and Edinburgh.
MUNDER, P. G., MODOLELL, M. and HOELZL WALLACH, D. F. (1971) *FEBS Lett.* **15,** 191–196.
MUNDER, P. G., MODOLELL, M. and FISCHER, H. (1973) in: *Non-specific Factors Influencing Host Resistance* (edited by BRAUN, W. and UNGAR, J.) pp. 259–266. Karger, Basel.
ROBOCK, K. (1968) *Staub* **28,** 148–156.
ROBOCK, K. (1974) *Beitr. Silikoseforsch.* **26,** 111–262.
ROBOCK, K. and KLOSTERKÖTTER, W. (1973) *Staub* **33,** 60–63.
ROBOCK, K., BECK, E. G. and MANOJLOVIC, N. (1973) *Silikoseber. NRhein-Westfalen* **9,** 91–98.

DISCUSSION

S. J. ROTHENBERG: How were the dusts administered and what were the particle sizes?

Dr MUNDER: All these studies have been carried out *in vitro* not *in vivo*. We obtained all our SiO_2 modifications, etc., from Dr Robock who standardized the dusts we used very thoroughly. The details can be found in the papers by ROBOCK *et al.*, cited in the references.

W. T. ULMER: Lecithin (surfactant) protects the cell from attack by quartz. Do you think that with time, the lecithin film on the quartz surface is dissolved *in vivo*? Do other substances, viz. serum, albumin, etc., have a similar protective effect?

Dr MUNDER: We covered silica particles with 1-^{14}C labelled lecithin and could not find any significant degradation by macrophages during a 48-h incubation period. Therefore, we do indeed believe that the *in vivo* contact of SiO_2 particles with the lecithin-containing surfactant may also change the cytotoxic activity of these dusts. Other substances like serum, albumin or triglycerides had no significant protective effect in our system *in vitro*.

INVESTIGATION OF ALVEOLAR MACROPHAGES FROM RATS EXPOSED TO COAL DUST*

EULA BINGHAM, WILLIAM BARKLEY, RAMAN MURTHY and CHARLES VASSALLO

University of Cincinnati,
College of Medicine,
Department of Environmental Health,
Ohio, U.S.A.

Abstract—Rats were exposed to the inhalation of coal dust from either Utah (low prevalence coalworkers' pneumoconiosis (CWP)) or Pennsylvania (high prevalence CWP). Rats were sacrificed, the lungs removed and lavaged to obtain free cells. The number of alveolar macrophages recovered from rats inhaling these two coal dusts (exposures up to 4 months) was not remarkably different from the number recovered from rats inhaling filtered room air. This is in contrast to results obtained after intratracheal intubation of the dust. The capacity of the lavaged cells to phagocytize and kill bacteria decreased after exposure to either dust. The activity of certain enzymes also decreased.

INTRODUCTION

It is a widely accepted fact that the inhalation of coal dust contributes to the pathological and the physiological changes seen in the lungs of some coal miners. Coalworkers' pneumoconiosis can be defined as the accumulation of coal dust in the lungs and the response of tissue to its presence. HEPPLESTON (1947) has suggested that in essence the initial inceptive and crucial lesion in coalminers' pneumoconiosis is a mantle of macrophages burdened with coal-mine dust enmeshed in fibrous tissue around the respiratory bronchiole and lobular arteriole.

Since alveolar macrophages possess phagocytic properties, they are the first line of defence against inhaled particles which reach the deep lung, and are likely to be the first cells damaged by these particles. THOMAS (1965) reported that proteolytic enzymes are involved in inflammatory processes and cell injury. It is possible that macrophages which have engulfed coal particles may undergo regressive changes and eventually be lysed, thus releasing their load of lysosomal enzymes into the extracellular fluid. The enzymes may cause necrosis of vicinal cells and, according to VIGLIANI and PERNIS (1961), there is a proliferation and collection of new macrophages, fibroblasts, mast cells and pyroninophilic cells in the proximity of the injury.

Many hypotheses have been postulated to explain the fibrogenic process and most

* This work was supported by a Contract no. HSM 99–73–55 and the Grant no. OH 00357–04 from the National Institute for Occupational Safety and Health, and is part of the Center for the Study of the Human Environment no. ES 00159.

of them involve macrophages, either in the necrotic processes or in the production of factor(s) which bring the identical end result of fibrosis.

LABELLE and BRIEGER (1959) investigated the clearance of dust from the lungs as related to the number of free cells washed out. Their work, mainly from acute exposures, demonstrated that an increased number of alveolar macrophages enhanced pulmonary clearance of insoluble particles. BRAIN and FRANK (1968) described a reproducible technique for washing free cells (mostly alveolar macrophages) from the lung. Utilizing this technique, BINGHAM *et al.* (1968) demonstrated that the total number of cells recovered may be altered by the inhalation of certain metallic particles. Because it is apparent that coal-mine dusts have variable chemical and physical properties, it was of interest to expose animals to the same concentration of two coal dusts from mines where workers experience great differences in the risk of developing pneumoconiosis. Whether or not biological responses to two coal dusts would be different had not been investigated experimentally. The investigations to be described were designed to determine whether the inhalation of coal dust by rats altered: (1) the number of free cells washed from the lungs using a standard technique; (2) the type of cells as compared to those of control rats; (3) the phagocytic and bactericidal activities of the lavaged cells; (4) the activity of certain enzymes of the lavaged cells.

METHOD

Two bituminous coal-dust samples were provided by the National Institute for Occupational Safety and Health. Coal-dust samples were taken from a mine in Utah, where there is a low prevalence of coalworkers' pneumoconiosis, and from a mine in Pennsylvania that has a high prevalence of disease (LAINHART, 1969). The coal samples were micronized and supplied to us. The inhalation chambers were 27-in. stainless-steel cubes and the coal was fed into the chambers using a Wright dust feeder. The size distribution of the dusts in the chamber was determined using an Andersen impactor.

It should be pointed out that by this time we had chemically analysed the coals and were aware that the coals differed considerably in their content of metals. These data have been reported by NORD and BINGHAM (1973). Drs Pfitzer and Horstman (personal communication) found during the dust exposures that it was necessary to feed about 4 times as much Utah coal as Pennsylvania coal to obtain similar nominal concentrations and particle sizes.

Young adult albino rats (Greenacres control-flora) were subjected to the inhalation of coal dust at two concentrations, 2 mg/m^3 or 15 mg/m^3, for 6 h per day, 5 days per week and for periods up to 4 months. In addition, a group of aged rats (24 months old) were subjected to the inhalation of coal dust (2 mg/m^3). The size distribution of the two dusts in the chamber was determined using an Andersen impactor.

Cells were harvested from control and exposed rats using the procedure described earlier by Brain and Frank and modified by BINGHAM *et al.* (1968). The total cell count was determined with a Coulter Counter and periodically checked with a haemocytometer and a light microscope. The washings which remained were combined and centrifuged. Slides were made from some of the cell pellets for histochemical studies and the remaining pellet used for enzyme assays.

The phagocytic activity was determined by the method described by VASSALLO *et al.* (1973) using cells harvested from both control and exposed rats.

For comparison with inhalation studies, four groups of young rats, six per group, were subjected to intratracheal injection of Utah coal dust, Pennsylvania coal dust, carbon, or saline and the free cells harvested from the lungs after 24 h and counted.

RESULTS AND COMMENT

The size distribution of the two coal samples is presented in Table 1. The mass median aerodynamic diameter of Pennsylvania coal dust was 1.2 μm while the Utah coal dust was 1.6 μm.

The number of alveolar macrophages recovered from rats inhaling Pennsylvania or Utah coal dust at 2 mg/m^3 is presented in Fig. 1. Initially there was an increase in the number of cells recovered from about 50% of the young rats inhaling coal dust. The

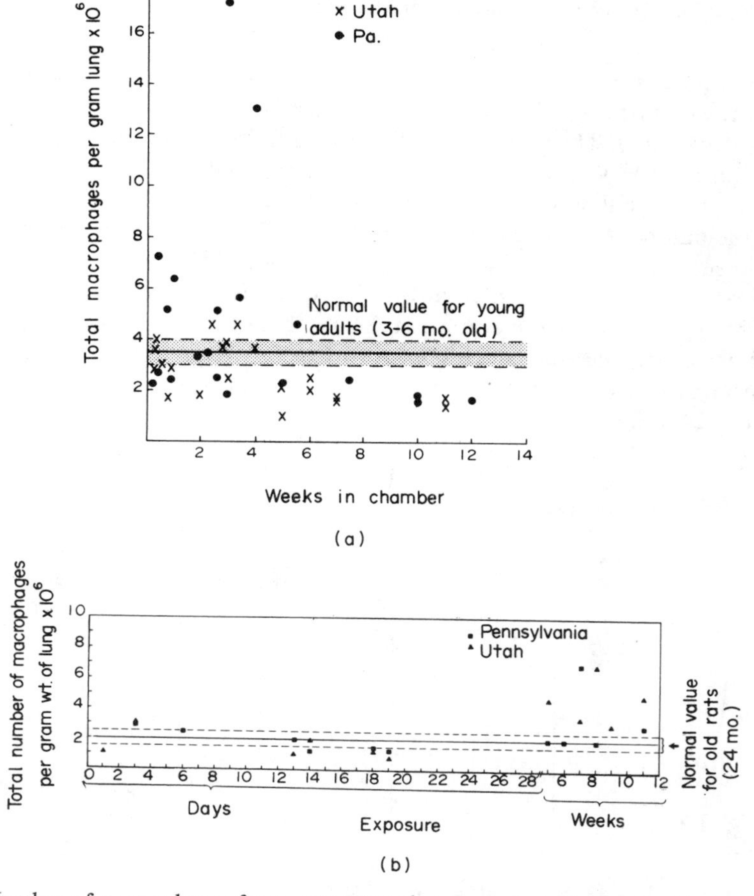

FIG. 1. Number of macrophages from rats exposed to coal dust (2 mg/m^3). (a) Young rats (3–6 months). (b) Old rats (24 months).

TABLE 1. PARTICLE SIZE DISTRIBUTION OF COAL DUST

Stage	MMAD[b] (μm)	Cumulative percentage of collected particulates[a]			
		Pennsylvania		Utah	
		total	respirable	total	respirable
1					
2	5.4	96.3	69.1	91.8	59.0
3	3.0	85.4	66.4	75.0	54.8
4	1.5	60.3	53.9	46.4	40.5
5	1.0	34.5	34.5	22.7	22.7
6	0.5	15.4	15.4	8.8	8.8
7	0.2	5.3	5.3	3.3	3.3

[a] Twenty-nine Andersen impactor samples; total volume sampled 102 m^3.
[b] Mass median aerodynamic diameter of particles collected on the stage.

majority of these animals inhaled Pennsylvania coal dust. In relation to the length of exposure the number of cells recovered from experimental rats gradually decreased to below control values. The number of cells washed from the old rats is about 2.0 ± 0.5 cells/g of lung $\times 10^6$. When old rats were subjected to coal dust, there was no difference between experimental and control data.

Since the number of cells did not increase markedly as had been reported by Brain in experiments with intratracheal injection, we performed similar injections. The results of these experiments are presented in Fig. 2. The initial increase is in agreement with Brain, who observed a great elevation in the number of macrophages washed out 24 h after intratracheal injection of carbon particles. Similar results are seen when coal dust, carbon, or saline (control) are injected intratracheally and the macrophages washed out 24 h later.

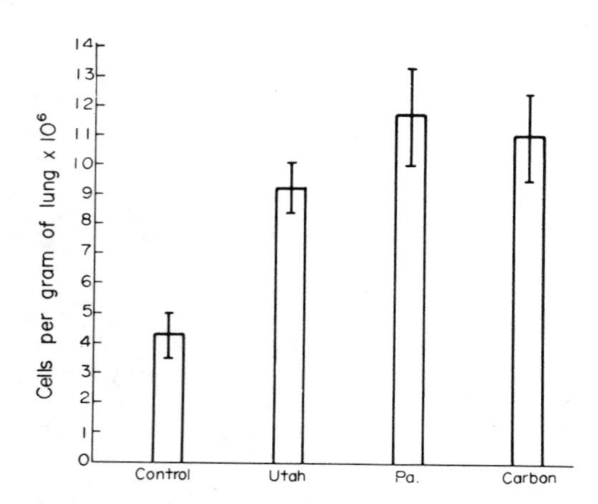

FIG. 2. Recovery of free cells 24 h after intratracheal injection of various particulates. Mean $\pm$ standard error.

The size of the cells washed from each experimental group exposed to inhalation of coal dusts is presented in Table 2.

TABLE 2. CELL SIZE DISTRIBUTION OF ALVEOLAR MACROPHAGES EXPOSED TO COAL DUST (2 mg/m³)

Exposure	Total number of cells counted	Cell size		
		<10 μm	10–20 μm	>20 μm
Control	200	138.0 ± 10.4	52.7 ± 7.1	8.7 ± 3.5
Pennsylvania	200	157.8 ± 8.8	43.8 ± 7.3	1.5 ± 0.6
Utah	200	175.5 ± 7.8	26.5 ± 7.6	0.3 ± 0.2

The activities of acid phosphatase, lysozyme, and β-glucuronidase were decreased in cells washed from rats exposed to inhalation of Pennsylvania or Utah coal dust. Esterase activity was increased in cells harvested from rats exposed to Utah coal dust; cells from rats exposed to Pennsylvania coal dust did not exhibit a significant increase in esterase activity. (Refer to Table 3.)

TABLE 3. ENZYME ACTIVITY* OF ALVEOLAR MACROPHAGES EXPOSED TO COAL DUST (2 mg/m³)

Enzyme	Enzyme activity		
	Control	Pennsylvania coal dust	Utah coal dust
Esterase	1.03 ± 0.04	0.98 ± 0.20	1.40 ± 0.18
Acid phosphatase	13.94 ± 4.45	3.93 ± 0.12	2.88 ± 0.12
Lysozyme	21.35 ± 6.29	6.41 ± 0.04	5.57 ± 0.67
β-Glucuronidase	0.13 ± 0.04	0.05 ± 0.01	0.03 ± 0.01

* Enzyme activity is expressed as specific activity = (μmoles of product released per mg of protein).

The capacity of the free cells harvested from coal dust exposed rats to ingest and kill bacteria is presented in Figs. 3 and 4. It can be seen that inhalation of either coal at either concentration resulted in a statistically significant decrease in the capacity of the macrophages to ingest and kill bacteria.

In conclusion then, even though these two coals differ in the production of disease in miners, and are distinctly different chemically in their content of metals, and are dissimilar in physical properties which became evident during the preparation of inhalation exposures—the differences in responses of macrophages have been similar. This does not mean that even small differences may be important over long periods of exposure or that we have even measured a critical biological response. A final point is that CHRISTIAN and coworkers (1973) in our Department have reported a significant difference in the toxicity of water extracts of these coals for cell cultures.

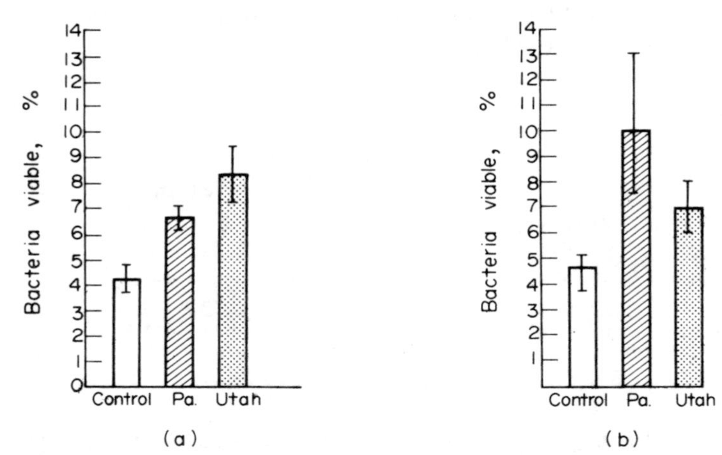

FIG. 3. Percentage of *Staphylococci* viable after phagocytosis by alveolar macrophages. Mean ± standard error. (a) 2 mg/m³ coal dust. (b) 15 mg/m³ coal dust.

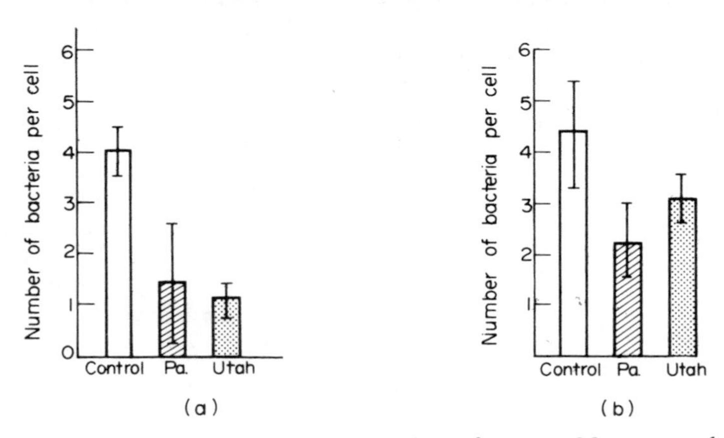

FIG. 4. Uptake of *Staphylococcus* by alveolar macrophages from rats. Mean ± standard error. (a) 2 mg/m³ coal dust. (b) 15 mg/m³ coal dust.

REFERENCES

BINGHAM, E., PFITZER, E. A., BARKLEY, W. and RADFORD, E. P. (1968) *Science, N.Y.* **162,** 1297–1299.

BRAIN, J. D. and FRANK, N. R. (1968) *J. appl. Physiol.* **25,** 63–69.

CHRISTIAN, R. T., CODY, T. E., CLARK, C. S., LINGG, R. and CLEARY, E. J. (1973) *A.I.Ch.E. Symp. Ser.* **70,** 15–21.

HEPPLESTON, A. G. (1947) *J. Path. Bact.* **59,** 453.

LA BELLE, C. W. and BRIEGER, H. (1959) *A.M.A. Archs ind. Hlth* **20,** 100–105.

LAINHART, W. S. (1969) *J. occup. Med.* **11,** 399.

NORD, P. J. and BINGHAM, E. (1973) in: *Trace Substances in Environmental Health VI* (edited by HEMPHILL, D. D.) Columbia, Missouri.

THOMAS, L. (1965) in: *The Inflammatory Process* (edited by ZWEIFACH, B. W., GRANT, L. and MCCLUSKEY, R. T.) Academic Press, N.Y.

VASSALLO, C. L., DOMM, B. M., POE, R. H., DUNCOMBE, M. L. and GEE, J. B. L. (1973) *Archs envir. Hlth* **26,** 270–274.

VIGLIANI, E. C. and PERNIS, B. (1961) *Bull. Hyg.* **36,** 1.

DISCUSSION

P. COLE: How long after harvesting the alveolar macrophages did you perform the bacterial killing assay?

Dr BINGHAM: Within 30 min.

P. COLE: Did you use antibiotics in the culture medium during the assay? This is a technical point which has bedevilled work in this kind of system for many years (COLE, P. J. and BRONTOFF, J. *Nature, Lond.* 1975, **256,** 515–517).

Dr BINGHAM: Dr Vassallo, at the Cincinnati Veterans Administration Hospital, did these assays and has published details. Antibiotics were *not* used.

G. BOULEY: Can the fall in the phagocytic capacity of the macrophages of dusted rats in relation to the controls be explained by an increase in the immature macrophages in the dusted animals?

Dr BINGHAM: I think that is entirely possible. The macrophages do appear to be somewhat smaller and perhaps less mature. They have not, as it were, manufactured their bag of enzymes ready for delivery.

S. E. DEVIR: I wonder if the coal dust dispersed by the Wright dust feeder used in your inhalation study really represented the airborne particles the coal miner inhales. The drastic procedures of grinding, pressing, shearing and finally air blasting the coal particles, carried out with the Wright dust feeder, probably change the shape and the size distribution of the original airborne coal-dust samples, taken from the mines. Do you assume that these parameters (shape and size) will have no effect on the number of alveolar macrophages recovered from the lung of the rats in your experiments?

Dr BINGHAM: I think that is a valid point. These two batches of coal were supplied to us by NIOSH and they have, I believe, made some extensive measurements on the shape and physical characteristics of the particles. I cannot say more.

A. G. HEPPLESTON: I wonder whether the low macrophage recovery after coal inhalation may reflect the low rate of pulmonary accumulation of dust. When coal was given as a single intratracheal mass the greater stimulus presumably caused an increased outpouring of alveolar macrophages.

Dr BINGHAM: I would assume that is correct. However, we have washed out and counted macrophages from rats receiving higher exposures up to 15 mg/m^3 and have found an initial increase but not in every animal. Some animals do have apparently an outpouring of macrophages from the stimulus early in the exposure period. However, the number then returns to control levels. It is interesting that we have this levelling off.

J. M. G. DAVIS: This paper lays emphasis on numbers of macrophages washed from the lung after coal-dust inhalation. In the disease of pneumoconiosis, however, the major feature is the fact that many dust-containing macrophages become "fixed" within the lung. After 4 months' dust inhalation, therefore, the important cells may be those that cannot be washed from the lung.

Dr BINGHAM: You may be right, I do not have data on that.

T. L. OGDEN: Why was it that four times as much of one of the dusts as the other had to be dispersed to maintain equal concentrations? Was the dust obtained by grinding coal, or collecting airborne dust?

Dr BINGHAM: I think there were larger particles of the Utah coal that had to be separated out with a cyclone. The procedure was, of course, artificial because it is not that way in the mine. We were trying to have as close as possible the same nominal concentrations of the two coal dusts and as close as possible the same particle size distribution, to get at the question of whether or not there are chemical differences that could account for the difference in prevalence of disease.

H. AYER: There were no systematic measurements made of coal dust in American mines prior to 1969. Therefore, the relative concentration to which miners in the two areas were exposed is not known. Neither is it known whether the physical state of the dust in the coal mines of the areas resembles that dispersed into the dust chambers.

M. BUNDY: Do you know whether the Pennsylvania coal was anthracite from Eastern, or middle type from central or Western Pennsylvania?

Dr BINGHAM: It was from a mine near Johnstown, Pennsylvania.

M. BUNDY: Middle type. Further to Mr Ayer's remarks, the dust levels in Utah before 1969 were probably not as high as in Pennsylvania, although they were above the present standard level. Dust levels alone cannot, therefore, account for the difference in prevalence and incidence of CWP in the two regions; it can only be explained by differences in the coal.

Dr BINGHAM: And in people, I might add.

D. K. CRAIG: I cannot let the comments regarding the possibility of the Wright Dust Feed Mechanism (WDFM) modifying the nature of the dust particles go unchallenged. The scraper blade, revolving slowly, carves a 33-μm thick slice of dust off the dust pack and this is then dispersed with compressed air. Providing the packing of the dust into the WDFM cylinder in the first place (at a pressure of the order of 250 kg/cm^2) does not modify the dust, and there is no evidence that it does, it is extremely unlikely that the coal dust would be altered by using the WDFM as the aerosol generator. In fact, the main problem with this device is that it is often not efficient enough in dispersing the dust.

In our studies, we have investigated the possibility that the Wright dust feeder might alter the nature of a softer powdered material than coal, namely talcum powder. We were unable to detect any such differences. Similar studies conducted elsewhere support our conclusions.

Dr BINGHAM: I am happy to hear that. I do know that the people concerned took much time and trouble to find the best method of dispersing the coal dust. They thought it was most appropriate at that time, but it has been 5 years since those experiments were begun.

THE EFFECT OF INCREASED PARTICLES ON THE ENDOCYTOSIS OF RADIOCOLLOIDS BY PULMONARY MACROPHAGES *IN VIVO*: COMPETITIVE AND TOXIC EFFECTS*

JOSEPH D. BRAIN and GRACE C. CORKERY

Department of Physiology,
Harvard University School of Public Health,
Boston, Mass., U.S.A.

Abstract—We have developed a technique for measuring the rate of particle ingestion by pulmonary macrophages *in vivo*. This technique has been used to examine the impact of pre-exposure to ferric oxide, colloidal carbon, and coal dust on the endocytosis of a test particle, colloidal gold. Our technique for estimating endocytosis is as follows: Syrian golden hamsters received intratracheal instillations (0.15 cm^3/100 g body weight) of a suspension of colloidal ^{198}Au (~30 nm diameter). Two hours following instillation, each hamster was sacrificed and its trachea cannulated. The lungs were lavaged 12 times with saline solutions, and the number of cells and gold particles in each wash determined. Analysis of the washout curves permits the calculation of the fraction, λ, of the colloidal particles which has been ingested at a time, t.

This method was then used to measure the influence of inhaled or intratracheally instilled particles on the endocytosis of the gold particles. Hamsters breathed ferric oxide aerosol spontaneously or were given intratracheal instillations of colloidal carbon or coal dust. Immediately following the exposure, the ability of the macrophages to ingest a test particle was assayed by the technique described above. In all instances, colloidal gold endocytosis measured at 2 h was significantly depressed. However, when challenged by the gold colloid 24 h after exposure to the inhaled or instilled particles, only the coal dust group exhibited depressed endocytosis. We conclude that all dusts studied competitively inhibit endocytosis, but only some exhibit a toxic effect on macrophage function.

INTRODUCTION

Despite continuous exposure of the lung to particulates characteristic of occupational and urban environments, the surfaces of the respiratory tract are relatively free of foreign matter. This is the result of the complex system of respiratory defence mechanisms which both prevents particle entry and removes particles that have been peposited. The alveolar macrophages are usually credited with keeping the alveolar surfaces clean and sterile. Alveolar macrophages are large, mononuclear, phagocytic cells found on the alveolar surface. They do not form part of the continuous epithelial

* This investigation was supported by grants ES–00583 and ES–00002 from the National Institute of Environmental Health Sciences.

layer, which is made up of pulmonary surface epithelial cells (type I pneumonocytes) and great alveolar cells (type II pneumonocytes). Rather, the alveolar macrophages rest on this lining. These cells are largely responsible for the remarkable bactericidal properties of the lung (GREEN and KASS, 1964), but here our concern is directed toward their ability to ingest non-living, insoluble dust and debris.

Rapid endocytosis of insoluble particles prevents particle penetration through the alveolar epithelia and facilitates alveolar-bronchiolar transport. SCHILLER (1961) and later SOROKIN and BRAIN (1975) found little evidence that macrophages laden with dusts can re-enter the alveolar wall; only free particles appear to penetrate. Thus phagocytosis plays an important role in the prevention of the entry of particles into the fixed tissues of the lung. Once particles leave the alveolar surface and penetrate the tissues subjacent to the air–liquid interface (type I and II cells, interstitial and lymphatic tissues), their removal is slowed. Pathological processes, such as fibrosis, may also impair their clearance from these compartments. The probability of particle entry into a fixed tissue in which it would have a long biological half-life is reduced if the particle is phagocytized by a free cell. Therefore endocytosis emerges as a central theme of macrophage activity.

The project described here is one of a series of experiments designed to study the impact of particle exposure on macrophage structure and function. Previously, we have described how particle exposure can increase the number of macrophages (BRAIN, 1971). Current studies in our own laboratory and others have revealed that particle exposure also increases the lysosomal enzyme content of macrophages and may result in release of these enzymes (SOROKIN and BRAIN, 1975). In this report we consider the impact of particle exposure on the subsequent phagocytosis of a test particle, colloidal gold. We present here tentative evidence for two effects: competition and cytotoxicity. In the first instance, we refer to a reversible, competitive inhibition of endocytosis. The phagocytic machinery is limited in its capacity and, if presented with a substantial challenge by one particle species, it is then less able to deal with another particle species. In the second instance, we refer to an impairment of endocytosis caused by the physical presence of particles which damage the cell and its phagocytic apparatus. Since other factors may also affect phagocytic efficiency, the rate of endocytosis may also be determined by the sizes and concentrations of particles reaching the alveoli and the extent of the adaptive macrophage response. Nonetheless, the ability to quantitate endocytosis and to study variations in the rate of endocytosis are essential to our understanding of respiratory defence mechanisms. Only then can the role of differing environmental conditions on endocytosis be understood. Endocytosis has been much studied, but most techniques which are available measure phagocytosis *in vitro*. Attempts to quantitate phagocytosis *in vivo* are considerably less frequent. Hepatic macrophages have been studied as the major component of the reticulo-endothelial system and the rate of disappearance of various particulate materials from the circulation is well described. In contrast, the rate at which phagocytosis occurs in the living lung is not well known. Serial sacrifice and visual observation can give some clues, but the studies reported here incorporate another approach to estimating endocytosis *in vivo*. This report now presents a brief description of the methods we used and then considers the impact of ferric oxide, colloidal carbon, and coal dust on the endocytosis of radioactive gold colloid.

METHODS AND MATERIALS

Animals

Three- to four-month-old male Syrian golden hamsters (Charles River Breeding Laboratories, Wilmington, Mass., and Denen Animal Farms, Gloucester, Mass.) of average weight, 135 g, were used. Intratracheal instillations of particles were administered while the animals were anaesthetized with sodium methohexital (Brevital Sodium, Eli Lilli & Co.), 0.52 g/kg body weight, i.p. A blunt 19-gauge needle was then introduced into the trachea and the appropriate fluid instilled. Sodium methohexital is a rapidly metabolized barbiturate, and the animals usually regained consciousness in 5 to 10 min. The volume instilled was 0.15 cm^3/100 g body weight. The technique of intratracheal instillation, the variables associated with it, and the resulting distribution patterns have recently been described in considerable detail (BRAIN *et al.*, 1976).

Lung Lavage

The lungs were lavaged by techniques similar to those already described (BRAIN and FRANK, 1968; BRAIN, 1971). The hamsters were anaesthetized with pentobarbital sodium (Nembutal Sodium, Abbott Laboratories), 0.185 g/kg body weight, and then exsanguinated by either cutting the aorta or by bilateral kidney excision. The lungs were collapsed by piercing the diaphragm through the abdominal incision just beneath the xyphoid process to avoid nicking the pulmonary pleura. With the lungs still in the body, the trachea was exposed and cannulated with an 18-gauge needle and polyethylene tubing (PE190). The lungs were washed internally (twelve 1-min wash cycles) with 3 cm^3 of wash solution. During the first six washes, a balanced salt solution containing divalent cations was used. During washes 7 through 12, physiological saline (0.85% NaCl) was used in combination with gentle massage of the thorax.

Particle Preparation

The iron oxide (Fe_2O_3) was administered by aerosol during a 3 h exposure period. The animals were unanaesthetized and breathed spontaneously. Submicronic particles were produced from the combustion of iron pentacarbonyl, $Fe(CO)_5$, in a furnace heated to 600°C (BRAIN *et al.*, 1974b). The result is a heterogenous agglomerate aerosol which penetrates into the airways and lungs. This aerosol is readily generated and can be administered accurately in a variety of particulate concentrations (BRAIN *et al.*, 1974b). This aerosol can be readily identified in tissue sections (both as prepared for light and electron microscopy) (SOROKIN and BRAIN, 1975). These iron oxide particles serve admirably as test particles; they also have added relevance to human biology since certain workers in steel refineries, foundries and machine shops are also exposed to iron oxide.

The colloidal carbon administered by intratracheal instillation was prepared from a commercially available carbon black dispersion (Pelikan no. C11/1431a, Hanover, Germany). This preparation contains 10% carbon black (particle diameters of 200 to 500 Å), 4.3% fish glue and 0.9% phenol in water. It does not contain shellac or other components which make some indian ink preparations highly toxic. It has been widely used by a number of investigators as an extravascular label for leaky blood vessels.

The coal dust, supplied by the U.S. Bureau of Mines, was from Experimental Mine no. 1, Braceton, Pennsylvania. More than 99% of it penetrates through a 200 mesh screen. To further reduce the particle size, only those particles penetrating a 325 mesh screen (44 μm aperture) were used. The dust was prepared as a suspension in physiological saline and was ultrasonically dispersed just prior to instillation to minimize agglomeration.

The ^{198}Au colloid was prepared by diluting Auretope-198 (Abbott Laboratories, Chicago) in physiological saline, 1: 10 or 1: 20. Each gold injection had an activity of about 2 μCi and contained approximately 2 μg of gold colloid (mean size 30 nm, range 5–50 nm). These particles are similar to those used by GOSSELIN (1956) for *in vitro* studies of endocytosis in rabbit peritoneal macrophages and by ROSER (1970) for *in vivo* studies of endocytosis in rodent hepatic macrophages.

Analytical Techniques

Aliquots of the lung washes were taken for both cell and radioactive analysis. The number of cells per washing was measured with a Spencer haemacytometer. Washes 1 and 2 as well as washes 7 and 8 were counted separately. However, subsequent pairs (3–4, 5–6, 9–10 and 11–12) were pooled and analysed together. One ml aliquots of the well-shaken washes were assayed for radioactivity. The samples were placed in disposable plastic tubes and counted on an automatic gamma well counter (Nuclear Chicago, Model 4230). The washed lung and trachea were excised after the lavage procedure and counted for radioactivity. Both the number of cells and the amount of radioactivity recovered were expressed as a percentage of the total obtained. Thus, both the cells per wash and the radioactivity per wash sum to 100% for all twelve washes. This proved to be a useful way of normalizing the data, an essential step if the shapes of the washout curves were to be analysed.

RESULTS AND DISCUSSION

The Lambda Technique

This approach utilizes curve-fitting techniques to obtain information regarding the progress of endocytosis in the lung (BRAIN *et al.*, 1974a). Figure 1a shows a washout curve obtained when the lungs were lavaged immediately after an intratracheal instillation of colloidal gold particles. The washout of the radioactivity exhibits an exponential appearance similar to that obtained for a substance being washed out of a container; that is, the amount coming out is less with each succeeding wash but is roughly proportional to the amount remaining in the container. As can be seen in Fig. 1b, the cell washout curve is characteristically different. During the balance salt solution (BSS) washes (1–6), relatively few cells are recovered. In washes 7–12, under the combined influence of physiological saline and gentle massage of the thorax, considerable numbers of macrophages are harvested. As has been discussed previously

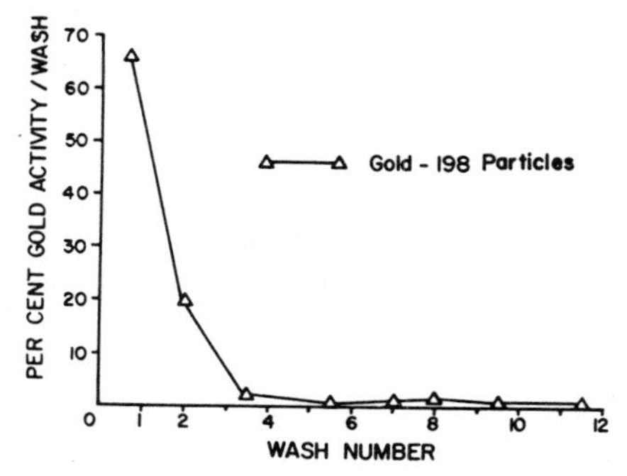

FIG. 1a. Washout curve for free gold particles. Hamster lungs were lavaged immediately after the intratracheal instillation.

(BRAIN and FRANK, 1973), this characteristic washout curve reflects the adhesive properties of pulmonary macrophages. Pulmonary macrophages are adherent to epithelial cell surfaces in the lung and adhesive forces holding them in place must be interrupted or overcome if the cells are to be recovered by the lavage procedure. Figure 1b clearly demonstrates the important role of calcium and magnesium divalent cations in these adhesive forces (BRAIN and FRANK, 1973). Endogenous divalent cations must be leached out by the washing procedure in order to permit harvesting of the pulmonary macrophages.

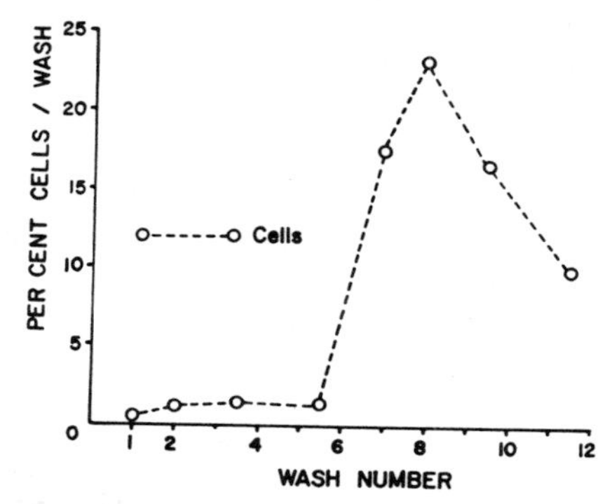

FIG. 1b. Washout curve for free cells (primarily pulmonary macrophages).

Figure 2 shows the shape of the gold colloid and cell washout curves 6 h following a ^{198}Au instillation. The cell washout curve is similar to Fig. 1b. However, the ^{198}Au curve has lost its exponential character and is now nearly identical to the cell washout curve. We believe that the gold particles and cells are now being harvested together, i.e. the gold particles must either be in or on the cells. Earlier studies (BRAIN *et al.*, 1974a) described a progression of gold washout curves as a function of time. The way in which the gold particles washed out gradually changed from that characteristic of free particles to that characteristic of the pulmonary macrophages. As time elapsed, the gold washout curve gradually approximated the macrophage washout curve. As will be summarized below, curve-fitting methods utilizing least squares techniques

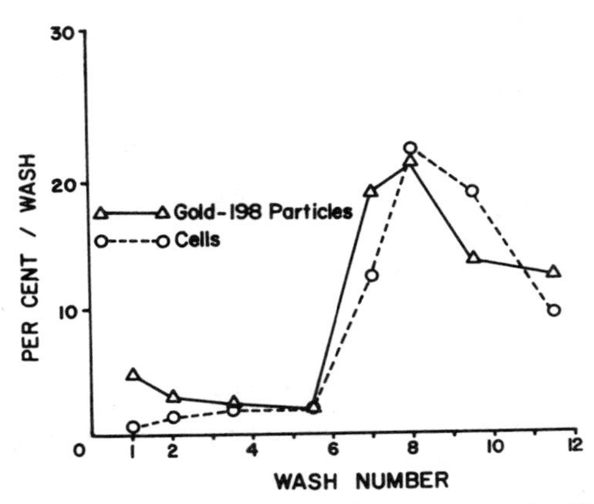

FIG. 2. Cell and gold washout curves 6 h following intratracheal instillation of gold particles.

permit the calculation of the fraction, λ, of the colloidal particles which have been ingested at any time, t.

As shown in Fig. 3, three data curves are used for the calculation of λ. The washout curve of the gold particles immediately after their instillation (plot of washout G_i against wash number i at $t = 0$) is similar to that already shown in Fig. 1a. G_i is based on the pooled data of eight animals which received intratracheal instillations of gold colloid and were immediately lavaged. In contrast, the C_i and X_i curves represent data obtained from a single animal. C_i, the cell washout at any time, t, gives a curve similar to Fig. 1b. The curve represents the gold washout X_i at any time t and can have a variety of shapes depending on the extent of endocytosis. In this case, both C_i and X_i are from an animal which received a gold instillation 2 h previously, thus t equals 2 h. Endocytosis is underway but not complete; therefore the X_i curve has a shape intermediate between those of G_i and C_i. From this we infer that some of the gold colloid is free and some is associated with the cells. Our hypothesis asserts that curve X_i is the sum of certain proportions of curves G_i and C_i. A certain fraction of the gold, λ, has been phagocytized and washes out with a characteristic pattern similar to C_i.

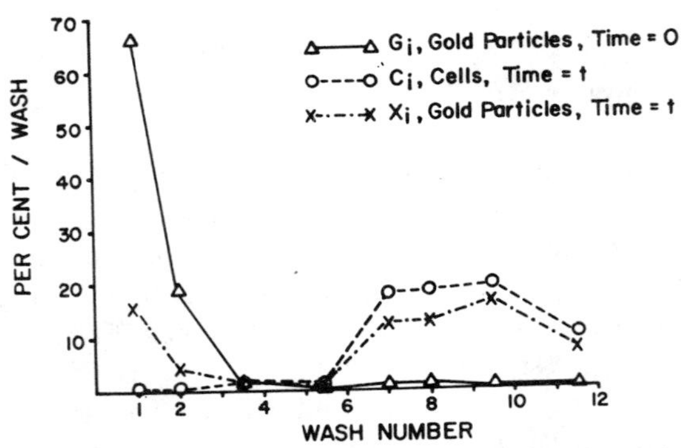

FIG. 3. The three data curves used in the computation of λ. G_i is the free gold washout curve at time = 0. C_i represents the cell washout curve at any time, t; X_i represents the gold washout curve at any time, t.

The remaining gold particles $(1 - \lambda)$ are still free and wash out like curve G_i. We then attempt, using curve-fitting techniques, to find the proportions of curve C_i and G_i which, when summed, yield a minimum deviation from the experimental curve, X_i. Therefore,

$$\Sigma X_i = \Sigma \lambda C_i + \Sigma(1 - \lambda)G_i \tag{1}$$

Using straightforward calculus, the computed point may be compared with the actual data point and the error minimized. The final result is

$$\lambda = \frac{\Sigma(G_i - X_i)(G_i - C_i)}{\Sigma(G_i - C_i)^2}. \tag{2}$$

This equation was used to calculate λ for each animal. It is important to remember that G_i represents pooled data, while C_i and X_i represent paired data from an animal at a particular time, t. There is a slight increase in the values of G_i in washes 7 and 8 and this probably reflects a tiny amount of particle endocytosis or adhesion which occurred during the 1 or 2 min it takes to sacrifice the animal and begin the lavage procedure.

Iron Oxide Exposures

Twelve hamsters received a 3-h exposure to the Fe_2O_3 aerosol. The mass concentration was approximately 160 μg/litre and the aerodynamic mass median diameter, as determined by an aerosol spectrometer, was 0.68 μm, $\sigma_g = 1.81$. Of the twelve animals exposed to iron oxide, half were given an intratracheal challenge with gold colloid immediately after the iron oxide exposure. The other six animals received their gold colloid instillation 24 h after the end of the iron oxide exposure. Table 1 summarizes

TABLE 1. IRON OXIDE

Group	Number of animals	λ at 2 h post-gold	P*	Cells recovered (10^6) 12 washes
Control. Gold only (no Fe_2O_3)	4	0.83	—	6.19 ± 1.23
Fe_2O_3 exposed, gold immediately after	6	0.63 ± 0.05	<0.01	5.27 ± 1.05
Fe_2O_3 exposed, gold 24 h later	6	0.79 ± 0.04	0.3–0.4	4.57 ± 1.12

* P is the probability that the difference between the control and experimental means occurred by chance as calculated by Student's t-test.

the data obtained. Morphological studies (SOROKIN and BRAIN, 1975) have shown that immediately following the iron oxide exposure macrophages are actively engaged in phagocytosis. Their preoccupation with the iron oxide aerosol challenge is shown by the drop in λ from 0.83 to 0.63 ($P < 0.01$). Thus, because of simultaneous presentation of ferric oxide and gold particles, the percent of the gold colloid which has been phagocytized after 2 h drops from 83% to 63%. Twenty-four hours following the

Fe_2O_3 exposure iron oxide phagocytosis is essentially complete. However, the iron oxide is still present within the cytoplasm of most macrophages (SOROKIN and BRAIN, 1975). In spite of the physical presence of the iron oxide within the cells, endocytosis of gold colloid is essentially normal. As can be seen from Table 1, approximately 79% of the gold colloid has been ingested 2 h after the gold instillation. This value is not significantly different from the control values. Also shown in Table 1 is the number of cells recovered. Naturally, the shapes of the washout curves of cells and radioactivity are required for the calculation of λ. These curves are not shown, but are available from the authors upon request.

Colloidal Carbon

These particles were given by intratracheal instillation. In one group of animals, a mixture of colloidal carbon and colloidal gold was administered. Two hours following the intratracheal instillation, the lungs were lavaged and the λ values were determined. In the second group of animals, the gold colloid was given 24 h following the colloidal carbon instillation. Again λ values were determined 2 h following the gold instillation. The data shown are for suspensions containing 0.3% carbon black.

As can be seen in Table 2, the impact of the colloidal carbon was dramatic. When gold colloid was given simultaneously with the carbon, the λ value fell precipitously.

TABLE 2. COLLOIDAL CARBON

Group	Number of animals	λ at 2 h post-gold	P*	Cells recovered (10^6) 12 washes
Control. Gold only (no carbon)	7	0.56 ± 0.04	—	5.27 ± 0.40
Colloidal carbon + gold mixture	6	0.11 ± 0.04	<0.001	3.77 ± 0.57
Colloidal carbon, gold 24 h later	7	0.68 ± 0.07	0.3–0.4	18.22 ± 1.22

* P is the probability that the difference between the control and experimental means occurred by chance as calculated by Student's t-test.

Only 11% of the gold was endocytized after 2 h as compared to 56% of the gold in the control animals. Twenty-four hours following the colloidal carbon instillation, the gold λ's have now risen to and, in fact, exceeded normals; 68% of the gold instilled has been ingested. This mild enhancement may reflect the greater number of macrophages available. The numbers of macrophages lavaged from the lungs have also been dramatically influenced by the colloidal carbon instillation. There is more than a three-fold increase in the number of macrophages recovered in the twelve washes 24 h after the carbon instillation. These results are similar to those reported earlier (BRAIN, 1971). Figure 4 shows the cell washout curves for the three groups of animals in greater detail. It can be seen that both the number of macrophages recovered with balanced salt solution, as well as the cells recovered with physiological saline and

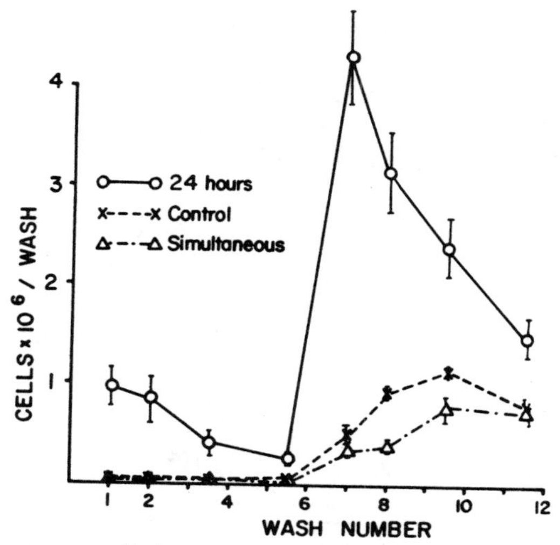

FIG. 4. Cell washout curves following intratracheal instillations of colloidal carbon.

massage, increase. The latter group reflects cells closely applied to the alveolar surface. The cells recovered in the first six washes may be more indicative of rounded cells and cells recovered from the airways (BRAIN and FRANK, 1973).

Figure 5 displays the shape of the radioactivity (gold) washout for the three groups of animals. The low value of λ for the animals receiving the colloidal carbon and gold mixture is clearly reflected in that washout (simultaneous). The washout of activity is much more like the washout of free gold than it is like the washout of the cells shown in Fig. 5. Since λ was depressed markedly, we repeated this experiment at other concentrations of instilled carbon. These data are summarized in Table 3. This table shows that there is indeed a dose-dependent competition of carbon with gold. All values

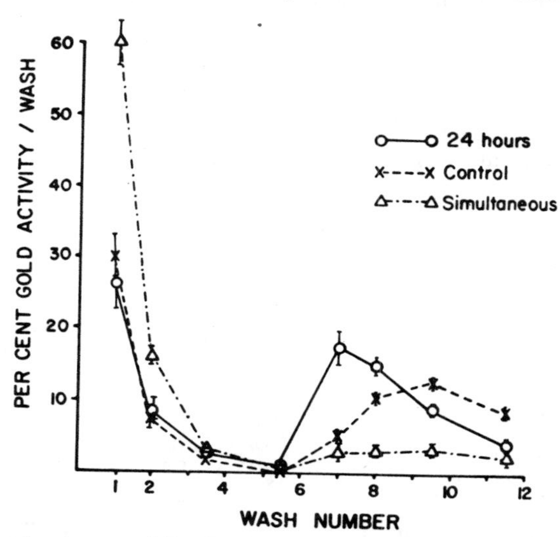

FIG. 5. Activity washout curves following intratracheal instillations of colloidal carbon.

shown in Table 3 represent simultaneous challenge. No studies were performed 24 h following the carbon exposure. However, the data in Table 2 clearly show that although the mixture does depress λ, the presence of carbon in the cell 24 h later does not influence the rate of endocytosis. In fact, there may be an enhancement due to an increase in cell number and to activation of the macrophages.

TABLE 3. VARYING DOSES OF COLLOIDAL CARBON

Group	Number of animals	λ at 2 h post gold	P*	Cells recovered (10^6) 12 washes
Control. Gold only (no carbon)	7	0.77 ± 0.06	—	5.67 ± 2.01
1.0% carbon + gold mixture	7	0.05 ± 0.02	0.001	2.58 ± 0.31
0.1% carbon + gold mixture	7	0.45 ± 0.07	0.001	5.88 ± 0.50
0.01% carbon + gold mixture	7	0.74 ± 0.05	0.6–0.5	6.16 ± 0.82

* P is the probability that the difference between the control and experimental means occurred by chance as calculated by Student's t-test.

Coal Dust

Table 4 shows the results of intratracheal instillations of coal dust. The gold was administered ½ h following the instillation of 1% coal dust and thus the macrophages were confronted with the gold particles while still phagocytizing the coal. The λ values showed a marked reduction. The percentage of gold ingested fell from 85% to 48%. Most interesting is the fact that the suppression of endocytosis persisted. Measured 24 h later, when coal phagocytosis is essentially complete, the percentage of gold ingested remained at only 45%. Although the initial suppression was more modest than that provided by colloidal carbon, there was no recovery. We believe this suggests not only true competition but also a cytotoxic effect of the coal dust.

It is interesting to note that the colloidal carbon initially has a more potent competitive effect than does the coal dust. We believe that this reflects the difference in particle size; the colloidal carbon is much smaller and the same mass amount will presumably require a greater amount of endocytic activity. Earlier we showed that the ability of

TABLE 4. COAL DUST

Group	Number of animals	λ at 2 h post gold	P*	Cells recovered (10^6) 12 washes
Control. Gold only (no coal dust)	6	0.85 ± 0.04	—	6.62 ± 0.96
1% Coal dust, gold 1/2 h later	6	0.48 ± 0.10	<0.01	4.92 ± 0.81
1% Coal dust, gold 24 h later	6	0.45 ± 0.08	<0.01	7.73 ± 1.12

* P is the probability that the difference between the control and experimental means occurred by chance as calculated by Student's t-test.

particles to elicit increases in macrophage number is also a function of particle size (Brain, 1971). The same effect may also be reflected here.

It should also be noted that control values for λ in Table 2 are significantly lower than those from the control animals described in Tables 1, 3 and 4. The animals from Table 2 were obtained from Lakeview Breeding Colonies (Charles River Breeding Co., Wilmington, Mass.), while those shown in Tables 1, 3 and 4 were obtained from Denen Animal Farms, Gloucester, Mass. The differences in λ values may represent differences in the strain or environment of the animals. In any event, it is important to note that parallel controls should be carried out during the course of each experiment. Animals studied at one time should not be compared with controls obtained earlier.

CONCLUSIONS

Curve-fitting techniques can be applied to data obtained from multiple lung lavages to estimate the percent of particles ingested by pulmonary macrophages at various times and under differing environmental conditions. Thus the λ technique offers a useful way of measuring endocytosis in the lungs; it is applied here to study particle competition and cytoxicity. Our results suggest that all particles, if given in sufficient quantities, can depress λ during the phagocytic period. However, if the particles are non-toxic, the rate of endocytosis should return to normal if the gold test particles are given after the phagocytic period is over. In contrast, particles which are cytotoxic, such as silica, not only depress λ when measured during the phagocytic period, but the depression persists after the phagocytosis is over. We believe that this approach may be a useful screening procedure for ascertaining the degree of toxicity for a variety of inhaled dusts.

Most pulmonary disease is either initiated by, or at least complicated by, the inhalation of particles and gases. Pollutants characteristic of occupational and urban environments, bacteria, viruses and other infectious particles, allergens and antigens all may cause or aggravate pulmonary disease. Furthermore, the magnitude of these effects is strongly influenced by the number of particles deposited, their site of deposition and especially their ultimate fate. The ability of pulmonary macrophages to ingest particles is an essential aspect of that fate and quantitation of ingestion under a wide range of environmental conditions is a prerequisite to an improved understanding of the effects of inhaled particulates.

REFERENCES

Brain, J. D. (1971) *Inhaled Particles III* (edited by Walton, W. H.) pp. 209–225. Unwin Bros., Old Woking, Surrey.
Brain, J. D. and Frank, R. (1968) *J. appl. Physiol.* **25,** 63–69.
Brain, J. D. and Frank, R. (1973) *J. appl. Physiol.* **34,** 75–80.
Brain, J. D., Mets, M. B. and Cashman, G. E. (1974a) *Fed. Proc.* **33,** 365 (Abstract).
Brain, J. D., Valberg, P. A., Sorokin, S. P. and Hinds, W. C. (1974b) *Envir. Res.* **7,** 13–26.
Brain, J. D., Knudson, R. E., Sorokin, S. P. and Davis, M. A. (1976) *Envir. Res.* **11,** 13–26.
Green, G. M. and Kass, E. H. (1964) *J. exp. Med.* **119,** 167–176.
Gosselin, R. (1956) *J. gen. Physiol.* **39,** 625–649.
Roser, B. (1970) *J. reticuloendothel. Soc.* **8,** 139–161.
Schiller, E. (1961) *Inhaled Particles and Vapours* (edited by Davies, C. N.) pp. 342–347. Pergamon Press, Oxford.
Sorokin, S. P. and Brain, J. D. (1975) *Anat. Rec.* **181,** 581–625.

DISCUSSION

J. FERIN: Your results are in agreement with the results of our work on the effect of asbestos on TiO_2 clearance. We found that asbestos pre-exposure to TiO_2 aerosol inhalation, depending on the dose, depressed the clearance of the TiO_2 test particles.

What do you think would happen if you pre-exposed animals to gold particles prior to your gold-testing procedure: would gold particles compete with gold particles? This may be important when comparison of single versus multiple exposures is made.

Dr BRAIN: I am not certain that our two experiments can be easily compared. You examined clearance by measuring the disappearance of a quantifiable material from the lungs. We examined the rate at which particles in the lung are ingested by macrophages. Phagocytosis and pulmonary clearance are, no doubt, related but they should not be equated.

In answer to your question, if the initial exposure is to gold colloid and that is followed by a challenge with gold colloid there is no difference. We deliberately chose radioactive gold so that we can easily measure very tiny amounts; the amount introduced is in the microgram range. This is so small that it places an insignificant load on the phagocytic machinery. One has to go to higher concentrations of gold colloid before the gold begins to compete with itself.

J. BRUCH: Do you think that the λ-test is a direct assay for measuring the phagocytic potential of the alveolar macrophage? The gold particles are very small (0.03 μm) and seem to be ingested by a *pinocytotic* process. The particle size of the coal dust seems to be larger than that of the colloidal carbon or iron oxide. For comparison, similar weights and particle sizes should be used.

Dr BRAIN: Yes, by endocytosis I mean all kinds of ingestive phenomena which range from phagocytosis to pinocytosis. We have found that λ values depend little on particle size. In experiments with chromium-labelled microspheres which are 2 to 4 μm in diameter and with chromium labelled red cells, the λ values and the potential for competition is similar. Gold colloid is cheaper than many other radiolabelled particles and so we frequently use it. Thus, the numbers might vary a little but the qualitative conclusions would be identical even if I had presented data obtained with larger particles.

P. D. OLDHAM: May I ask a question about the ingenious method you use to estimate λ? The washouts are carried out in sequence on the same animal, so that each animal has its individual curve; these may vary in shape, in particular in the position of the maximum, from one animal to another. Could this seriously affect the value of λ obtained?

Dr BRAIN: The analysis of λ is based on three curves. Two are from an individual animal: we use the animal's own cell washout curve and his own particle washout curve at time t, because each animal has its own peculiar washout curve. We did calculate λ using average data from a whole group of animals but the variability is much greater. What cannot be measured for each animal is the way free gold washes out; that must be based on average values from a group of animals. We assume that free gold washes out with an exponential curve identical to that of the group.

M. KUSCHNER: I should like to congratulate you on this outstanding piece of work. It appears to be the beginning of the development of the type of quantitative evaluation of macrophage function similar to that employed by Bennacerraf in measuring reticulo-endothelial function. Is not the estimation of λ in part dependent on numbers of macrophages? If this is so, must we not be concerned about how certain materials influence the numbers of macrophages?

Dr BRAIN: It is likely that λ is dependent on the number of phagocytic cells available. Recently, we had a group of control animals with individual values of λ which were surprisingly variable. We ran a correlation coefficient between λ and the number of cells recovered by lung lavage. They correlated very well ($r = 0.85$). This suggests that much of the variability in λ for a given group of animals can be explained by the variability in the number of macrophages. This is not unexpected since increased numbers of macrophages should increase the probability of particles being phagocytosed. In spite of this effect, it is important to realize that variations in cell number or in the percent of instilled gold that is recovered do not cause artefacts in the calculation of λ. This is because the data are always normalized by expressing them in terms of percent recovered; we examine only the shape of the washout curves. For example, in the colloidal carbon animals there was an increase in the number of cells out recovered and also a considerable change in the shape of the washout curves (Fig. 4). There were many more cells recovered in the first six BSS washes which suggests that not only were there more cells but also that it was easier to recover them purely by mechanical forces. In spite of those changes, if one waits until the phagocytosis of the gold is completed the gold washout still mimicks the cell washout curve. Thus even when the shape of the cell washout curve changes dramatically, if phagocytosis is complete, the gold washout curve follows it.

L. MAGOS: How do you standardize the particle size and dose of the dust to be tested for cytotoxicity?

Dr BRAIN: The size and quantity of the dusts used are listed in the text. At this stage, we have mainly been interested in determining whether results with the λ method correlate with what is known about particles that are known to be toxic or non-toxic. We have also applied our technique to other situations such as oxygen toxicity. However, if one used this method to compare the risks of mining Utah coal and Pennsylvania coal, for example, then one would be faced with all the problems that have been well discussed at this meeting, such as whether the particle size is representative. At this point, we are not using this assay to make realistic predictions about occupational dusts and their relative toxicity.

O. G. RAABE: It is not obvious to me that the washout curve for "free" gold several hours after instillation will be the same as immediately after instillation; this assumption is implicit in the method of calculating λ.

On another point, have you changed the number of washes used before switching from the calcium–magnesium washes to the physiological saline, to see if the gold and cell washout are equally affected? This would provide additional evidence that the gold was associated with the cells.

Dr BRAIN: Yes, you are correct. The method assumes that non-ingested gold colloid at any time t washes out like non-ingested gold at time zero. Although indirect evidence suggests this is a reasonable assumption, we can think of no direct way of testing it. To the extent that the assumption fails, our λ values may not be precise. It is important not to take the λ values too literally. If λ equals 0.67 we are not certain that exactly 67% of the particles have been ingested. The method provides an indirect estimate of a parameter which is difficult to measure directly and there may be some errors. On the other hand, if λ falls from 0.67 to 0.27 we are confident in asserting that phagocytosis has been depressed.

We have done experiments similar to that suggested by your second question. If one washes 12 times rather than 6 times with BSS, then the cell yield remains low until one finally switches to physiological saline which lacks divalent cations. If there has been enough time for considerable phagocytosis, then the particle washout curves follow the same pattern. That the particles are inside the cells is also suggested by two other independent approaches. If we use larger particles (2–4 μm plastic spheres), then microscopy yields estimates similar to the λ technique. Nucle pore filters can also be used to separate cells and ingested particles from free particles in the lavage fluid. This approach also corroborates λ estimates.

P. COLE: I am not certain that you have excluded the possibility that 24 h after iron exposure the ^{198}Au is being endocytosed by macrophages recently entering the lung rather than those initially exposed to the iron. Similarly, 24 h after coal exposure, perhaps there is little traffic to the lung thus accounting for the "blockade" effect on ^{198}Au endocytosis.

I use colloidal ^{198}Au uptake *in vitro* as a test of endocytosis of small particles in a different system and wonder whether you could use a combination test "dusting" your macrophages *in vivo*, then lavaging the cells and challenging them with ^{198}Au after 24 h in culture so ensuring that the cells exposed to dust are the same ones challenged with ^{198}Au.

Dr BRAIN: I would agree with the possibility that you raise. With some exposures, the increase in macrophages recoverable by lung lavage clearly reflects an influx of new cells. Differences in the ability of particles to recruit more macrophages may influence the percent of particles ingested (λ).

We are now carrying out some of the experiments you suggested in the second part of your question. We are harvesting macrophages from pre-exposed animals and then using those macrophages for *in-vitro* assays. One can also use a totally *in-vitro* assay to look at competition.

G. PATRICK: Did the liquid used in the intratracheal instillations of colloidal carbon and of coal dust contain divalent cations? If not, this might affect the adhesion of macrophages to the alveolar wall.

Dr BRAIN: Only 0.15 cm^3 of saline is instilled per 100 g body weight. Although there were no divalent cations present in the instilled fluids we think it very unlikely that this had any influence on alveolar macrophage adhesion. This assertion is supported by the control groups. Controls for the colloidal carbon and coal dust received intratracheal instillations of saline alone. This had no effect on λ or on the number of macrophages recovered.

G. PATRICK: In the case of colloidal carbon (Tables 2 and 3), did the hamsters in the control group receive the vehicle in which carbon was suspended for the experimental groups? This vehicle should presumably contain 0.9% phenol and 4.3% fish glue.

Dr BRAIN: It is important to remember that the colloidal carbon was diluted by factors of 100 to 10 000. Then only 0.15 cm^3/100 g body weight was instilled. Thus the amount of phenol or fish glue instilled is small.

Nonetheless, your question is an important one and we have also wondered whether the depression in λ was due to the colloidal carbon itself or to the carrier material. We are attempting to answer this question by exposing the animals to the vehicle only as you suggest. It is interesting that the carbon, although non-toxic, was much more dramatic in its competitive effects. We attribute that to the much smaller size and therefore to the exceedingly high particle number. The effect appears to be more dependent on particle number than on mass.

A. G. HEPPLESTON: Do you think the quantity of the primary particles ingested by the individual alveolar macrophages affects their subsequent uptake of colloidal gold?

Dr BRAIN: Definitely yes. Table 3 shows that clearly. λ values fall from 0.74 to 0.05 as the number of carbon particles instilled is increased. We have also seen a dose-dependent relationship for depression in λ, for iron oxide from 400 μg/litre down to 25 μg/litre. The depression in λ is definitely related to dose as one might expect.

It is important to realize that competition occurs at relatively high mass loadings. The macrophage does have considerable reserve capacity and it is quite difficult to overwhelm it. To put it in perspective, we might consider the iron oxide pre-exposures. The animals breathed 3 h in a chamber containing 160 μg/litre. The threshold limit value for iron oxide is 10 mg/m^3; therefore the animals were exposed to a concentration 16 times the permissible level. However, it is only for 3 h and not for a 40-h week.

A. G. HEPPLESTON: Have you employed a test particle of larger size than colloidal gold and, if so, have the results been modified in any way?

Dr BRAIN: We have used chromium-51 labelled microspheres which are 2–4 μm in diameter (3M Company, United States). We have also used chromium-labelled red cells and in both instances the results were similar.

SESSION 7

Thursday, 25th September

RADIOACTIVE PARTICLES

POLONIUM-210: LEAD-210 RATIOS AS AN INDEX OF RESIDENCE TIMES OF INSOLUBLE PARTICLES FROM CIGARETTE SMOKE IN BRONCHIAL EPITHELIUM

EDWARD P. RADFORD

Department of Environmental Medicine, Johns Hopkins University School of Hygiene and Public Health, Baltimore, U.S.A.

and

EDWARD A. MARTELL

National Center for Atmospheric Research, Boulder, U.S.A.

Abstract—Lead-210 and its granddaughter polonium-210 are both natural constituents of cigarette smoke, the ^{210}Pb being enriched in insoluble particles derived from sintered tobacco trichome tips.

These particles are stripped of the polonium on combustion, and thus the polonium begins ingrowth at the time of inhalation. Polonium-210 is found in bronchial tissues of smokers, and evidence shows that ^{210}Pb is present at these sites in excess of the polonium. On the assumption that all polonium arises from ingrowth from the insoluble particles, one may calculate from the polonium–lead ratio the mean residence time of these particles. The half-life of polonium (138 days) is almost ideal for this purpose, and its alpha radiation makes measurements of very low concentrations possible. This technique is the first available to assess residence time for inhaled particles in the bronchial epithelium, an important datum because of the vulnerability of bronchial tissues to disease. Measurements from three smokers and two non-smokers show that ^{210}Pb from natural aerosols also is concentrated at bronchial bifurcations, but little ^{210}Po is associated with this soluble lead. This fact makes estimates of residence time in bronchial epithelium of smokers (3–5 months in these preliminary data) likely to be low.

UP TO THE present, models of the deposition, retention and clearance of insoluble particles from pulmonary tissues have emphasized processes within the lung parenchyma, with the bronchi being considered primarily as conduits through which mucociliary clearance occurs. There is recognition that preferential deposition of some inhaled particles occurs by impaction at special locations in the bronchial tree, such as at bifurcations of the trachea and major bronchi, and there is also evidence that localized regions of the epithelium may have inefficient ciliary clearance because of splitting of the mucociliary stream at bifurcations, development of squamous metaplasia and loss of ciliary function in small areas, or other mechanisms affecting mucociliary competence. For these reasons, one would conclude that in some regions of the bronchial epithelium, especially at bifurcations, localized concentrations of insoluble inhaled particles might accumulate, both by direct deposition or after entrainment in the mucociliary stream and subsequently becoming trapped in regions of inefficient clearance. Especially in relation to development of bronchial cancer—certainly one of the most serious consequences of inhalation of particles—the failure of current lung-clearance models to take account of the retention of materials in the bronchial epithelial structures is a serious limitation of these models.

One reason for this situation is that little quantitative information has been available on the distribution of particles in bronchial structures. This paper describes a method to study the retention of particles in the bronchial tissues of cigarette smokers, with the aid of insoluble radioactive particles found in cigarette smoke (MARTELL, 1974). These particles are derived from the combustion of tobacco trichome tips consisting of a resinous material. These tips have a high specific activity of naturally-occurring lead-210 (^{210}Pb, a daughter of ^{222}Rn) and upon burning produce fused residual particles, some of which are inhaled with the smoke. Over 95% of the ^{210}Pb activity in mainstream smoke is firmly bound within these fused particles averaging about 1 μm in diameter. These particles are resistant to dissolution in nitric and hydrochloric acid and are unaffected by prolonged exposure to aqueous solutions similar to biological fluids (MARTELL, 1975).

Previous work has indicated that higher concentrations of polonium-210 (^{210}Po), a daughter product of ^{210}Pb, do occur in the bronchial epithelium of smokers when compared to concentrations in alveolar tissues (LITTLE *et al.*, 1965; LITTLE and RADFORD, 1967). The counting techniques for measuring ^{210}Po in small tissue samples used in this earlier work had a relatively high background, which limited the sensitivity of the measurements. Thus an indirect method of calculating the ^{210}Po concentration in bronchial epithelium was necessary. Nevertheless the concentration of ^{210}Po appeared to be up to 1000 times greater at bronchial bifurcations than in lung tissue or blood of smokers. HOLTZMAN and ILCEWICZ (1966) showed that ^{210}Po was also elevated in alveolar tissues of smokers compared to non-smokers, but they did not evaluate its concentration in bronchial samples. With the aid of more sensitive analytical and counting methods available at the National Center for Atmospheric Research, it is now possible to measure the distribution of both ^{210}Po and ^{210}Pb in small samples of bronchial tissue.

This method of evaluating particle residence time in small tissue volumes basically depends on measurement of the ratio of polonium activity to lead activity, the buildup of polonium daughter being the measure of time since the particle was inhaled. Lead-210 has a physical half-life of 21.5 years, long in relation to biological processes, while the half-life of ^{210}Po, 138.4 days, is nearly optimum for determining residence times up to a year or two, as will be shown below.

THEORY

Assumptions

1. Insoluble particles in cigarette smoke containing high specific activity of ^{210}Pb are stripped of its daughter ^{210}Po at the time of smoking. Data validating this assump-

tion are presented below. The half-life of the intermediate daughter ^{210}Bi is so short (5 days) that its presence or absence is of no practical significance (^{210}Bi is assumed to be absent in our estimation of residence times, below).

2. As ^{210}Pb decays in the body after inhalation, the daughters remain with the ^{210}Pb, within the insoluble particles. The radiochemical data for smoke condensate reheated to 650°C are consistent with complete retention of ^{210}Po which has grown into the insoluble smoke particles between the dates of smoking and analysis (see below).

3. Polonium-210 is inhaled by smokers in a volatile form, separated from its parent ^{210}Pb, and does not remain long in pulmonary or bronchial tissues; its contribution to ^{210}Po activity in small specimens of bronchial epithelium tissue is negligible. This assumption is supported by the finding that alveolar parenchyma and bronchial subepithelial tissues in smokers contain low concentrations of ^{210}Po (LITTLE *et al.*, 1965) and by the estimates of pulmonary clearance of ^{210}Po when smokers stop smoking (LITTLE and McGANDY, 1968).

4. Soluble ^{210}Pb will not contribute significantly to smoke-derived activity in bronchial tissues. Lead-210 inhaled by smokers is derived from two sources: ^{210}Pb in smoke, over 95% in the insoluble particle fraction, and that associated with natural aerosols whose ^{210}Pb activity arises from decay of atmospheric ^{222}Rn. This latter activity is present on the aerosol surfaces in a chemical form which should be readily soluble in lung fluids (POET *et al.*, 1972). If present in bronchial tissues, this soluble ^{210}Pb activity will cause the estimates of residence time to be underestimated if no correction is made for it, because the ^{210}Po daughter from this source will be less effectively retained in the tissue than for the insoluble particles. Thus the measured ^{210}Po/^{210}Pb ratio will be lower than for the insoluble particles alone. The contribution of this source of ^{210}Pb can be estimated from measurements in non-smokers.

Derivation of Relationship of ^{210}Po/^{210}Pb *Activity Ratio to Mean Residence Time of Particles*

We wish to find expressions for the relative frequency, $F(t)$, of particles which, at death, have been present for time t, and for the ^{210}Po/^{210}Pb activity ratio of each particle as a function of time, $R(t)$. Note that $\int_0^\infty F(t)\mathrm{d}t = 1$. Given these functions, with certain assumptions we can express the mean activity ratio $\bar{R}$ for the ensemble of insoluble particles in a tissue sample as:

$$\bar{R} = \int_0^\infty R(t)F(t)\mathrm{d}t \tag{1}$$

This expression for $\bar{R}$ is valid if the ^{210}Pb activity of the particles is relatively constant over time, as is the case because of its long physical half-life. In addition, $\bar{R}$ is useful as a measure of the retention of the ensemble of particles only if the ^{210}Pb activity is relatively uniformly distributed among them. This latter assumption is implicit in what follows.

$R(t)$ is determined strictly by physical processes of growth and decay, under assumption 2, with initial conditions given by assumptions 1 and 3. The age distribution,

$F(t)$, of the retained particles will depend on the model of clearance from bronchial tissues adopted for insoluble particles. This function can be expressed in terms of the mean residence time, which is the quantity desired.

The physical decay scheme of ^{210}Pb and its daughters ^{210}Bi and ^{210}Po is:

$$^{210}\text{Pb} \xrightarrow{\beta} {}^{210}\text{Bi} \xrightarrow{\beta} {}^{210}\text{Po} \xrightarrow{\alpha} {}^{206}\text{Pb}.$$
$$T_{1/2} = 21.5\ \text{yr} \quad T_{1/2} = 5.013\ \text{d} \quad T_{1/2} = 138.4\ \text{d} \quad \text{Stable}$$

Denoting the amounts of ^{210}Pb, ^{210}Bi and ^{210}Pb present at any time by A, B, and C, and the decay constants for each transition by p, q, and r, respectively, we have

$$A \xrightarrow{p = 0.03224\ \text{yr}^{-1}} B \xrightarrow{q = 50.50\ \text{yr}^{-1}} C \xrightarrow{r = 1.8293\ \text{yr}^{-1}}$$

The initial conditions defined by assumptions 1 and 3 are: $A = A_0$, $B = 0$, $C = 0$ at time $t = 0$, with A_0 the initial insoluble particle ^{210}Pb concentration. The amounts of the various elements will be determined by the usual differential equations (assumption 2):

$$\dot{A} = -pA,$$
$$\dot{B} = pA - qB,$$
$$\dot{C} = qB - rC.$$

Solution of these equations for A and C, the isotopes of interest, gives

$$A = A_0 e^{-pt} \tag{2}$$

$$C = A_0 \frac{p}{r}(K_A e^{-pt} + K_B e^{-qt} - K_C e^{-rt}), \tag{3}$$

where
$$K_A = \frac{q}{q-p} \times \frac{r}{r-p},$$

$$K_B = \frac{q}{q-p} \times \frac{r}{q-r},$$

$$K_C = \frac{q}{q-r} \times \frac{r}{r-p}.$$

Note that $K_A + K_B - K_C = 0$, thus the initial conditions are satisfied.

We wish to obtain the activity ratio of ^{210}Po to ^{210}Pb. The activity of ^{210}Pb is Ap, and of ^{210}Po it is Cr, thus $R \equiv Cr/Ap$. From equations (2) and (3):

$$Ap = A_0 p e^{-pt}, \tag{2a}$$

$$Cr = A_0 p(K_A e^{-pt} + K_B e^{-qt} - K_C e^{-rt}) \tag{3a}$$

and
$$R = K_A + K_B e^{-(q-p)t} - K_C e^{-(r-p)t}. \tag{4}$$

Equation (4) is therefore the expression for $R(t)$ for any particle.

We now consider the deposition and clearance of the particles in pulmonary tissues, a dynamic process, which will determine the length of time the particles will be present in tissues of interest. For any particular region of the lungs or bronchi we define a mean residence time, T, the average length of time any insoluble particle may remain in that tissue. It is the purpose of this method to determine T by measurement of mean R for the tissue.

In mathematical terms we can express the number of particles N at a location:

$$N = f_1(D,t) - f_2(N,t)$$

where f_1 is a function describing the arrival or deposition D of particles at the location, and f_2 is a function describing the release of particles from the location. The two functions can have any continuous or discontinuous character, and on biological grounds we have no *a priori* basis for selecting the form of these functions. If deposition takes place intermittently or if smoking habits have changed significantly, then obviously the mean residence time of particles will be altered. We proceed on the assumption that smoking and smoke-particle deposition are relatively constant.

The mean residence time also depends on the particles actually being localized in a particular tissue for a substantial period. Without aggregation in a subregion, the mean residence-time concept does not have any meaning except in terms of retention of the particles in the respiratory tract as a whole. The fact that the concentration of ^{210}Po in bronchial epithelium is 100 $\times$ or more that found in other pulmonary tissues (LITTLE *et al.*, 1965) strongly indicates that aggregation with relatively prolonged retention is most probable there.

For simplicity we assume that the probability of release or loss of a particle from the tissue location follows a Poisson stochastic process. Thus the probability of a particle remaining for a time t after it is deposited in the region is given by

$$P(t) = e^{-st}, \tag{5}$$

where s is a rate constant, the reciprocal of T. To normalize the cumulative retention of all particles, we multiply by a constant k such that $\int_0^\infty kP(t)dt$ will equal unity. If $kP(t) \equiv F(t)$, the fraction of particles retained for time t, then

$$F(t) = se^{-st}. \tag{6}$$

This completes the definition of the two functions required to determine $\bar{R}$, the mean $^{210}Po/^{210}Pb$ ratio for insoluble particles.

From equations (1), (4) and (6):

$$\bar{R} = \int_0^\infty (K_A + K_B e^{-(q-p)t} - K_C e^{-(r-p)t}) se^{-st} dt, \tag{7}$$

$$\bar{R} = K_A + \frac{sK_B}{q-p+s} - \frac{sK_C}{r-p+s}.$$

Substituting $T = 1/s$ we have, therefore,

$$\bar{R} = K_A + \frac{K_B}{T(q-p)+1} - \frac{K_C}{T(r-p)+1}. \tag{8}$$

Equation (8) contains only known constants, $\bar{R}$ which is measured, and T which is to be determined. The numerical values for the constants, expressed per month, are: $p = 0.002687\ \text{mo}^{-1}$, $q = 4.209\ \text{mo}^{-1}$, and $r = 0.1524\ \text{mo}^{-1}$; $K_A = 1.0185$, $K_B = 0.0376$ and $K_C = 1.0561$.

Thus
$$\bar{R} = 1.0185 + \frac{0.0376}{4.206T + 1} - \frac{1.0561}{0.1498T + 1}. \tag{9}$$

T is in units of months, and Fig. 1 shows T plotted against $\bar{R}$ from equation (9). It can be seen that if particle residence times are between a month and about 2 years,

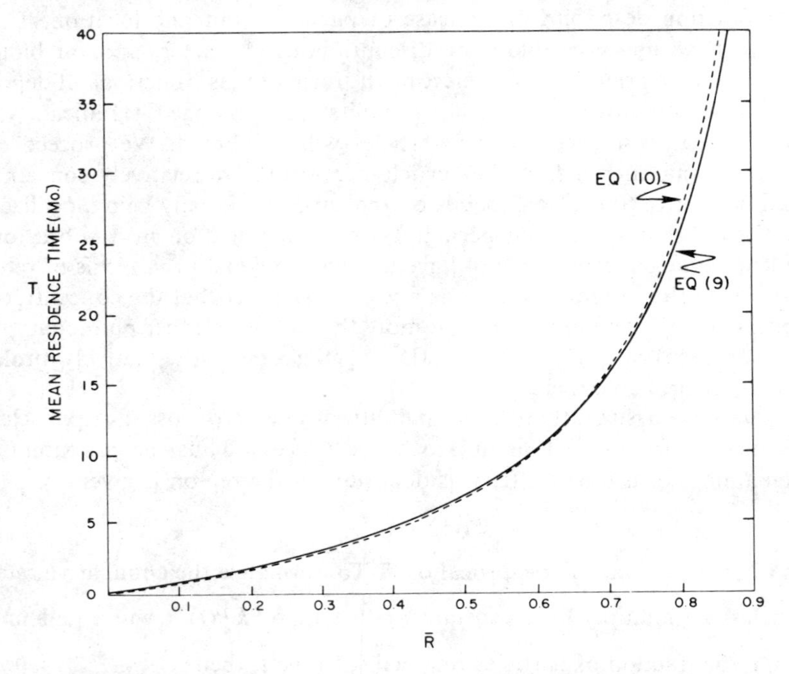

FIG. 1. Mean residence time, T, of insoluble smoke particles in lung tissue samples determined from mean $^{210}Po/^{210}Pb$ activity ratio, $\bar{R}$. Solid line derived from equation (9); dashed line from equation (10).

the method has good resolution. If equation (9) is simplified by neglecting the second term and assuming the constants nearly 1 are unity, we have

$$T = \frac{1}{r - p}\left(\frac{\bar{R}}{1 - \bar{R}}\right) = 6.68\left(\frac{\bar{R}}{1 - \bar{R}}\right). \tag{10}$$

This approximate equation is adequate to describe the relationship within the limits of the assumptions, and is also shown on Fig. 1.

The above derivation makes no assumptions about the rate of deposition of insoluble particles in relation to the rate of decay of the daughters. One can also derive a simpler expression, on the assumption that steady state conditions exist in a tissue, i.e. that the ^{210}Pb is constant and that the rate of production of daughters equals their rate of loss by physical and biological processes. This is the approach used by POET *et al.* (1972) in investigating the residence time of particles in the atmosphere by measurements of these isotopes. Their expression for $\bar{R}$, with the notation used here, is

$$\bar{R} = \frac{T^2 qr}{(Tr+1)(Tq+1)}. \tag{11}$$

If $Tq \gg 1$, that is for $T > 2$ or 3 months, equation (11) reduces to

$$\bar{R} = \frac{Tr}{Tr+1}, \text{ or } T = \frac{1}{r}\left(\frac{\bar{R}}{1-\bar{R}}\right). \tag{12}$$

Equations (11) and (12) give a relationship of T to $\bar{R}$ which is close to those shown in Fig. 1. This fact indicates that the assumption of either a steady state or an unsteady state makes little difference in the estimate of residence time calculated from $\bar{R}$. The relationship of T to $\bar{R}$ is determined almost entirely by the physical half-life of ^{210}Po.

MATERIALS AND METHODS

Preparation of Tissue Samples

Analytical results have been nearly completed on lung and bronchial tissue samples from three smokers and two non-smokers obtained at autopsy at the Maryland Medical Examiner's Office. All autopsy specimens have been removed within 12 hours of death, and isolation of tissue samples was made immediately on receipt in our laboratory. Pertinent information on the five subjects is given in Table 1.

TABLE 1. DATA ON SUBJECTS WHOSE TISSUES HAVE BEEN ANALYSED TO DATE

Subject no.	Age	Sex	Serum SCN$^-$ μg/ml	Cause of death
Smokers				
1	52	M	5.8	Congestive heart failure
2	16	M	6.3	Homicide, exsanguination
3	41	M	9.8	Myocardial infarction
Non-smokers				
A	72	F	1.7	Struck by car
B	32	F	3.3	Acute narcotic poisoning

Measurement of serum thiocyanate (method of BOWLER, 1944) is the best objective datum we have found of the degree of cigarette-smoke inhalation in individuals coming to autopsy. Because of the slow clearance of thiocyanate from the body (Radford, Kaufman and Steinberg, unpublished observations), it is relatively unaffected by conditions just before death, and thus reflects integrated smoking experience up to 2 weeks prior to death. From the data in Table 1 we confirm that subjects A and B were non-smokers (normal SCN^- derived from diet ranges from 1 to 4 μg/ml), subjects 1 and 2 were light to moderate smokers, and subject 3 was a heavy smoker.

Tissue samples were obtained by opening the trachea and bronchi down to third-order branches longitudinally. After the lumen was gently blotted with absorbent gauze, epithelium was scraped from the trachea, carina, main stem and secondary bronchi and from selected bifurcations. In addition whole tracheal and bronchial sections were taken with and without epithelium intact, and samples at bifurcations ("blocks") were taken by making cuts 1 mm deep and 1 mm wide, with removal of these slices by sharp dissection. Lung parenchymal samples were taken so as not to include bronchi over 1 mm in diameter. Scrapings and small samples were placed on slides, and larger samples in screw-top jars, and wet weight was measured as soon as possible. After the samples were air-dried overnight, they were sealed and sent to the National Center for Atmospheric Research. Here they were air-dried at 45°C for 24 h and final dry weights were obtained.

Radiochemical and Counting Methods

Details of the procedures of radiochemical separation and purification of ^{210}Pb, ^{210}Bi and ^{210}Po as well as the ^{210}Po plating method used and low-level β and α counting techniques are described elsewhere (POET *et al.*, 1972). For assay of these three radioisotopes in tissue specimens, some of the separation steps were modified. Each tissue specimen was digested for 1–2 h in concentrated HNO_3, followed by small additions of concentrated H_2SO_4 and HNO_3 alternately, to complete the solution of charred residue. Lead and bismuth carriers and ^{208}Po or ^{209}Po alpha calibration spikes were added at the beginning of the first HNO_3 digestion step. When the tissue sample was completely in solution in sulphuric acid, lead was precipitated as the sulphate by diluting the acid to 18 N. This lead carrier precipitate was separated, purified for yield determination and reserved for 6 months, for ingrowth of ^{210}Po and determination of ^{210}Pb by separation, plating and alpha counting. The supernate of the 18 N sulphuric acid solution was diluted to 9 N and the Bi and Po were coprecipitated as sulphides. The sulphides were redissolved in HCl and the polonium was separated by plating on silver at 70°C for 8 h.

The assay of both ^{210}Pb and ^{210}Po in very small tissue specimens from smokers and non-smokers, in some cases as little as 1 mg dry weight of tissue, placed unusual demands on the procedures of low-level measurement. For these low activity samples ^{210}Pb was determined by ^{210}Po assay after ^{210}Po growth in the separated purified lead carrier fraction. However, for the first sets of tissue specimens processed, the low but detectable concentration of both ^{210}Pb and ^{210}Bi present in the commercially available lead carrier was comparable to or in excess of that in some of the tissue specimens. This difficulty was eliminated as the result of a successful search for lead carrier of exceptional radiochemical purity (lead from galena crystals). In addition some of the specimens had activity ranging down to one count per day or less under the ^{210}Po alpha peak, an activity level comparable to our early background level. It was found that the background for the silicon surface barrier detectors used is essentially zero for new crystals which are carefully handled, giving about one count in 10 days under the ^{210}Po peak. The crystal contamination which builds up under the peak for each

Po isotope is, for a given geometry, directly proportional to the total count for that isotope, and decays during storage with the half-life of the given isotopes. Thus the crystal contamination is attributable almost entirely to direct contamination of Po isotopes from the plated sample and spike due to recoil processes accompanying alpha-decay.

It now appears that we can make substantial improvements in the precision and sensitivity of measurements indicated by our preliminary results, by several means, as follows: (a) use of lead carrier of high radiochemical purity; (b) use of new barrier detectors or detectors reserved for low activity samples; (c) use of longer counting times per specimen. We have recently added more counting equipment to permit longer counting times.

It is reasonable to conclude that with an alpha counting efficiency of about 15% (due largely to counting geometry), amounts of ^{210}Po and ^{210}Pb down to 0.001 pCi (or 1 femtocurie) can be readily detected. Such activity will yield only about 1 count/2 days, thus long counting times will be required to obtain accurate measurements.

RESULTS

^{210}Po/^{210}Pb Ratio in Cigarette-smoke Condensate

Cigarette tobacco contains ^{210}Pb and ^{210}Po in physical equilibrium, due to the long time for curing and storage of the tobacco after harvesting (2 years or more). The activity of these isotopes in cured tobacco is generally about 0.4 pCi/g. When a cigarette is smoked, the mainstream smoke contains about 10% of the cigarette ^{210}Po, and about 5% of the ^{210}Pb (Radford and Hunt, 1964; Martell, 1974). Thus the ^{210}Po/^{210}Pb ratio in whole mainstream smoke condensate is about 2 (Holtzman and Ilcewicz, 1966; Martell, 1974), this value varying by type of tobacco and probably also smoking parameters. Isolation of the insoluble fraction of smoke condensate (about 0.01% of the total condensate by weight) has shown that over 95% of the ^{210}Pb activity is present in the small insoluble particles.

Table 2 shows results of analysis of total mainstream condensate for Kentucky tobacco obtained by use of standard smoking machines and supplied by Dr John

Table 2. Radiochemical Data for Whole Mainstream Smoke Samples of Kentucky 1R1 Blended Tobacco, Smoked on 6/6/75 and Analysed on 7/9/75

Ashing conditions	Measured radioactivity pCi/g condensate ± s.d.			
	^{210}Pb	^{210}Bi	^{210}Po	^{210}Po/^{210}Pb
Wet ashed	0.62 ± 0.014	0.76 ± 0.074	1.62 ± 0.150	2.61 ± 0.25
Dry ashed 650°C	0.55 ± 0.045	0.47 ± 0.017	0.051 ± 0.007	0.093 ± 0.015

Benner, University of Kentucky Tobacco and Health Research Institute. The analyses were carried out 33 days after smoking. One aliquot was wet ashed, to prevent ^{210}Po loss, and a second was dry ashed at 650°C, a temperature well below the temperature of a burning cigarette and also below the temperature at which fusion of the insoluble smoke particles takes place.

The ratio of ^{210}Po to ^{210}Pb was 2.61 at the time of analysis in this sample, showing that the more volatile polonium escapes into mainstream smoke more readily than the ^{210}Pb parent. Bismuth-210 was approximately in equilibrium with ^{210}Pb, as would be expected. When the condensate was heated to 650°C, however, 97% of the ^{210}Po was lost, while ^{210}Pb remained essentially unchanged. This result strongly supports the conclusion that ^{210}Po will be stripped from the lead parent at the time of smoking (assumption 1, above).

The residual ^{210}Po activity left after heating is close to the amount that would be expected from ingrowth from ^{210}Pb in the insoluble particles. From physical growth the $^{210}Po/^{210}Pb$ ratio expected would be 0.121; the observed value of 0.093 has a measurement error such that it does not differ significantly from the theoretical value. In any case, if the ^{210}Po remaining is trapped within the insoluble particles even after this rather severe treatment, assumption 2 is also supported. Further work is in progress evaluating the ^{210}Po content of the insoluble smoke fraction as a function of time after smoking and with various solvent treatments.

$^{210}Po/^{210}Pb$ Ratios in Bronchial Tissues of Smokers and Non-smokers

Table 3 shows the analytical results in the two non-smokers. Polonium activity was found to be very low in bronchial samples from both non-smokers, and in all instances was close to background measurements. In contrast ^{210}Pb was definitely present. Unfortunately a few samples in Subject B were lost during measurements of ^{210}Pb. It is clear that in no cases where ^{210}Pb was measured did the $^{210}Po/^{210}Pb$ ratio of epithelium significantly exceed 0.05, the $^{210}Po/^{210}Pb$ ratio characteristic of natural aerosols. Lung parenchymal samples showed variable but low ^{210}Po concentrations, and the $^{210}Po/^{210}Pb$ ratios were also highly variable. In the two samples of bronchial wall very low ^{210}Po concentrations were observed. It is evident from the results in these non-smokers that despite some aggregation of ^{210}Pb in bronchial bifurcations, evidently from ^{210}Pb in natural aerosols, very little ^{210}Po is associated with this lead, supporting the conclusion that soluble ^{210}Po not trapped within insoluble particles does not remain at the regions of high lead concentration (assumption 3). The presence of significant ^{210}Pb in epithelial samples shows that correction for this source of lead will be necessary in smokers (assumption 4).

Table 4 shows the results of analyses of bronchial tissues, lung parenchyma and hilar lymph nodes of the three smokers. The data in Table 4 demonstrate some important results, even though the high background due to lead carrier activity limits the precision of the measurements in these cases. First, polonium activity is significant in the epithelial scrapings and blocks, especially at the bronchial bifurcations. This finding is in sharp contrast to the results in the non-smokers (Table 3). The ^{210}Pb activity is also higher than in the non-smokers, but the difference is less striking, even for the small epithelial samples, evidently because of the presence of ^{210}Pb inhaled independently of smoking. It is also important that even with the high background, an analytical problem which has now been solved, it is possible with the new methods

TABLE 3. ANALYTICAL RESULTS ON BRONCHIAL TISSUES OF TWO NON-SMOKERS

Description	Dry weight (mg)	^{210}Po (pCi/g d.w.)	^{210}Pb (pCi/g d.w.)	$\bar{R}$ $^{210}Po/^{210}Pb$
SUBJECT A, female aged 72				
Tracheal epithelium	3.03	0[b]	4.1 ± 0.9[a]	0
Carinal epithelium	2.08	0.2 ± 1.3	5.2 ± 1.9	0.04 ± 0.25
Left main stem bronchus wall incl. epith.	98.6	0.032 ± 0.023	0.20 ± 0.05	0.16 ± 0.12
Epithelium LUL 1° + 2° bifurcations	0.92	0	20 ± 7	0
Block RML 2° bifurcation	1.31	0	14 ± 11	0
Block RML 3° bifurcation	1.62	0	4.5 ± 2.5	0
Block LUL 2° bifurcation	1.45	0	8.2 ± 2.8	0
Epithelium RLL 3 bifurcations	2.19	0	7.1 ± 3.5	0
Hilar parenchyma RUL	1387	0.013 ± 0.002	0	—
Peripheral parenchyma RUL	1358	0.016 ± 0.004	0.023 ± 0.006	0.72 ± 0.25
SUBJECT B, female aged 32				
Tracheal epithelium	10.82	0	0.8 ± 0.3	0
Carinal epithelium	1.40	1.3 ± 3.9	7.1 ± 2.6	0.18 ± 0.55
Left main stem bronchus wall with epith.	44.8	0	Sample lost	
Block LUL 1° bifurcation	1.53	0	5.9 ± 2.7	0
Block LUL 2° bifurcation	4.94	1.5 ± 1.5		
Block LUL 3° bifurcation	5.14	0	Samples lost	
Epithelium LLL 3 bifurcations	6.63	0		
Block LLL 2° bifurcation	10.92	0.8 ± 0.5		
Lymph nodes, carina	320.8	0.006 ± 0.007	0.054 ± 0.013	0.11 ± 0.14
Lymph nodes, hilus	400.2	0.064 ± 0.014	0.062 ± 0.024	1.02 ± 0.45
Hilar parenchyma	1113	0.034 ± 0.006	0.019 ± 0.006	1.75 ± 0.66
Peripheral parenchyma	1510	0.001 ± 0.001	0.022 ± 0.008	0.04 ± 0.07

[a] Values are mean ± s.d. of error.
[b] Zero values reported if measured quantity less than background.
LUL = left upper lobe, LLL = left lower lobe, RUL = right upper lobe,
RML = right middle lobe, RLL = right lower lobe.

TABLE 4. ANALYTICAL RESULTS ON LUNG TISSUES OF SMOKERS

Description	Dry weight (mg)	^{210}Po (pCi/g d.w.)	^{210}Pb (pCi/g d.w.)	$\bar{R}$ $^{210}Po/^{210}Pb$
SUBJECT 1, male aged 52				
Tracheal epithelium	1.87	6.3 ± 3.4	40 ± 12	0.16 ± 0.10
Carinal epithelium	0.83	14.2 ± 5.5	21 ± 19	0.68 ± 0.66
Epithelium, left main bronchus	3.69	4.3 ± 1.7	14.8 ± 8.6	0.29 ± 0.20
Epithelium, right main bronchus	4.20	3.0 ± 1.1	8.2 ± 3.1	0.36 ± 0.19
Epithelium RLL 1° bifurcation	3.09	2.7 ± 1.5	9.3 ± 6.6	0.29 ± 0.26
Epithelium LUL 1° bifurcation	0.78	8.7 ± 6.4	64 ± 35	0.14 ± 0.13
Epithelium LLL 2° bifurcation	2.54	4.3 ± 2.2	17.4 ± 8.9	0.25 ± 0.20
Parenchyma, peripheral RML	189	0.0024 ± 0.0024	0.055 ± 0.019	0.04 ± 0.04
SUBJECT 2, male aged 16				
Tracheal epithelium	3.33	0.27 ± 0.55	1.8 ± 1.8	0.15 ± 0.33
Tracheal wall with epithelium	275.6	0.031 ± 0.018	0.038 ± 0.026	0.83 ± 0.75
Carinal epithelium	1.07	0.13 ± 1.69	12 ± 4	0.01 ± 0.015
Epithelium, left main bronchus	4.72	0.48 ± 0.48	1.3 ± 0.8	0.38 ± 0.44
Epithelium, right main bronchus	1.68	7.3 ± 2.4	N.A.	
Left main bronchus wall with epith.	172.2	0.008 ± 0.016	0.079 ± 0.039	0.10 ± 0.21
Epithelium 1° bifurcation	2.18	0.63 ± 0.83	N.A.	
Block, RML 2° bifurcation	1.97	6.9 ± 3.7	16.7 ± 2.8	0.51 ± 0.20
Block, RLL 3° bifurcation	1.03	2.2 ± 4.4	21.2 ± 11.4	0.10 ± 0.21
Lymph nodes, hilus	348.7	0.036 ± 0.014	0.40 ± 0.10	0.09 ± 0.04
SUBJECT 3, male aged 41				
Carinal epithelium	1.44	1.1 ± 1.1	3.8 ± 3.2	0.3 ± 0.4
Epithelium, 2 bifurcations, UL & LL	2.03	0.18 ± 0.78	3.6 ± 2.0	0.05 ± 0.18
Blocks, 2 bifurcations UL & LL	7.12	0.22 ± 0.28	<2	<0.4
Epithelium UL 2°, 3°, 4° bifurcations	5.57	0.14 ± 0.43	2.8 ± 0.7	0.05 ± 0.15
Bronchial wall without epithelium	169.6	0.009 ± 0.009	0.15 ± 0.03	0.06 ± 0.07
Lymph nodes, carina	90.9	0.038 ± 0.028	0.15 ± 0.05	0.25 ± 0.21
Lymph nodes, hilus	237.7	0.041 ± 0.013	0.048 ± 0.017	0.86 ± 0.48
Parenchyma, hilus	1888	0.041 ± 0.006	0.016 ± 0.004	2.5 ± 0.7
Parenchyma, peripheral	1460	0.066 ± 0.006	0.026 ± 0.006	2.5 ± 0.6

N.A. Analysis not yet completed.

to detect by direct measurements these isotopes in samples as small as less than a milligram dry weight.

Values for $\bar{R}$, the $^{210}Po/^{210}Pb$ ratio, are highly variable with large error ranges, but the epithelium and bifurcation blocks generally show values around 0.3 to 0.4. In contrast, the tracheal and bronchial walls (with or without epithelium) show low values. Of special interest are the ratios for lung parenchyma in Subject 3 of 2.5, close to that observed in smoke condensate (Table 2). This result supports the conclusion that polonium from cigarette smoke absorbed on soluble smoke particles is taken up predominantly in alveolar tissues with large surface area, where it remains until cleared into the blood or via mucociliary clearance. Because of its low absolute concentration, however, it is unlikely to affect the concentration of polonium in bifurcations or other regions containing insoluble particles, where the measured ^{210}Po concentration is 50 to 1000 times higher. In contrast to subject 3, the parenchymal sample analysed for subject 1 showed low ^{210}Po concentration. This man died of congestive heart failure and may have stopped smoking long enough before death to result in clearance of most of the alveolar polonium.

The analyses of lymph nodes gave highly variable results for the $^{210}Po/^{210}Pb$ ratio with relatively high values for subject 3 and a low value for subject 2. This low value may be due to the fact that he was a young man who had not smoked long. Obviously further data are needed to determine whether the method is suitable for determining residence time of particles in hilar lymph nodes.

DISCUSSION

These are preliminary data, presented at this time to show how the method may be applied. Obviously much additional work will have to be done with lung tissues of smokers, non-smokers and former smokers of different ages, with the aid of the better analytical and counting techniques now available, before we can be certain of the interpretation of these measurements. These preliminary results, however, encourage us that the method has definite potential for determining residence time of insoluble particles in bronchial tissues and possibly lymph nodes of smokers.

Validity of the Assumptions

Assumptions 1 and 2 appear to be supported by the results to date, and further work related to them is under way. Assumption 3 appears to be reasonable and has qualitative support from the low concentrations of ^{210}Po found in the lung and bronchial wall samples of the smokers. Assumption 4 is clearly not strictly valid, and the presence of ^{210}Pb from natural sources in non-smokers in relatively high concentrations will require correction of data of smokers for this additional source of ^{210}Pb which is not associated with its daughter ^{210}Po.

Estimates of Mean Residence Times

From Table 4 and Fig. 1, the data indicate that for bronchial epithelium the particles appear to have residence times of about 3 to 5 months ($\bar{R} = 0.3$ to 0.4), although the errors of these estimates are large. As pointed out in discussion of assumption 4, these estimates are probably low because of the contribution of ^{210}Pb from natural aerosol which is independent of smoking. Thus the measured activity ratio is lower than would be the case from the assumption that all ^{210}Pb is present in the insoluble particles. These results confirm the view that insoluble particles contribute a large part of the polonium activity and alpha dose at these sites, and account for the fact that local bronchial concentrations of ^{210}Po and ^{210}Pb can exceed their concentration in whole smoke condensate.

Concentrations of Polonium

The results of these measurements for smokers confirm those of LITTLE *et al.* (1965) and show that concentrations of ^{210}Po greater than 1 pCi/g wet weight ($>$5 pCi/g dry weight) are commonly found in epithelium of bifurcations of smokers. Even though these concentrations have been measured directly in our present work, we believe that the crude nature of the separation of tissues taken with the small volume of epithelium actually present makes it likely that local doses are much higher than would be predicted from the mean concentration if the particles are principally within the epithelial layer.

On the assumption that the ^{210}Pb activity of a single insoluble particle in smoke is about 3×10^{-6} pCi (MARTELL, 1974), then a 2-mg sample of tissue at a bifurcation containing 1 pCi ^{210}Pb/g wet weight, or 0.002 pCi in the sample, will contain about 600 particles. If these are localized in a relatively small region in the epithelium, the radiation dose around this cluster would be expected to be well above that calculated for uniform distribution in the epithelium, about 200 rem in 25 years (LITTLE *et al.*, 1965). The significance of these local radiation doses in relation to lung cancer production remains a matter of considerable controversy. But the fact that the polonium is supported by its long-lived parent ^{210}Pb at the regions of high concentration at the bifurcations lends added weight to the role of this natural radiation source in the genesis of bronchial cancer in smokers (LITTLE and RADFORD, 1967; HOLTZMAN, 1967).

Acknowledgements—We are indebted to Dr Russell Fisher, the Chief Medical Examiner of Maryland, for assistance in obtaining autopsy specimens, and to Dr John Benner of the University of Kentucky Tobacco and Health Research Institute for tobacco and smoke condensate samples. The careful analytical work of S. E. Poet is also gratefully acknowledged. Thanks are also due to Mrs Eve Steinberg and Mr Bruce Pitt, who assisted with collection of tissue samples.

Radiochemical measurements were carried out at the National Center for Atmospheric Research, sponsored by the National Science Foundation.

REFERENCES

BOWLER, R. G. (1944) *Biochem. J.* **38,** 385–388.

HOLTZMAN, R. B. (1967) *Science, N.Y.* **155,** 607.

HOLTZMAN, R. B. and ILCEWICZ, F. H. (1966) *Science, N. Y.* **153,** 1259–1260.

LITTLE, J. B. and MCGANDY, R. B. (1968) *Archs envir. Hlth* **17,** 693–696.

LITTLE, J. B. and RADFORD, E. P. Jr., (1967) *Science, N.Y.* **155,** 606–607.

LITTLE, J. B., RADFORD, E. P., Jr., MCCOMBS, H. L. and HUNT, V. R. (1965) *New Engl. J. Med.* **273,** 1343–1351.

MARTELL, E. A. (1974) *Nature, Lond.* **249,** 215–217.

MARTELL, E. A. (1975) *Am. Scient.* **63,** 404–412.

POET, S. E., MOORE, H. E. and MARTELL, E. A. (1972) *J. geophys. Res.* **77,** 6515–6527.

RADFORD, E. P. Jr., and HUNT, V. R. (1964) *Science, N.Y.* **143,** 247–249.

DISCUSSION

C. N. DAVIES: You have presented a long and complex argument, supported by delicate experiments, which leads to the conclusion that bronchial carcinoma in smokers derives from highly insoluble particles about 1 μm in diameter which are claimed to exist in tobacco smoke. This theory is devoid of supporting experimental evidence in two respects: (1) the presence of the α-active particles in tobacco smoke has not been demonstrated. (2) The mechanism by which these highly insoluble particles, if present, are able to deposit and remain static at bronchial bifurcations is not explained. If your arguments are to become acceptable I think it essential that experiments on the tobacco smoke aerosol should be undertaken to cover these two points. Work with condensate is not enough; there is loss of volatile constituents and the possibility of forming particles in the course of laboratory manipulation.

Prof. RADFORD: I would indeed feel more comfortable to have evidence of ^{210}Pb enriched particles in smoke rather than in condensate. To fill in all the gaps in the chain running from the tobacco trichome tip to the bronchial epithelium is important and this preliminary report attempts to deal with some of these gaps. If our estimates are correct, there are only about 10 000 insoluble particles in the smoke from one cigarette, so we are looking for a needle in a haystack, but I agree with what you are saying. With regard to the mechanisms by which these particles may remain trapped in the bronchial epithelium, they are separated from lymphatics by the basement membrane, which may be relatively impermeable, and the only mechanism for their release may be by physical movement as the stem cells divide and take up a surface position on the epithelium. This may be a very inefficient way for particles close to the basement membrane to be removed, compared with tissues to which macrophages or other phagocytic cells have ready access.

R. THOMAS: You previously indicated that the lead-rich particles were 5 μm diameter, but now you report 1 μm. How do you account for this?

Dr MARTELL: The observed size range for separated, insoluble cigarette-smoke particles was about 0.1 to 5.0 μm diameter, with a median diameter of about 1 μm. It is possible that the separation procedure used to isolate these particles from main-stream smoke condensate had some influence on their nature and size distribution of the particles. Direct measurements of the properties of these insoluble smoke particles produced by tobacco trichome combustion are needed. However, it should be kept in mind that these insoluble radioactive particles make up less than 0.01% of dry, whole smoke condensate and thus there is only about one such insoluble particle per 10 million smoke particles.

Prof. RADFORD: The only constituent of tobacco smoke with a high enough specific activity of ^{210}Pb to account for the measured specific activity in bronchial bifurcations is the small insoluble particle component.

$^{239}PuO_2$ AEROSOL INHALATION WITH EMPHASIS ON PULMONARY CONNECTIVE TISSUE MODIFICATIONS*

H. METIVIER, R. MASSE, D. NOLIBÉ and J. LAFUMA

Commissariat à l'Energie Atomique, Département de Protection Laboratoire de Toxicologie Expérimentale, Montrouge, France

Abstract—Inhalation studies were undertaken in which plutonium dioxide ($^{239}PuO_2$) was administered to either unanaesthetized Wistar rats or anaesthetized baboons. In both groups of animals some deaths occurred from acute lung damage resulting from cell necrosis particularly to vascular tissue followed by alveolar oedema. At later stages, marked interstitial pneumonitis and interstitial fibrosis occurred and deaths resulted from respiratory insufficiency preceded by high arterial blood pCO_2 and low pO_2. In rats as many as 50% of the animals finally developed lung neoplasms but only two such tumours were found in baboons. Attempts were made to correlate biochemical parameters with observed tissue damage and animal mortality.

INSOLUBLE $^{239}PuO_2$ remains in the lung for a long time and the energy emitted by ^{239}Pu disintegration is entirely absorbed in the lung, mainly in discrete volumes of tissue surrounding the particles (BAIR *et al.*, 1973). The biological effects are related to the dose: the main hazards have been reviewed by BAIR (1974): (1) acute toxicity, with first severe inflammatory reactions, haemorrhages and necrosis destroying the functional tissue of the lung; (2) subacute respiratory insufficiency associated with large modifications of arterial blood gases; (3) pulmonary fibrosis, when survival time is half the life-span; (4) carcinomas as late effects.

Biochemical quantitation of fibrous tissue in the whole lung as a function of time and initial burden should help to understand pathological evolution and allow full histopathological analysis. However, few biochemical analyses of connective tissues after inhalation of radionuclides have been carried out so far (TSVELEVA and LINBINZON, 1968; PICKRELL *et al.*, 1973). A sequential study of the deleterious effects following administration of $^{239}PuO_2$ aerosols to rats and baboons was therefore carried out, with emphasis on biochemical modifications of the pulmonary connective tissue and their relationship with histopathological findings and causes of death.

MATERIAL AND METHODS

Unanaesthetized conventional Wistar rats and anaesthetized baboons (phencyclidine 2.0 mg/kg) were administered $^{239}PuO_2$ by means of an inhalation device

* This work was performed with the technical assistance of N. Legendre, G. Rateau, I. l'Hullier and M. Beauvallet.

(METIVIER *et al.*, 1974a). The particles ($\rho = 11.4$) had a count median aerodynamic diameter (CMAD) of 2.06 μm ($\sigma = 1.28$) for a real diameter of 0.6 μm. The oxide was obtained by burning peroxide at 1000°C. The inhaled activity was determined by X-ray counting of ^{239}Pu daughters with use of a proportional counter (LANSIART and MORUCCI, 1964).

Arterial oxygen tension (pO_2), carbon dioxide tension (pCO_2) and pH were measured using a Radiometer BMS 3 analyser. Arterial blood samples were drawn by a capillary tube from catheterized carotid (rats) or femoral (baboons) arteries 30 min after anaesthesia. Animals were sacrificed by section of abdominal aorta (rats) or carotid artery (baboons). Exsanguinated lungs were removed and weighed.

Rats' azygos lobes and several baboons' pulmonary samples were used for conventional histological analysis.

The samples for biochemical measurements were dried and defatted in ethanol, acetone and acetone/ether mixture. Collagen extracted by 5% trichloracetic acid at 90°C (NEUMAN and LOGAN, 1950) was determined by hydroxyproline measurement (STEGEMANN, 1958). Whole proteins were determined, after HCl 6 N hydrolysis, by amino acid ninhydrin colorimetry (RUBINSTEIN and PRYCE, 1959), mucopolysaccharides by sodium borohydride alkaline solution extraction (LAROS *et al.*, 1972) and total uronic acids according to BITTER and MUIR (1962).

EXPERIMENTS ON RATS

1. *Pulmonary Retention*

Lung clearance of inhaled plutonium was obtained by measuring the lung burden at death after removal of thoracic lymph nodes. The values obtained were fitted best by the exponential model and long term retention half-time was estimated at about 160 days (Fig. 1) for rats having inhaled 100–150 nCi of $^{239}PuO_2$ per gram of fresh lung. Whatever might be the dose of inhaled $^{239}PuO_2$, lung clearance was always lower than obtained with atoxic particles (CHRETIEN and MASSE, 1973); this could be ascribed to inhibition of migration of macrophages (NOLIBÉ *et al.*, 1974). Similar decrease of lung clearance was only observed by NENOT (1971) in rats which had inhaled high doses of acid solution of ^{239}Pu. Lower clearance seems therefore to depend on absorbed α-dose by single cells since the number of macrophages engulfing PuO_2 particles is much smaller than that of cells engulfing "soluble" plutonium aerosols.

2. *Dose Mortality Relationship, Biological Effects*

Survivals of 195 rats were plotted as a function of the estimated initial alveolar burden (measured 7 days post-exposure) (Fig. 2). Ninety-four rats died between 55 and 200 days post-exposure due to respiratory insufficiency after inhalation of doses over 300–400 nCi and two toxicological processes were observed: inflammatory reactions, haemorrhages and necrosis destroying the functional tissue but without modifications of blood gases at rest. Early death was also due to the development of

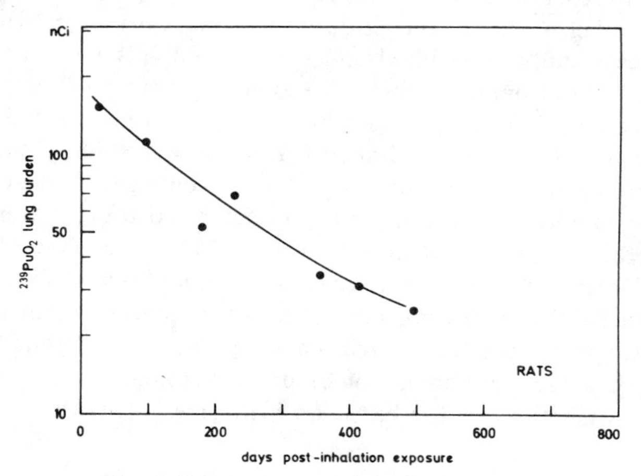

FIG. 1. Pulmonary retention of $^{239}PuO_2$ in rats.

fibrosis, associated with respiratory insufficiency and preceded by high arterial blood pCO_2 and low pO_2. In animals dying during the first 3 months, strong increase of reticular fibres together with cellular infiltrations of the interstitium were observed. Some alveolar foci filled with fibrin particles were especially abundant near the hyalinized arteriolae. Many veinous thromboses occurred, pneumocytes Type II proliferation foci were scarce. There was a strong trend towards the formation of honeycombing type lacunae. Later lesions were non-homogeneous: surrounding true

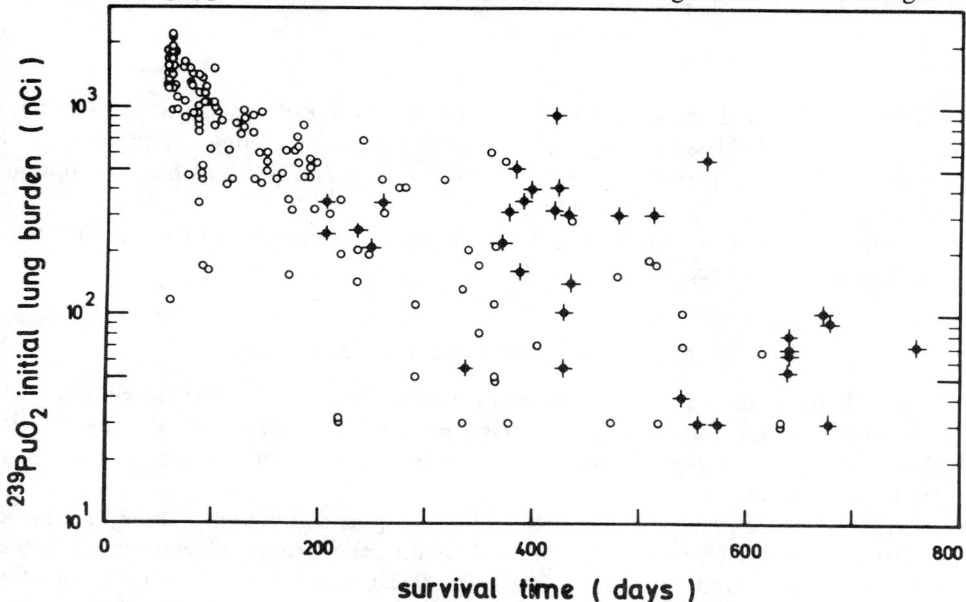

FIG. 2. $^{239}PuO_2$ initial lung burden *vs.* survival time of rats (○, no carcinoma; +, one or two carcinomas identified).

scars appeared in the foci of particles trapped or surrounding squamous metaplasia or adenomatosis. At other places the interstitium was either normal or hypovascularized and slightly fibrous or infiltrated with plasma cells, eosinophils and mast cells. In some places interstitium was atrophic leading to focal emphysema.

Death occurring after 200 days was also of respiratory origin but the modifications of blood gases were not distinguished at rest. Fibrosis was slightly more developed, increasing respiratory rates were noticed 1–2 weeks only before death, weight loss (10–30 %) was the major clinical sign predicting death. Histological analysis showed lung carcinomas (one or more foci) in 50 % of rats (35 % from 200 to 400 days, 65 % after 400 days). Death could not be ascribed to cancers because few were seriously invasive (less than 15 %) and death occurred in rats without carcinomas at the same time. In thirty-five rats with lung carcinomas eighty-nine different tumours were identified, more than two carcinomas of different histological types were observed (Table 1). The classification used is based on histogenesis (MASSE *et al.*, 1974). The

TABLE 1. HISTOLOGY OF LUNG TUMOURS

BRONCHOGENIC CARCINOMAS		50.5 %
squamous cells		
bronchogenic adenocarcinomas		
anaplastic (great cells)		
BRONCHIOLO-ALVEOLAR CARCINOMAS		40.5 %
SARCOMAS		9.0 %
lymphoreticular sarcomas	5.6	
haemangiosarcomas	3.4	

percentages observed are similar to those obtained with different types of α-emitters (LAFUMA *et al.*, 1974) except for the higher percentage of sarcomas. The location of tumours was often peripheral, no extrathoracic metastasis was observed and no spontaneous carcinoma in 100 control rats.

Seventeen rats with initial lung burdens between 10 and 50 nCi are still alive 500 days after exposure.

3. *Pulmonary Connective Tissue Modifications*

One of the consequences of plutonium dioxide inhalation is the development of pulmonary fibrosis (ABRAMS *et al.*, 1946; BAIR *et al.*, 1973) that occurred in the 200–400-days group and in the last period of survival time, in conjunction with death from neoplasia.

Quantitation of fibrous tissue in the whole lung as a function of time or inhaled burden by chemical analysis was studied in different groups of rats: early effects (50 and 100 days) and late effects (200 and 400 days) as a function of dose, effect of ageing for an initial dose giving 50 % of lung carcinomas, and study of connective tissue at death for each rat whatever the type of death.

Early effects

Study of early effects as a function of dose showed a quick increase of wet or dry lung weight, from the 3rd week post-exposure, this process was significant for doses above 100 nCi. To this increase there corresponded a first increase of whole protein values 50 days post-exposure from 0 to 50% of control values, then an increase of collagen and uronic acids amounts between 50 and 100 days after inhalation. Blood gas modifications at rest could only be observed 100 days post-exposure (Fig. 3). The first reaction—increase of lung weight and whole proteins—can be explained as cellular infiltration before reaction of the fibrous components of connective tissue. These local cellularity changes might play on the distribution of perfusion, and asso-

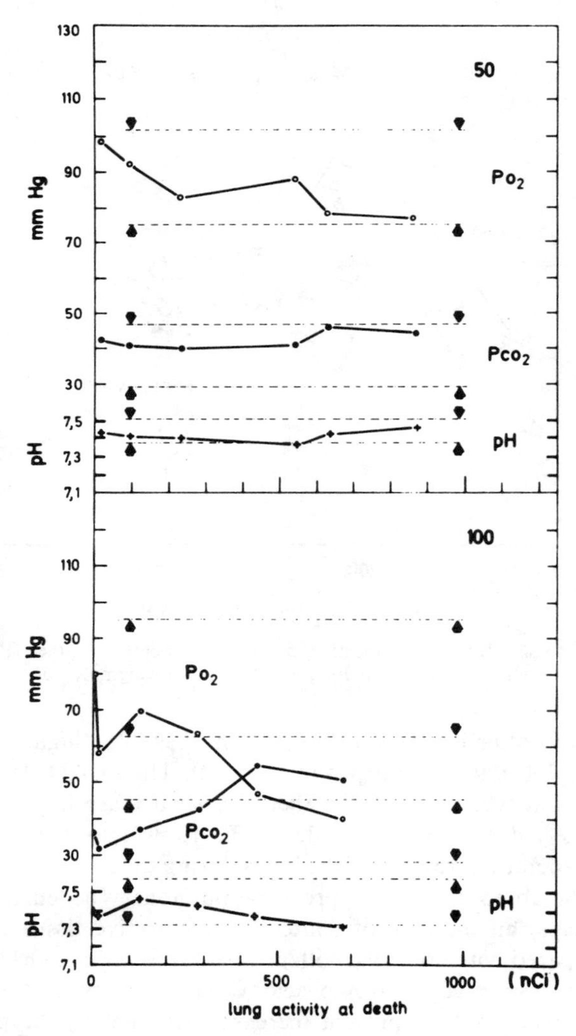

FIG. 3. Blood gas modification *vs.* lung burden 50 and 100 days post-exposure. Arrows show extreme values for controls.

ciated with a small increase of fibrous components could lead to modification of active surface area and blood gas values.

The 50% carcinoma group

Initial lung burdens in this group ranged from 150 to 200 nCi with expected life-span from 300 to 500 days post-exposure. Each group included eight or six exposed rats and three or four controls. Rats with invading cancers at autopsy were not included in the study.

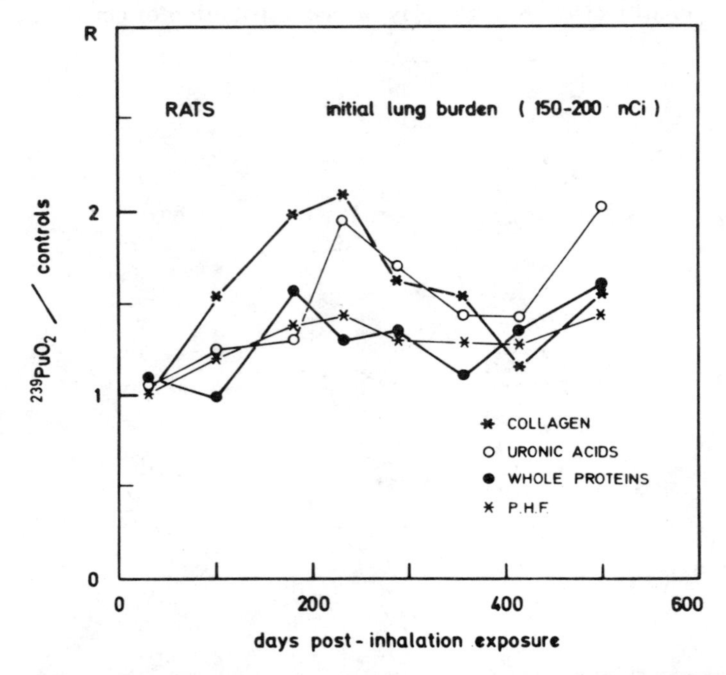

FIG. 4. $^{239}PuO_2$/control ratios for connective tissue components *vs*. time. (PHF—pulmonary hypertrophy factor—is lung weight/animal weight $\times 10^3$.)

One hundred days after inhalation, lung weight was 20% higher than in controls and reached 44% 230 days post-exposure (Fig. 4). Up to 400 days post-exposure recovery of the organ seemed to occur, then a new increase happened by 500 days post-exposure largely due to oncoming death. There was no increase of the relative content of the dry (defatted) residue of the lungs during the entire investigation period, which indicated the absence of any appreciable pulmonary oedema. During the first period (till 200 days) an increase of content of connective tissue components was observed. As compared with controls, collagen values were 55 and 110% higher after 100 and 230 days respectively. Uronic acid values were twice the control values 230 days post-exposure. Whole protein increase was smaller, the part of the non-collagenous component of the lung being probably weak in this increase. From 230 to 400 days the drop of all these component values cannot be evaluated as a sign of organ recovery since death occurred with the same frequency, and histological observations showed diffuse fibrosis, metaplasias, scars, cell infiltrations and emphysema (Fig. 5). Incomplete correlation between histological and biochemical data from 300 to 400 days post-exposure suggests modification or redistribution of connective tissue components.

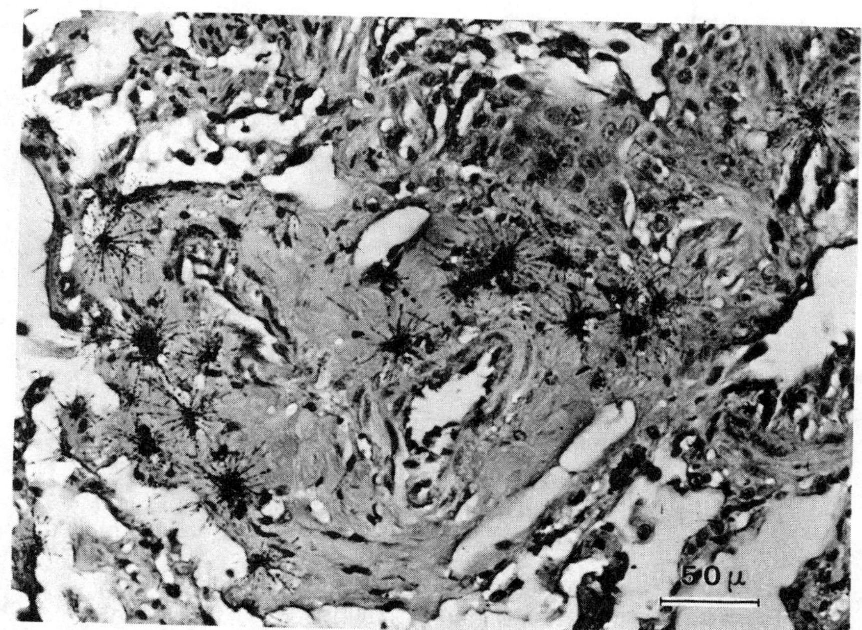

FIG. 5. Scar around arteriola disruption of alveolar walls and focus of metaplasia arising from a bronchus. Paraffin embedding. Autoradiography, HES stain.

As DAGLE *et al.* (1975) showed for popliteal lymphadenitis, plutonium-induced fibrosis can be first a general response to necrotic cells through a possible release of phospholipids (HEPPLESTON and STYLES, 1967; BURREL and ANDERSON, 1973) and finally, cavitation occurs either as a result of direct breakdown of collagen or failure of collagen synthesis. Also sequestration of plutonium particles occurring in the scar tissue could reduce the alpha radiation potential damage to surrounding parenchymal cells. Further increase observed after 400–500 days could be explained either by tumour induction or as a last reaction of parenchymal tissue before death as shown by the increase of uronic acids. During the investigation period no significant modifications of blood gases were observed.

Biochemical values at death

Values at death (from 60 to 430 days) whatever the toxicity hazards, were plotted (Fig. 6) as ratio of exposed animal values (mean of four or five rats) to values in controls sacrificed at the same age. Values of collagen, whole proteins and uronic acids have obviously increased with scattered results during the first 150 days. Blood

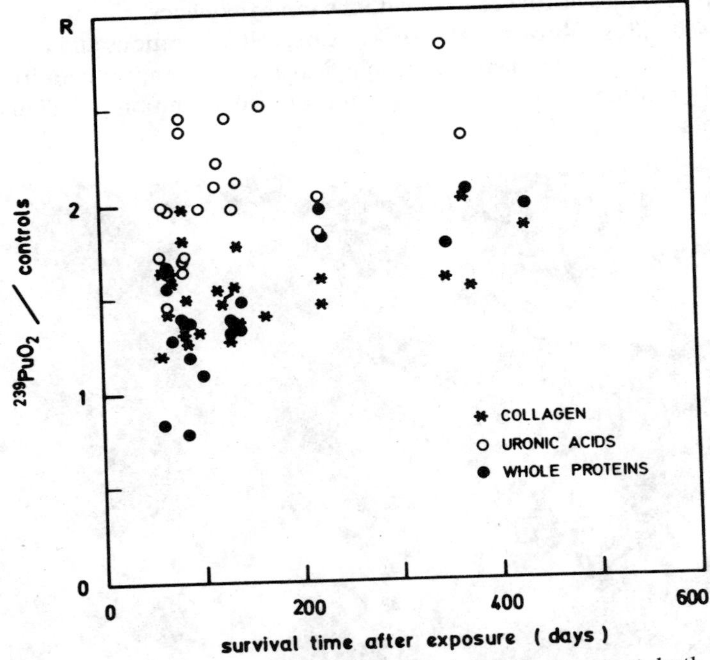

FIG. 6. $^{239}PuO_2$/control ratios for connective tissue components at death.

gas values are altered, not significantly, however, since animals were sacrificed when moribund. Fresh lung weights versus animal weights were always 100 to 200% higher than control values; however, death occurrence seemed to correspond to a limit of functional lung weight without carcinoma. Whole uronic acids always increase more than other values, likely due to higher synthesis of mucopolysaccharides.

BABOON EXPERIMENTS

Following inhalation of $^{239}PuO_2$, and during a short period of observation (less than 100 days), clearance half-times of 202 and 421 days were measured for two groups with less than 50 and more than 100 nCi/g initial lung burdens (METIVIER *et al.*, 1974b); these values were higher than those observed with atoxic particles (METIVIER *et al.* 1974c). Further observations based on twenty-seven baboons sacrificed later, verified these results, giving 500 days. However, if clearance half-times are calculated with the values obtained after 100 days, deep lung clearance values are higher, about 500–800 days, in agreement with those obtained by BAIR and PARK (1968) with beagle dogs, and with atoxic particles in man (GRAHAM *et al.*, 1972). The main fraction of plutonium removed from the lung after bronchial and tracheal mucociliary processes was deposited in thoracic lymph nodes, 1 and 5%, 100 and 400 days post-exposure respectively (Fig. 7). Skeletal and liver burdens were always below 1% of initial lung burden. Translocations to thoracic lymph nodes was slower in baboons (Fig. 8) than in dogs (SANDERS, 1972; SANDERS and PARK, 1972). As observed in dogs (PARK *et al.*, 1972)

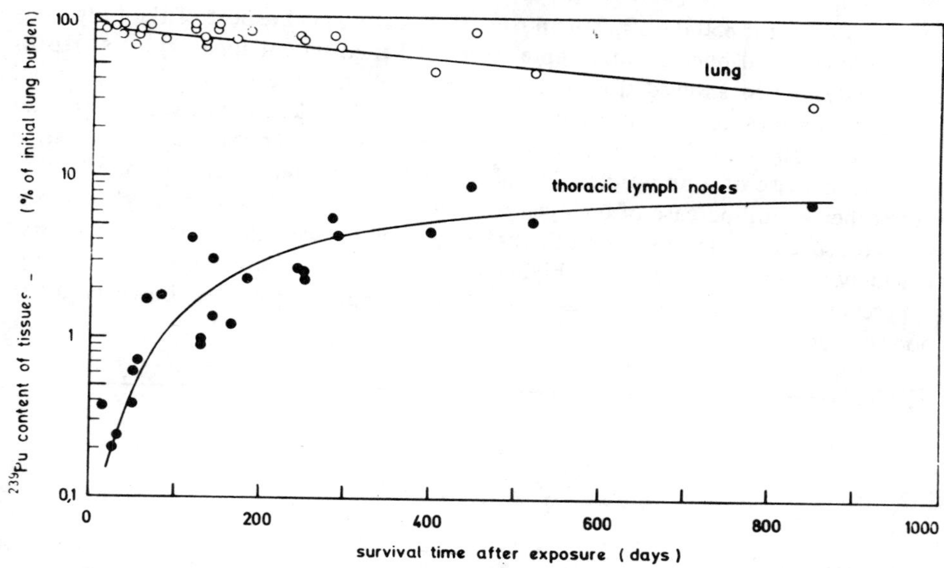

FIG. 7. Distribution of plutonium in baboons following inhalation of $^{239}PuO_2$.

the variation of survival times as a function of plutonium deposits in lung is well represented by the power function (Fig. 9). To date, no death has been observed beyond 850 days; twenty-five baboons are still alive, with initial lung burdens ranging from 1 to 50 nCi/g of fresh lung. Baboons are 3 times as sensitive as dogs to acute internal irradiation; this might be correlated with translocation to lymph nodes that should be regarded as a detoxication process.

During the first 50 days death was caused by alveolar oedema that followed vascular

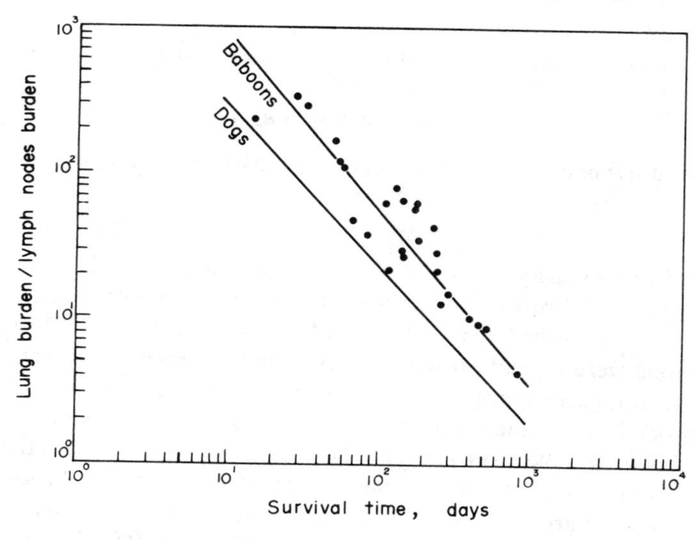

FIG. 8. Lung and lymph node burdens *vs.* death occurrence.

injuries. Later, until 850 days post-exposure, the histological aspect of the lungs was typical of interstitial pneumonitis, septa were thickened by collagen deposits. Histological analysis also showed fibrinous exudates, and inflammatory cell infiltration. Hyaline membranes, foci of vacuolated macrophages and desquamated pneumocytes Type II (Fig. 10) were to be found in the alveoli. Whatever the survival times, a significant increase of lung weights was always observed after inhalation of $^{239}PuO_2$. On the other hand, increase of collagen was difficult to show, as lung weights on the day of exposure were unknown and the baboons' weights were different. Collagen was also widely scattered in lobes; the higher the survival time the wider the scattering. The percentage of collagen increase versus lung weight cannot be shown either in baboons or in rats.

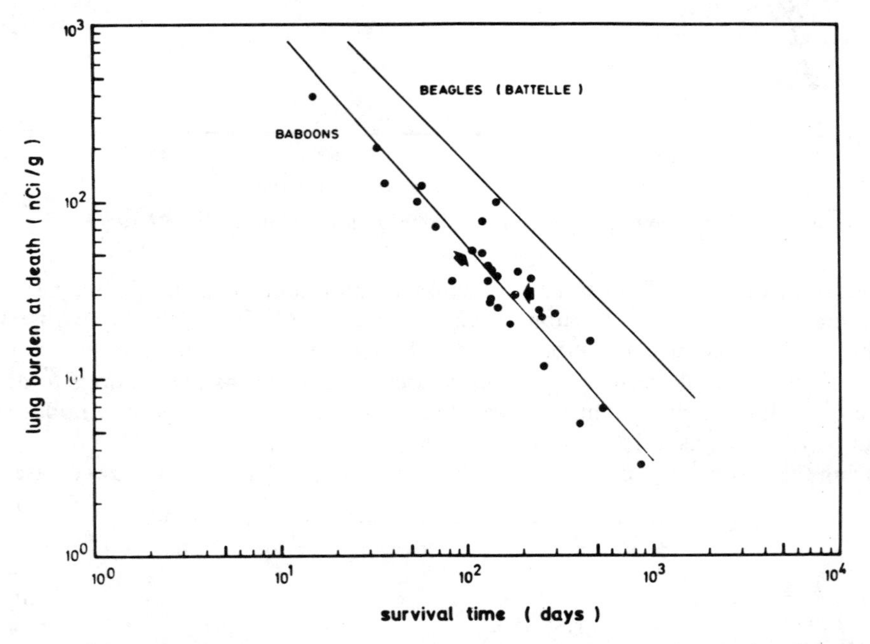

FIG. 9. Lung burden at death *vs*. survival time of baboons and beagles. (Beagle data by courtesy of W. J. Bair.)

As observed by CLARKE and BAIR (1964) foci of squamous metaplasia were observed early in many parts of bronchi and alveoli. However, in two animals, lung cancers were histologically identified (METIVIER *et al.*, 1974b) at 100 and 180 days post-exposure. Lesions were typical growth and extended for about 1 cm into the parenchyma; two histological types were observed: slightly differentiated epidermoid carcinoma, bronchogenic adenocarcinoma. Meaning of these lesions still remains unclear. As shown by BRIGHTWELL and HEPPLESTON (1973) for urethane-induced pulmonary adenomas, they might be true cancers sterilized by ^{239}Pu α-radiation or non-extensive atypical growth since larger growth was observed neither in the animal dead 850 days after inhalation nor in animals alive 1000 and 1600 days post-exposure

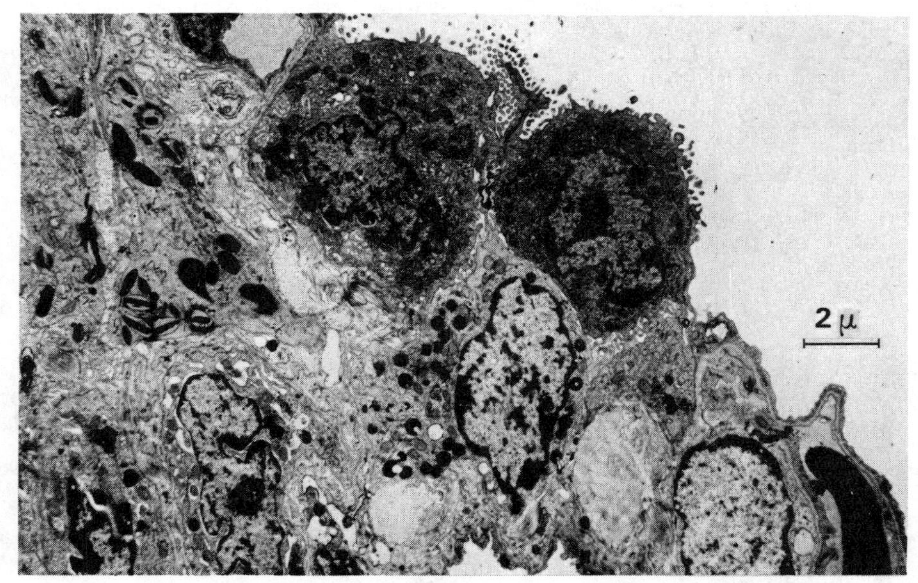

FIG. 10. P_{II} type cells hyperplasia, a few collagen deposits and infiltration of the septum by mast cells, histiocytes and eosinophils. Araldite embedding.

(30–40 nCi/g initial lung burdens), which has been checked by roentgenography every year.

CONCLUSIONS

The toxicity of plutonium is well known; life-span shortening is induced by inhalation together with the advent of carcinomas but is not correlated with lung carcinomas. By itself the study of the connective tissue of rats and baboons cannot explain the occurrence of death, though some components such as uronic acids are sensitive reactives of irradiated lung. The increase of uronic acid may involve a chronic inflammatory state in agreement with histological data, showing permanent cellular infiltration of mast cells and plasmocytes into alveolar walls, at all the doses studied so far. Death cannot be correlated with "pulmonary fibrosis" either. In baboons, histopathological findings, up to 850 days, mainly point to interstitial pneumonia rather than fibrosis.

A qualitative modification of collagen may be considered in order to explain discrepancies between histological and biochemical findings, but lack of modification of blood gases in animals at rest with low $^{239}PuO_2$ lung burdens does not lead to loss of gas permeability in the alveolae. The causes of death in rats still require further investigation.

REFERENCES

ABRAMS, R., SEIBERT, H. C., FORKEL, L., GREENBERG, D., LISCO, H., JACOBSON, L. O. and SIMMONS, E. L. (1946) *Acute Toxicity of Intubated Plutonium*. Report CH-3875, Metallurgical Laboratory, University of Chicago.

BAIR, W. J. (1974) *Advances in Radiation Biology* (edited by LETT, J. T., ADLER, H. and ZELLE, M.) vol. 4, pp. 255–315. Academic Press, New York.

BAIR, W. J. and PARK, J. F. (1968) *Proceedings of the First International Congress of Radiation Protection. Rome, 1966* (edited by SNYDER, W.) vol. I, pp. 181–197. Pergamon Press, Oxford.

BAIR, W. J., BALLOU, J. E., PARK, J. F. and SANDERS, C. L. (1973) *Uranium, Plutonium and Transplutonic Elements* (edited by HODGE, H. C., STANNARD, J. N. and HURSH, J. B.) p. 503. Springer, Berlin.

BITTER, T. and MUIR, H. M. (1962) *Analyt. Biochem.* **4,** 330–334.

BRIGHTWELL, J. and HEPPLESTON, A. G. (1973) *Br. J. Radiol.* **46,** 180–182.

BURREL, R. and ANDERSON, M. (1973) *Envir. Res.* **6,** 389–394.

CHRETIEN, J. and MASSE, R., (1973) *Journées méd. ann., Broussais la Charité. Acquisit. méd. réc.*, pp. 117–146.

CLARKE, W. and BAIR, W. J. (1964) *Hlth Phys.* **10,** 391–398.

DAGLE, G. E., PHEMISTER, R. D., LEBEL, J. L. JAENKE, R. and WATTERS, R. L. (1975) *Radiat. Res.* **61,** 239–250.

GRAHAM, L. S., UPHAM, T., STECKEL, R., POE, D. N. (1972) *Physics Med. Biol.* **17,** 874.

HEPPLESTON, A. G. and STYLES, J. A. (1967) *Nature, Lond.* **214,** 521–522.

LAFUMA, J., NENOT, J. C., MORIN, M., MASSE, R., METIVIER, H., NOLIBÉ, D. and SKUPINSKI, W. (1974) *Experimental Lung Cancer, Carcinogenesis and Bioassays International Symposium, Seattle, June 1974* (edited by KARBE, E. and PARK, J. P.) pp. 443–453. Springer, Berlin.

LANSIART, A. and MORUCCI, J. P. (1964) in *Assessment of Radioactivity in Man. Heidelberg, May 1964*, vol. 1, pp. 131–140. I.A.E.A., Vienna.

LAROS, C. D., KUYPER, C. M. A. and JANSSEN, H. M. J. (1972) *Respiration* **29,** 458–467.

MASSE, R., LAFUMA, J., METIVIER, H., NOLIBÉ, D., FRITSCH, P., NENOT, J. C., MORIN, M., SKUPINSKI, W., CHAMEAUD, J., PERRAUD, R. and CHRETIEN, J. (1974) *Colloques Inst. natn Santé Rech. méd.* **29,** 307–324.

METIVIER, H., RATEAU, G., MASSE, R. and NOLIBÉ, D. (1974a) *Description d'un Dispositif permettant la Contamination d'Animaux de Laboratoire par Inhalation d'Aérosols Radioactifs.* Note CEA-N-1722. Commissariat à l'Energie Atomique, Montrouge.

METIVIER, H., NOLIBÉ, D., MASSE, R. and LAFUMA, J. (1974b) *Hlth Phys.* **27,** 512–514.

METIVIER, H., NENOT, J. C., MASSE, R., NOLIBÉ, D. and LAFUMA, J. (1974c) *C. r. hebd. Séances Acad. Sci. Paris, D* **278,** 671–674.

NENOT, J. C. (1971) *Inhaled Particles III* (edited by WALTON, W. H.) vol. 1, pp. 239–246. Unwin Bros., Old Woking, Surrey.

NEUMAN, R. E. and LOGAN, M. A. (1950) *J. biol. Chem.* **186,** 549–556.

NOLIBÉ, D., METIVIER, H., MASSE, R. and LAFUMA, J. (1974) *Revue fr. Mal. resp.* **2** (suppl. 1) 128–132.

PARK, J. F., BAIR, W. J. and BUSCH, R. H. (1972) *Hlth Phys.* **22,** 803–810.

PICKRELL, J. A., HARRIS, D. V., PFLEGER, R. C. and BENJAMIN, S. A. (1973) p. 180. Report LF 46. Lovelace Foundation, Albuquerque.

RUBINSTEIN, H. M. and PRYCE, D. J. (1959) *J. clin. Path.* **12,** 80.

SANDERS, C. L. (1972) *Hlth Phys.* **22,** 607–615.

SANDERS, C. L. and PARK, J. F. (1972) *Hlth Phys.* **22,** 815–822.

STEGEMANN, H. (1958) *Hoppe-Seyler's Z. physiol. Chem.* **311,** 41–45.

TSEVELEVA, I. A. and LINBINZON, R. E. (1968) *Radiobiologiya* **8,** 535–541 (U.S.A.E.C. Translation AEC-Tr-7o14, pp. 68–76).

DISCUSSION

G. BOULEY: What proportion of your rats died of infection?

Dr METIVIER: There were no deaths, as can be seen from the graphs.

H. SMITH: Did you observe metastases in the thoracic lymph nodes in either rats or baboons? Did you look for connective tissue changes in the thoracic lymph nodes?

Dr METIVIER: We have not observed any metastases in the thoracic lymph nodes of baboons so far. We have made no biochemical measurements on the connective tissue of the thoracic lymph nodes.

A. G. HEPPLESTON: In classifying lung tumours as carcinomas or sarcomas, was there clear evidence of local invasion or distant metastasis? If not, malignancy cannot be assumed.

You refer to the study by Dr Brightwell and me on the effect of inhaled $^{239}PuO_2$ on urethane-induced pulmonary adenomas in mice. It is not correct to assume, as you do, that α-irradiation sterilized "true cancers" in the pathological sense of malignancy, since, in my experience, pulmonary adenomas in mice are, and remain, benign neoplasms.

Dr METIVIER: To answer your second point, it seems well established that most bronchioalveolar or alveolar tumours in mice are really carcinomas since they are transplantable and sometimes give birth to metastasis. The problem is to know whether adenomas do exist! (STEWART, DUNN and SNELL, AEC-Conf-21, 1970, pp. 161–184). In rats, invasions were obvious into mediastinum, diaphragm and liver. Metastases occurred in the lymph nodes of the thoracic cavity. No other lymphatic metastases were observed; however, metastases were observed in kidneys with squamous cells and bronchiolo-alveolar carcinomas. All types of tumour described as malignant in this study were found to be transplantable.

As to your first point, there seems to be no doubt, as far as histology is concerned, about the characters of the tumours in the rat. With the baboon there are problems since the tumours are very small. We observed them at 100, 180 and 800 days and the lesions did not seem to progress in any way. It is rather difficult to conclude that it is a carcinoma, because it has no invasive character.

F. F. HAHN: Did you find any correlation either anatomical or biochemical between the pulmonary fibrosis and the pulmonary cancers?

Dr METIVIER: We observed the highest collagen rate during the first 200 days, then there was a drop that suggested recovery; we tried to find a relation between the biochemical result and the development of future cancers. This work is still in progress and we have been unable to demonstrate a clear-cut relationship. We would like to have biochemical tests to see if there is a relationship between fibrosis and cancer. From the anatomical point of view, metaplasia were often associated with scars but this relationship could not be established with invading tumours.

THERAPEUTIC EFFECT OF PULMONARY LAVAGE *IN VIVO* AFTER INHALATION OF INSOLUBLE RADIOACTIVE PARTICLES

DANIEL NOLIBÉ, HENRI METIVIER, ROLAND MASSE and JACQUES LAFUMA

Commissariat à l'Energie Atomique, Département de Protection, Laboratoire de Toxicologie Expérimentale, Montrouge, France

Abstract—Pulmonary lavages *in vivo* after inhalation of $^{239}PuO_2$ were conducted using more than 100 baboons. Results have permitted the definition of optimal conditions of lavage. It was shown that both lungs can be lavaged during the same sitting, and that the procedure could be applied up to 3 months after exposure with a significant efficiency. The treatment must be repeated several times because only 10–15% of the lung burden is removed during one sitting.

With a schedule of ten bilateral bronchopulmonary lavages (at days 1, 4, 9, then once a week) 58% of initial lung burden is removed. In addition, up to 30% is removed by an accelerated natural clearance after lavage. No chronic histological or physiological alterations of the lungs were observed after this procedure, which seems an efficient therapy for removing inhaled insoluble radionuclides.

EXPERIMENTAL studies in dogs (BAIR, 1974) and rats (METIVIER *et al.*, this Symposium, pp. 583–594) have shown that deposition of plutonium dioxide at doses above 300 nCi/g of lung caused early death due to inflammatory reactions, oedema, haemorrhage and necrosis of the lung tissue. At doses between 50 and 300 nCi/g of lung, death was due to respiratory insufficiency resulting from extensive fibrosis or interstitial pneumonitis (MASSE *et al.*, 1975). At doses below 50 μCi/g the incidence of neoplasia was more than 50% (LAFUMA *et al.*, 1974). In baboons early lung pathology appeared with initial lung burdens lower by a factor of 3 than in rodents or dogs (METIVIER *et al.*, 1974a).

Therefore it is particularly important to attempt a rapid removal of the retained particles, but previous techniques have not been successful (TOMBROPOULOS, 1964) and only bronchopulmonary lavage seems an effective therapy (MCCLELLAN *et al.*, 1972). For several years we have studied the effectiveness of this procedure on monkeys (KUNZLE-LUTZ *et al.*, 1970; NOLIBÉ, 1973a and b). Our research on lavage parameters and studies of effectiveness of the procedure are reported here. Lavage was first extended to the whole lung during the same sitting and the consequences on effectiveness observed. After determination of efficiency at different times following inhalation exposure the procedure was then repeated. In order to determine the schedule of treatment several bronchopulmonary lavage schedules, more or less delayed, were tested. Finally, effects of bronchopulmonary lavages on lung physiology, histology and translocation of insoluble radioactive particles were discussed.

MATERIAL AND METHODS

The experiments were conducted using baboons (*Papio papio*) of 4–10 kg body weight. As premedication acepromazine, 0.5 mg/kg, was given intramuscularly then anaesthesia was induced by chlorhydrate phencyclidine, 2 mg/kg, initially.

Procedures of $^{239}PuO_2$ inhalation have been reported previously (METIVIER *et al.*, 1974b). Dusts were administered by nose only or by tracheal catheter. $^{239}PuO_2$ particles ($\rho = 11.4$) had a count median aerodynamic diameter (CMAD) of 2.06 μm ($\sigma = 1.28$) for a real diameter of 0.6 μm; oxide was obtained by burning peroxide at 1000°C. After exposure the animals were housed in metabolism cages and faeces collected daily and measured. Radioactivity of the lavage fluid was measured and cell counts were performed on an aliquot.

Inhaled activity was determined, *in vivo*, initially and at time of lavage, by X-ray counting of ^{239}Pu daughters using a proportional counter (LANSIART and MORUCCI, 1964). The results were checked at death by summing the faecal, sacrifice lung burden, and lavage fluid activities to obtain the initial lung burden activity. Faecal activity for days 1–4 was not included. Ninety per cent of baboons had lung burdens ranging from 70 to 200 nCi/g of lung; only from 40 to 85% of the inhaled body burden was retained in deep lung, a variation due to differences in breathing patterns during exposure and upper respiratory clearance.

Arterial oxygen tension (pCO_2), arterial carbon dioxide tension (pCO_2) and acid pH were measured by a Radiometer BM S3 Analyzer on blood samples obtained by femoral arterial puncture. Heart rate, electrocardiograms, systemic arterial pressure and pulmonary frequency were measured with a physiograph DMP 4A.

Complete haemogram and blood chemical determinations were also established. At death, selected tissue samples from each lobe were prepared for light and electron microscopy.

STANDARDIZATION OF LAVAGE PROCEDURE

Pulmonary lavage was described by VAN GEMERT *et al.* (1957) and utilized in man with alveolar proteinosis by RAMIREZ *et al.* (1965). The right and left lungs were separated by a double lumen tube, and one lung was completely filled with isotonic saline solution while breathing was supported by the opposite lung. This basic method was slightly modified for use in the monkey. Pulmonary lavage was conducted under general anaesthesia. Proper positioning of the tube was checked by radiography. Before lavage, partial degassing was carried out in order to achieve denitrogenation, pure oxygen was passed for 5 min in the region to be washed then the tube was clamped from 3 to 5 min. The lung lavage technique is illustrated in Fig. 1. The saline solution at 38°C equal to the vital capacity was introduced slowly with a 100 ml syringe under controlled pressure; during this operation the monkey was tilted to a 25° head-up position. One minute after the operation the animal was tilted to a 25° head-down position and the liquid was drawn. Several successive irrigations were performed during one sitting whose total duration for one lung did not exceed 30–40 min.

Using this basic procedure, the effects of nature and pH of lavage fluid, degassing and number of irrigations on the effectiveness of one lavage were studied. Autoradiographs of lavage fluid after inhalation of plutonium dioxide showed that particles were rapidly phagocytized by alveolar macrophages (Table 1).

TABLE 1. PERCENT OF INHALED $^{239}PuO_2$ PARTICLES PHAGOCYTIZED BY ALVEOLAR MACROPHAGES

Time after inhalation	1 h	2 h	12 h	1 day	2	4	7	14	21	30	43
Percent of particles phagocytized	50	74	85	96	98	98	100	98	100	99	99

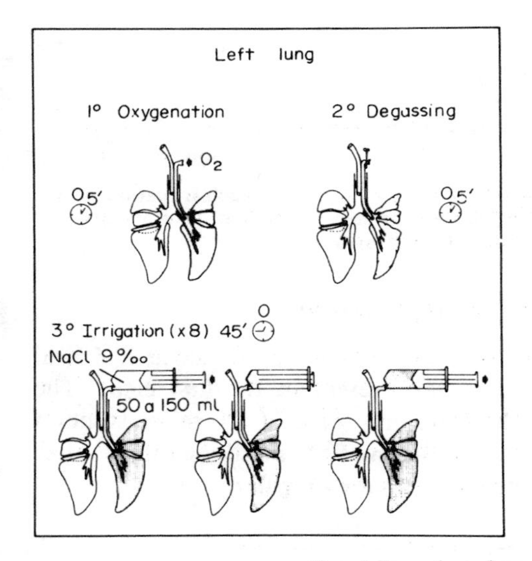

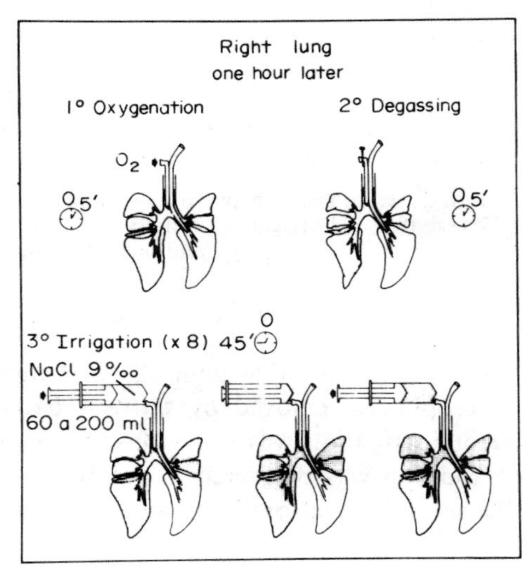

FIG. 1 Bronchopulmonary lavage procedure.

One day after inhalation 96 % of $^{239}PuO_2$ particles was found inside macrophages, and nearly 100 % at 43 days post-exposure. Lack of free particles in alveoli was seen with large variations of lung burdens (SANDERS and ADEE, 1968) despite the toxicity of $^{239}PuO_2$ particles on macrophages (NOLIBÉ, 1973c). The relative percentages of total number of macrophages and total activity removed during a lavage with thirteen successive irrigations are plotted for each irrigation in Fig. 2. The activity removed is proportional to the number of macrophages recovered in the fluid, except for the first lavage in which activity is more important: removal of macrophages with PuO_2 particles in the upper part of the tracheobronchial tree should be more rapid. In view of this result, the number of macrophages removed (from animals not exposed to PuO_2) was used as a test of lavage effectiveness in experiments to determine an appropriate schedule: no. of irrigations, nature and pH of washing fluid, oxygenation and gas absorption.

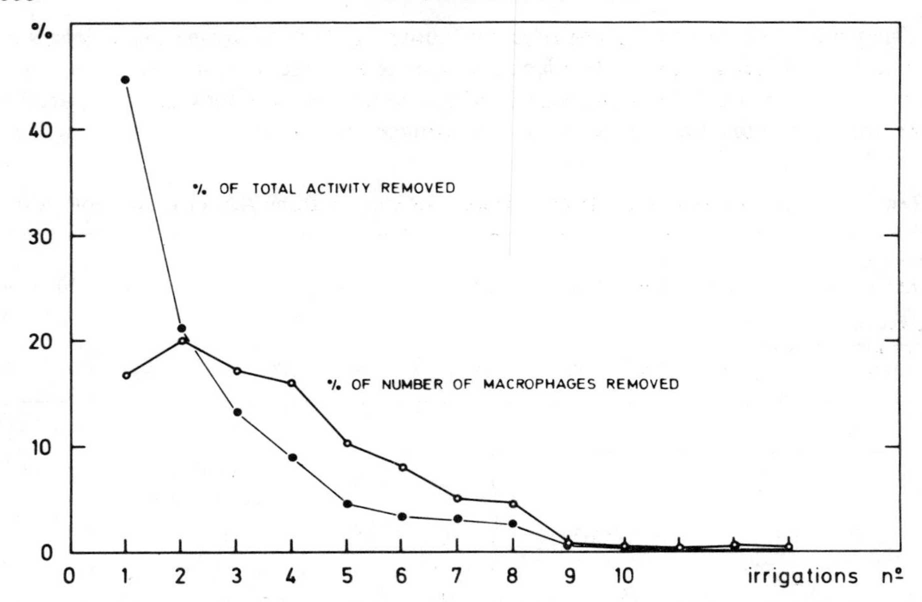

FIG. 2. Relationship between macrophages and radioactivity removed by each irrigation of a lavage (for each irrigation, activity and macrophages are expressed in per cent of total activity and macrophages removed by a lavage).

Number of Irrigations During a Lavage

Figure 3 shows that going beyond eight irrigations was not useful since 97.5% of macrophages removed by thirteen irrigations was present in the first eight. The second irrigation was more effective than the first: only 75% of the saline solution introduced was recovered in the first one and more than 95% in all the others; after the second irrigation the number of macrophages decreased regularly.

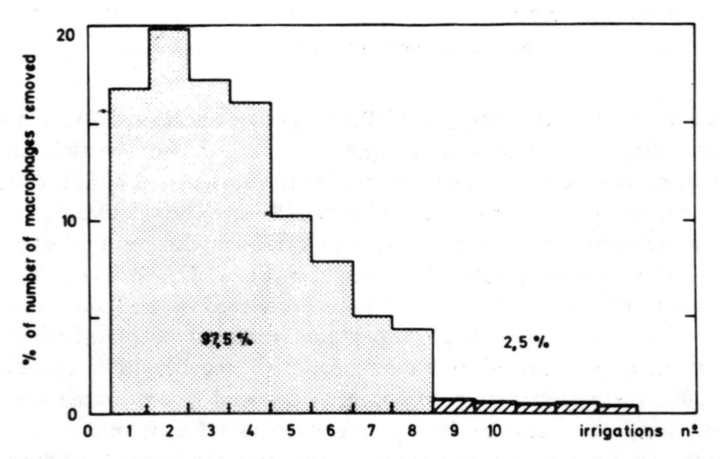

FIG. 3. Per cent of macrophages removed by each irrigation of a lavage (macrophages are expressed in per cent of total number of macrophages removed).

Nature of the Washing Fluid

In animal no. 1 eight irrigations were performed with isotonic saline 9 g/1000 ml and 30 days later with Hanks balanced solution. The inverse procedure was performed in animal no. 2. Five to eight times more cells were removed by isotonic saline solution (Table 2). This large difference in cell recovery seemed to be related to Ca^{++} and Mg^{++} that influenced the adherence of free cells to alveolar walls (BRAIN and FRANK, 1968).

TABLE 2. EFFECT OF NATURE OF WASHING FLUID ON NUMBER OF ALVEOLAR MACROPHAGES REMOVED

Animal no.	Time	Fluid of lavage	Number of macrophages removed ($\times 10^6$)
1	0	NaCl 9 g/1000 ml	49.6
	30 days	Hanks solution	15.8
2	0	Hanks solution	20.5
	30 days	NaCl 9 g/1000 ml	110.9

pH of Washing Fluid

The number of macrophages removed from right and left lungs by two different pH saline solutions were compared. During the same sitting the left lung was washed with an unbuffered (pH 6) isotonic saline solution and 1 h later the right lung was washed with isotonic saline buffered by sodium bicarbonate pH 8.8 as used in broncho-pulmonary lavage of human lungs by EKINDJIAN *et al.* (1972). Four times more cells were removed with the unbuffered solution. This result was verified, on the same animal, 30 days later with an inverse procedure (Table 3).

TABLE 3. EFFECT OF pH ON NUMBER OF ALVEOLAR MACROPHAGES REMOVED

		Number of alveolar macrophages removed ($\times 10^6$)	
		Left lung	Right lung
First lavage	isotonic saline pH 6	44	
	" " pH 8.8		11
(30 days later)			
Second lavage	isotonic saline pH 8.8	15	
	" " pH 6		59

Oxygenation and Gas Absorption

The lungs of the same animal were washed after oxygenation and degassing or without this treatment after a sufficient delay to eliminate the effect of the first lavage.

60×10^6 macrophages were obtained with oxygenation-degassing treatment (Fig. 4) and only 11×10^6 without. Thus it was shown that, after nitrogen washout by breathing in 100% oxygen and consumption of oxygen by clamping of the catheter, the liquid could reach the deep lung and alveoli.

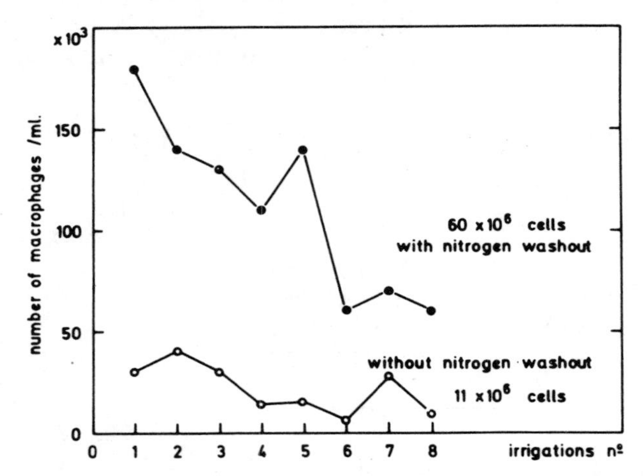

FIG. 4. Effect of degassing on the number of macrophages removed.

RESULTS

Extension of Bronchopulmonary Lavage to the Whole Lung

Nineteen baboons were lavaged once only, the animals were distributed into three groups in which the pulmonary volume treated during a sitting was one lobe (30%), one lung (60%) or two lungs. In each group, lavage was performed at different times post-exposure and the animals were sacrificed 1 day later. The mean effectiveness, in per cent of PuO_2 removed *versus* lung burden in the lavaged territory, was constant even if the volume treated during one sitting increased.

Single Bronchopulmonary Lavage at Various Times Post-exposure

Studies of effectiveness of a single lavage at various times post-exposure were performed with forty animals treated only once. It was observed (Fig. 5) that effectiveness decreased when the time interval between exposure and lavage increased. The important decrease during the first days after inhalation was due to removal of material initially deposited in the upper respiratory tract. Four days after exposure the fraction of the initial lung burden removed was 50% of that obtained after the first day; 1 month later 40% and 3 months later 25%. These data indicate that the lavage procedure could be applied up to 3 months with a significant removal of radioactivity, and showed that one lavage removed too small a fraction of the initial lung burden.

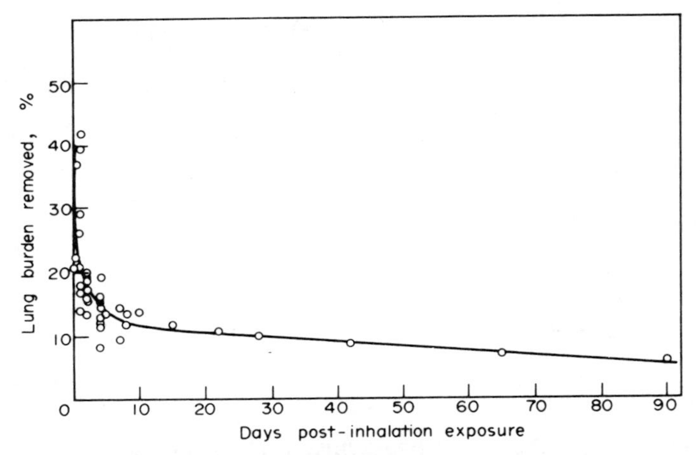

FIG. 5. Percentage of residual lung burden removed by a single lavage at various times post-exposure.

Multiple Bronchopulmonary Lavages

On a group of eleven animals lavages were repeated five times at days 4, 11, 18, 25 and 32 after inhalation. Mean effectiveness is reported in Table 4.

TABLE 4. EFFECTIVENESS OF REPEATED BRONCHOPULMONARY LAVAGES (11 ANIMALS)

Cumulative effectiveness in per cent of initial lung burden				
1 lavage	2 lavages	3 lavages	4 lavages	5 lavages
13.7 (8.2–20)	22.9 (15.9–27)	31.9 (22.3–37.7)	37.3 (26.8–43.8)	44.4 (36.5–48.7)

The total mean activity of $^{239}PuO_2$ recovered in the lavage fluid represented about 45% of the initial lung burden. These results are in good agreement with studies of MUGGENBURG *et al.* (1973). In order to diminish the delivered dose to the lung tissue the smallest period between two lavages was studied. Efficiency of lavage decreased to a lowest value when successive sittings were performed after a 6-h delay. A delay of 1 or 2 days significantly decreased effectiveness but after 4 or 7 days the fraction of the initial lung burden removed was kept at a high value. Effects of 2–3 days delay (fast treatment) and 1 week delay (slow treatment) are presented in Table 5 with a fifteen lavage schedule.

Slow treatment is significantly more efficient; the removed percentage of the lung burden decreased more rapidly with time in animals that had received several lavages than in baboons that had only one. The decrease was more important if the lavage schedule was accelerated (Fig. 6). The last five lavages had a weak effectiveness and were given up in the definitive schedule.

TABLE 5. COMPARATIVE EFFECTIVENESS OF TWO SCHEDULES OF FIFTEEN LAVAGES

	Mean initial lung burden per cent removed in lavages nos.		
	1 to 5	5 to 10	10 to 15
Fast treatment (3 animals)	41	7.1	3.2
Slow treatment (4 animals)	50.4	13	4.6

Effectiveness of an Optimal Treatment Schedule

Previous results allowed the optimal schedule to be chosen. It was tested on a group of nine animals in which inhalation was performed by tracheal catheter. Baboons were lavaged 10 times at days 1, 4, 9, then once a week; results are plotted on Fig. 7. A mean effectiveness of 58% was obtained with large individual variabilities from 47% to 67%; 21.6% was attributed to the first lavage; 26.9 to lavages 2–4 and only 9.6% were removed in the last five lavages. Comparison with survival times as a function of plutonium deposits in lung of controls at time of death (Fig. 8) suggests that lifespan should be significantly lengthened. Only three baboons were kept alive. The present situation is summarized in Table 6.

The other animals were sacrificed for pathological studies, three were sacrificed 60 to 200 days after the end of lavages and three after 12 to 14 months. One that was expected to die within 55 days was sacrificed after 200 days and no extensive pathology was observed. In the others, radiation pathology was less developed than in non-lavaged animals. Biological half-life of deep lung particles after the end of lavages was

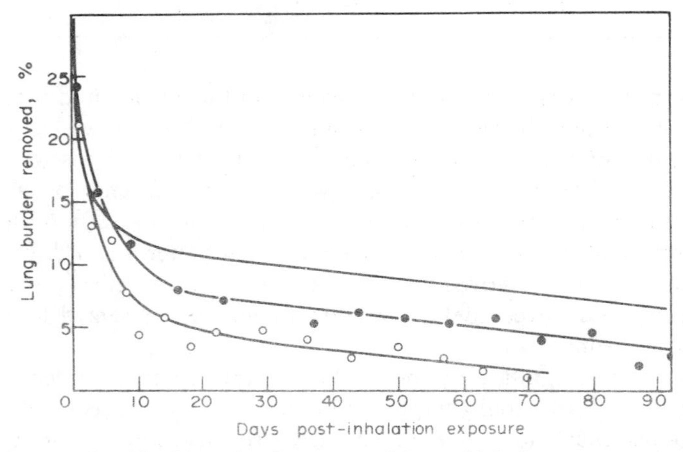

FIG. 6. Percentage of residual lung burden removed by multiple lavages at various times post-exposure, ——— single lavage, ○———○ fifteen lavages, at days 1–3–6–8–10–14–18–22 and once a week ●———● fifteen lavages, at days 1–4–9 and once a week.

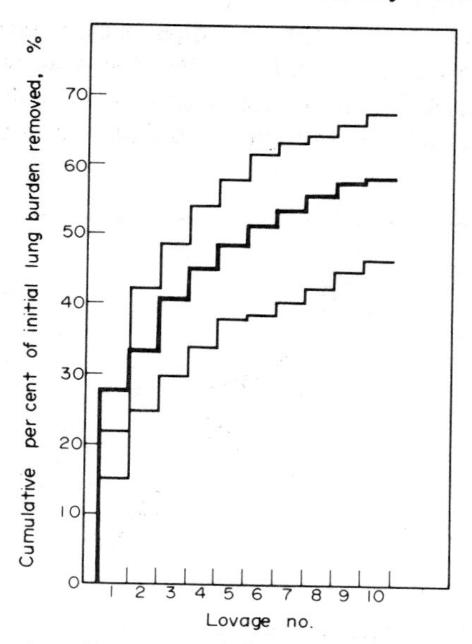

FIG. 7. Effectiveness of a ten-lavage schedule: lavages at days 1–4–9 then once a week (thick line: mean of nine baboons; thin line: ranges).

TABLE 6. SURVIVAL TIME AFTER LAVAGE

Initial lung burden (nCi/g)	Calculated survival time without lavage	Lung burden after lavage (nCi/g)	Calculated survival time with lavage	Observed survival time
60	500	20	1000	alive after 600 days
150	45	35	150	alive after 770 days
200	35	100	60	alive after 720 days

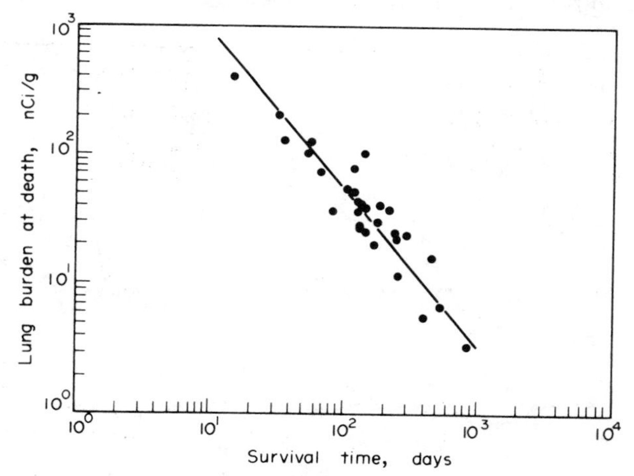

FIG. 8. Relationship between $^{239}PuO_2$ lung burden at death and survival time of baboons (activity is expressed by the ratio of lung activity, and weight of lung at death).

observed to equal those of controls: 500–900 days in three animals, but an important acceleration of the clearance half-time to 80–290 days was observed in three others. A greater lymph node burden increase was noticed in animals lavaged 15 times than in animals lavaged 5 times (Fig. 9) but again individual variations were observed.

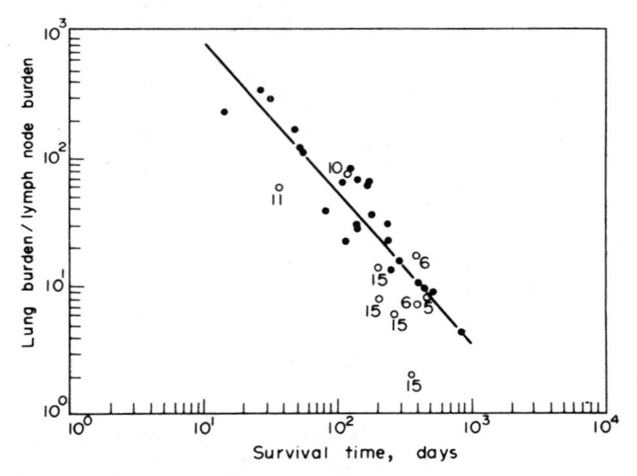

FIG. 9. Relationship between $^{239}PuO_2$ lymph node burden/lung burden ratio at death, and survival time of baboons. (● unlavaged baboons, ○ lavaged baboons with number of lavages).

Physiological Parameters during Lavage

Physiological studies were performed first during one lavage, secondly after an accelerated schedule of fifteen lavages within 70 days. Baseline values were performed on ten controls prior to lavage procedure.

Blood gas variations were observed during a lavage procedure (Fig. 10). During anaesthesia initial pO_2 85 mm Hg fell to 74 mm Hg, rose to 130 mm Hg when 100%

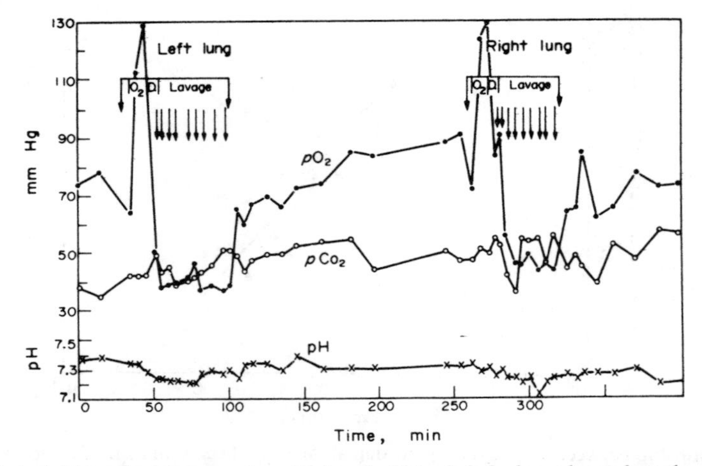

FIG. 10. Arterial blood gas tension (mm Hg) and pH (units) during a bronchopulmonary lavage.

oxygen was given and fell under 40 mm Hg when the left airway was clamped and during lavage of left lung. When the left airway was reopened the pO_2 increased to 65 mm Hg and was normal after 1 h of breathing room air. The same values were obtained during lavage of the right lung.

The arterial pH 7.39 in controls decreased to 7.25–7.20 during lavage and returned to 7.32 2 h after the end of left lavage, return to normal was slower after right lavage.

pCO_2 increased during lavage procedure and 2 h after complete lavage it had not returned to baseline. Heart rate decreased from 150 to 120 during anaesthesia then to 100 during lavage procedure, 1 h after lavage it returned to normal. No significant alterations were observed in the electrocardiogram tracings obtained during or following lavage procedure; respiratory frequency increased two- to three-fold during lavage but was normal 3 h after lavage.

^{131}I labelled albumin, or ^{24}Na was added to a 0.9% NaCl solution of lavage to measure the permeability of the alveolar membrane. Increased permeability was observed just after lavage but return to normal absorption was observed 2 days later.

During an accelerated schedule of fifteen lavages within 70 days, the mean recovery of lavage fluid remained constant for each lavage (90–95%) even when lavages were repeated every 2 days. Red and white blood cell counts, haematocrit, haemoglobin content, sedimentation rate showed no differences from controls.

pO_2 decreased and pCO_2 increased under baseline values when six lavages occurred during the first 14 days but were normal when lavages were performed only once a week, the same values were obtained in sham-lavage animals (anaesthesia, introduction of catheter, pure oxygen: 10 min, degassing: 10 min). However, arterial pH values for lavaged animals and sham lavaged animals were above the baseline values of controls between the 30th and 70th days of treatment. Blood gas values were similar to controls, 1, 6 or 12 months after lavage procedure.

Pathological Effects of Lavage

The short-term pathological effects of lavage were studied in control animals sacrificed immediately, 3 h, 6 h, or 1, 2 or 4 days after lavage of one lung, the non-lavaged lung was used as control. Similar studies were made on sham-lavaged animals. Long-term pathology was studied in animals sacrificed 3, 6 or 12 months after a complete and accelerated lavage procedure (fifteen lavages within 70 days).

Microscopic pathology. Immediately and a few hours after lavage, earlier effects on lung histology were haemorrhage, peribronchial and perivascular oedema, infiltration of neutrophilic granulocytes. Twenty hours after lavage some alveoli were filled with fibrinous exudate and foamy macrophages, infiltration of granulocytes and often megakaryocytes were still observed. None of these effects was extensive. After 2 days there were a large regression of these pathological signs and after 4 days the whole lungs were normal. No evidence of chronic lung pathology was observed several months after a complete schedule of fifteen lavages.

Ultrastructural pathology. During the first hours following lavage, changes in the ultrastructure occurred in alveolar epithelium, endothelium, basement membrane and interstitium. Three to six hours after lavage the alveolar epithelium was markedly swollen and even focally disrupted by areas of extensive swelling on pneumocyte I

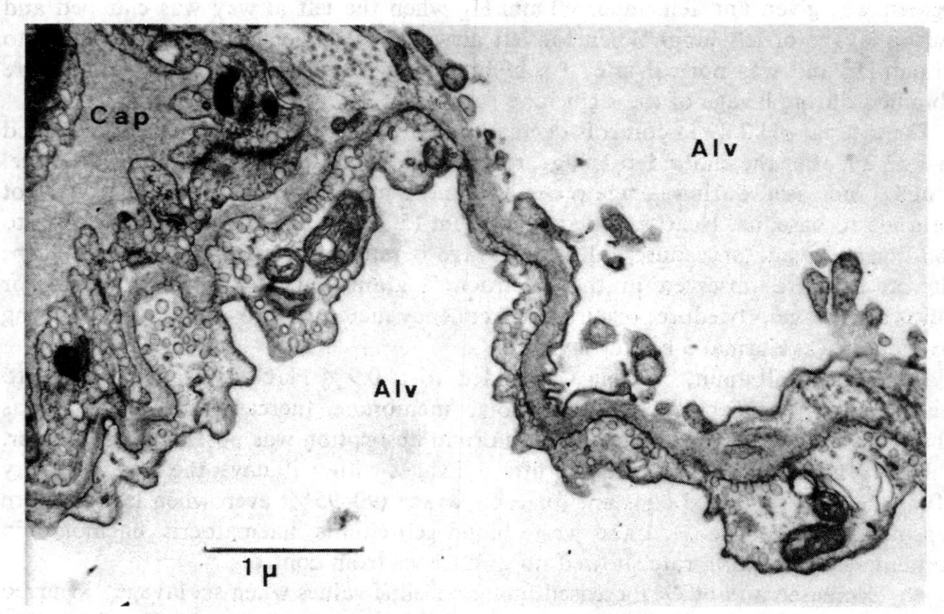

FIG. 11. Lung section 6 h after pulmonary lavage. Araldite section, uranyl lead staining. Destruction of pneumocytes I cytoplasm resulting in a bare basement membrane. Intense pinocytosis in endothelial cells. (Alv: alveolar space; Cap: capillary.)

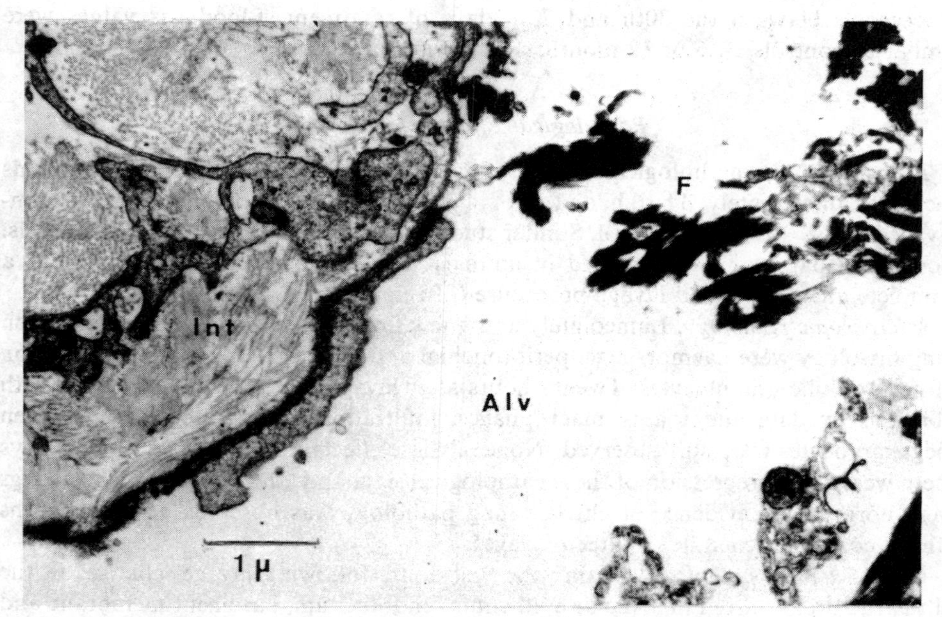

FIG. 12. Lung section 6 h after pulmonary lavage. Araldite section, uranyl lead staining. Formation of fibrin in alveolus in conjunction with destruction of pneumocyte I lining. Oedema in the interstitial tissue. (Alv: alveolar space. Int: interstitium. F: fibrin).

cytoplasm. Alterations were more important than those described by HUBER *et al.* (1971).

In many places large portions of bare basal membrane were seen due to disappearance of pneumocyte I or pneumocyte I cytoplasm (Fig. 11). Loss of lamellated bodies in pneumocytes II with occurrence of osmiophilic bodies of low density and increase of multivesicular bodies were often observed, some pneumocytes II were desquamed in alveoli. A strong pinocytosis was observed on capillary endothelial cells (Fig. 11). An interstitial oedema (Fig. 12) was also noticed with separation of the epithelial and endothelial basal membranes with sometimes accumulation of many dense bodies in the space thus created. Many alveoli were filled with fibrin (Fig. 12) or phagocytizing macrophages. Many of these observations were made on lungs after clamping of catheter and degassing in collapsed areas only; lavage could only increase this phenomenon. Ultrastructure was quite normal 48 h after treatment. No ultrastructural alterations were observed several months after lavage.

Comparison between animals sacrificed after plutonium inhalation and lavage or plutonium inhalation alone showed some interesting features (Figs. 13–14). It was observed, for similar cumulative doses, that lesions were less severe in treated animals. These differences are due to complete lack of hyaline membranes, lack of desquamative interstitial pneumonia, lack of metaplasic foci. Fibrosis was noticeably decreased in all the lobes in three out of six animals, and decreased in about half the lobes in the other animals, and remained important in one animal. In five out of six animals pneumocytes II hyperplasia and inflammatory infiltrations of the septa distributed in foci in the different lobes were still observed.

DISCUSSION

These results demonstrate that whole lung of baboons can be lavaged during the same sitting. This therapy may reduce PuO_2 lung burden more or less significantly according to the schedule used. In baboons receiving one lavage at various times post-exposure, decrease occurred in the fraction of the initial lung burden removed with increasing time intervals between exposure and lavage. The greatest effectiveness during the first week was directly related to the amount deposited in the upper respiratory tract and did not reflect removal from the deep lung. Some of the $^{239}PuO_2$ removed at the early times must have been removed more or less rapidly by natural processes, even if the animal had not been lavaged. After the first week the decrease was not important, and for lavages performed at 10, 30 and 90 days post-exposure effectiveness was respectively 12, 10 and 6%. These results have a great therapeutic importance and show that lavage can be performed a long time after inhalation with a good effectiveness. However, even if a significant percentage is removed after 3 months, the lavage therapy becomes less and less effective in reducing the total α dose delivered to the lungs. Lavages must be repeated several times because of the lack of effectiveness of one sitting and within the shortest time to reduce the delivered dose.

The time of the first intervention is difficult to specify. Early intervention may impair quick clearance of the upper tracheobronchial tree. However, our roentgenographic observations of lavages after inhalation of tantalum powder seem to indicate that particles are not drawn into the deep lung by the lavage fluid. We think that pul-

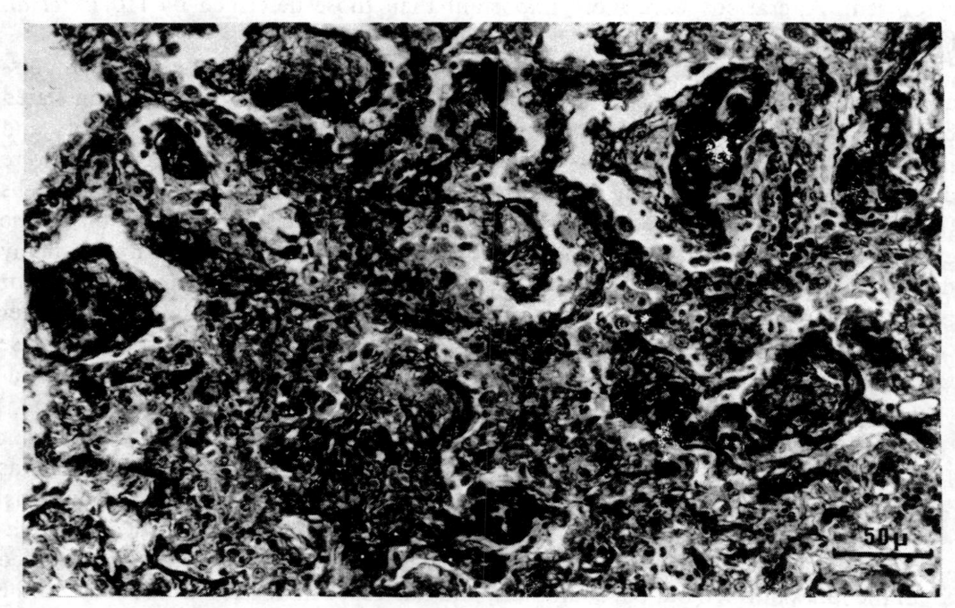

FIG. 13. Lung section 150 days after PuO_2 inhalation (no lavage); 3000 rad smeared dose (i.e. dose averaged over whole lung). Paraffin section, Mallory's haematoxylin stain. Hyaline membranes intra-alveolar fibrosis.

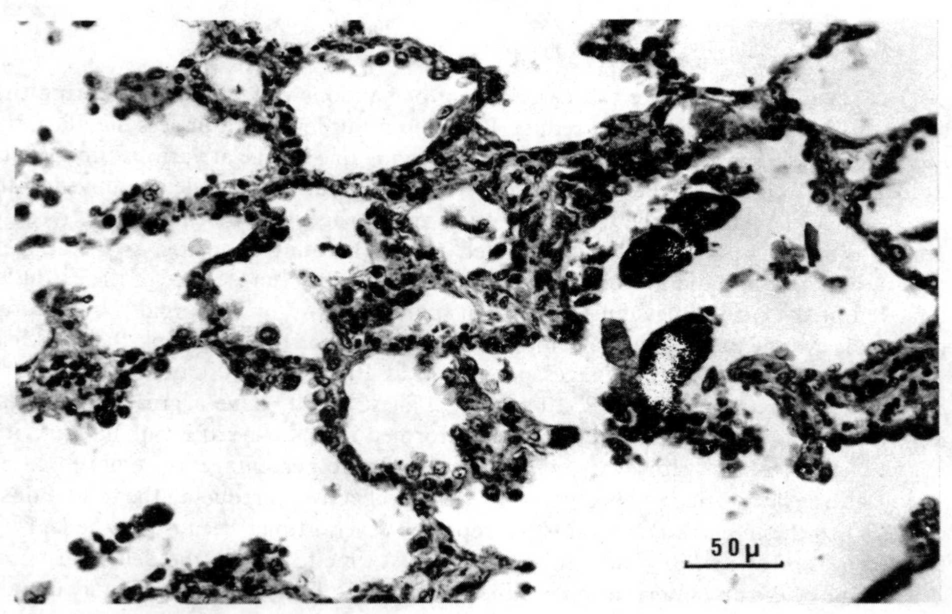

FIG. 14. Lung section 150 days after PuO_2 inhalation followed by pulmonary lavage; 3000 rad smeared dose. Paraffin section, HE stain. Lack of fibrosis and hyaline membrane with still discrete proliferation of pneumocyte II cells and inflammatory cells in the interstitium. A few giant cells.

monary lavage can be carried out 1 day after inhalation; this short delay is enough to allow for mucociliary clearance of a large fraction of the material deposited in trachea and bronchi.

In order to remove the greatest amount of the initial lung burden, lavages were repeated 15 times and several schedules tested. It was shown that an accelerated schedule decreased the percent of lung burden removed more rapidly than if animals had received one single lavage on the same day. With a slow schedule this decrease was less important but effective; it could be related to a decrease of the macrophages removed. A significant percentage of particles became inaccessible. This hypothesis is confirmed by an increase of the tracheobronchial lymph node burden in lavaged baboons (a more important increase was also noticed when lavages were more numerous) and by a decrease of deep lung clearance half-time in about 50% of lavaged animals. Ultrastructural lesions of alveolar epithelium and presence of fluid in the alveolus may increase interstitial clearance with two possibilities: excretion of particles at bronchi levels and elimination of particles by mucociliary clearance or retention in lymph nodes (CHRETIEN *et al.*, 1974).

Even when animals received fifteen lavages of the whole lung within 70 days (accelerated schedule) no chronic changes in pulmonary histology or physiology were seen from 3 weeks to 1 year after treatment. These results were also noticed by KYLSTRA (1958) and MUGGENBURG *et al.* (1972) after bronchopulmonary lavages of dogs.

We have only observed histological and physiological short-term alterations which disappear after 2 days, the most important are alterations of the alveolar epithelial lining. They are a consequence of atelectasia during degassing and anoxia during lavage; it is therefore recommended that degassing should not exceed 5 min. One day after lavage alveolar epithelium is reconstituted and no abnormal features are observed at long term.

The safety of repeated bronchopulmonary lavage is also supported by the low incidence of death during experimentation: only five deaths were registered after 800 lavages on more than 100 baboons, one from pulmonary haemorrhage, one from rupture of cuff and drowning, and three anaesthetic accidents. Another important feature is the observation that lesions were less important in lavaged animals than in PuO_2 controls (even if cumulative doses were similar). An important decrease of fibrosis and interstitial pneumonia was especially observed, probably related to removal of exudates liberated in alveoli by death of phagocytosing PuO_2 macrophages.

With a definitive schedule of ten bilateral bronchopulmonary lavages (at days 1, 4, 9, then once a week) a mean of 58% of initial lung burden is directly removed. This direct removal of $^{239}PuO_2$ is sometimes associated with an accelerated clearance. In favourable cases the whole of the elimination of the particles decreased the initial burden by a factor of 10. In spite of large individual variations this therapy results in a significant decrease of the radiation dose to the lungs that would result from accidental inhalation of insoluble radioactive particles. In that case, it was observed that the life-span of lavaged animals was significantly lengthened. This survival seemed longer than the calculated survival with the lung burdens at the end of lavages; it is due to a decrease of the development of radiation-induced disease, and accelerated post-lavage clearance; the importance of lavage therapy on neoplasia incidence is not known because of the long latency period of these diseases.

In conclusion, bronchopulmonary lavage is the only efficient therapy for removing inhaled insoluble radionuclides. It is a safe procedure, the main medical risk is associated with repeated anaesthesia of the subject. Before lavage the situation should be carefully studied to determine whether the hazard of radiation is greater than that of lavage.

REFERENCES

BAIR, W. J. (1974) *Advances in Radiation Biology* (edited by LETT, J. T., ADLER H. and ZELLE, M.) vol. 4, pp. 255–315. Academic Press, New York.

BRAIN, J. D. and FRANK, N. R. (1968) *J. appl. Physiol.* **25,** 63–69.

CHRETIEN, J., METIVIER, H., NOLIBÉ, D., LAFUMA, J. and MASSE, R. (1974) *Colloques Inst. natn. Santé Rech. méd.* **29,** 133–162.

EKINDJIAN, O. G., JARDILLIER, J. C., AKOUN, G. and AGNERAY, J. (1972) *Ann. Biol. clin.* **30,** 233–242.

HUBER, G. L., EDMUNDS, L. H. and FINLEY, T. H. (1971) *Am. Rev. resp. Dis.* **104,** 337–347.

KUNZLE-LUTZ, M., METIVIER, H., NOLIBÉ, D., SIMON-VERMOT, A., GIMBERT, J. L. and JOCKEY, P. (1970) *Archs Mal. prof.* **31,** 513–516.

KYLSTRA, J. A. (1958) *Acta physiol. pharmacol. neerl.* **7,** 163–221.

LAFUMA, J., NENOT, J. C., MORIN, M. MASSE, R., METIVIER, H., NOLIBÉ, D. and SKUPINSKI, W. (1974) *Experimental Lung Cancer, Carcinogenesis and Bioassays. International Symposium, Seattle, June 1974* (edited by KARBE, E. and PARK, J. P.) pp. 443-453. Springer, Berlin.

LANSIART, A. and MORUCCI, J. P. (1964) in *Assessment of Radioactivity in Man. Heidelberg, May 1964*, vol. 1, pp. 141–149. IAEA, Vienna.

MASSE, R., NOLIBÉ, D., FRITSCH, P., METIVIER, H. and LAFUMA, J. (1975) *Prog. resp. Res.* **8,** 74–90.

MCCLELLAN, R. O., BOYD, H. A., BENJAMIN, S. A., CUDDIHY, R. G., HAHN, F. F., JONES, R. K., MAUDERLY, J. L., MEWHINNEY, J. A., MUGGENBURG, B. A. and PFLEGER, R. C. (1972) *Hlth Phys.* **23,** 426.

METIVIER, H., NOLIBÉ, D., MASSE, R. and LAFUMA, J. (1974a) *Hlth Phys.* **27,** 512–514.

METIVIER, H., RATEAU, G., MASSE, R. and NOLIBÉ, D. (1974b) *Description d'un Dispositif Permettant la Contamination d'Animaux de Laboratoire par Inhalation d'Aérosols Radioactifs.* Note CEA–N–1722. Commissariat à l'Energie Atomique, France.

MUGGENBURG, B. A., MAUDERLY, J. L., PICKRELL, J. A., CHIFFELLE, T. L., JONES, R. K., LUFT, U. C., MCCLELLAN, R. O. and PFLEGER, R. C. (1972) *Am. Rev. resp. Dis.* **106,** 219–232.

MUGGENBURG, B. A., MIGLIO, J. J., MEWHINNEY, J. A., SLAUSON, D. O. and MCCLELLAN, R. O. (1973) *Inhalation Toxicology Research Institute Annual Report 1972–1973*, LF 46, pp. 255–260. Lovelace Foundation.

NOLIBÉ, D. (1973a) *C.r. hebd. Séances Acad. Sci. Paris, D* **276,** 225–228.

NOLIBÉ, D. (1973b) *C.r. hebd. Séances Acad. Sci. Paris, D* **276,** 681–684.

NOLIBÉ, D. (1973c) *C.r. hebd. Séances Acad. Sci. Paris, D* **276,** 65–68.

RAMIREZ, J. R., KIEFFER, R. F. and BALL, W. C. (1965) *Ann. int. Med.* **63,** 819–828.

SANDERS, C. L. and ADEE, R. R. (1968) *Science, N.Y.* **162,** 918–920.

TOMBROPOULOS, E. G. (1964) *Hlth Phys.* **10,** 1251–1257.

VAN GEMERT, A. G. M., KYLSTRA, J., VAN NOUYUS, F. and DEN HOTTER, G. (1957) *Acta physiol. pharmacol. néerl.* **5,** 445–455.

DISCUSSION

B. B. BOECKER: I note that the initial lung burdens were measured by external whole-body counting. How well did these measurements agree with the values obtained by summing the tissue and excreta data?

Dr NOLIBÉ: Values differ from 10 to 20% according to body weight.

O. G. RAABE: (i) In Table 1 you provide quantitative information obtained by autoradiography concerning phagocytosis. How were the cells and particles prepared and how were the quantitative measurements made? (ii) You describe ways in which the recovery of cells can be increased, using proper lavage fluid and N_2 washouts. Does the removal of plutonium also increase correspondingly?

Dr NOLIBÉ: (i) Sedimentation of cells was done under normal gravity in Petri dishes, cells were recovered on cover slips. The lavage fluid was put in Petri dishes at 37°C for 30 min; the attached cells were then fixed and covered with autoradiographic emulsion and the percentage of marked cells and free particles was thus obtained. The supernatant was controlled by counting after centrifugation. (ii) Recovery of PuO_2 does increase with the number of cells.

N. B. STOTT: The amount of activity administered was 70–100 nCi/g of lung. On a gram-for-gram comparison with human lung this represents roughly 7000 times the current I.C.R.P. permissible lung level. Have you any evidence that, at the lower levels of intake (which are much more likely to be encountered), your removal efficiencies will be maintained?

Dr NOLIBÉ: Rate of PuO_2 recovery was found to be independent of dose, between 2 and 200 nCi/g lung. Since cytotoxicity increases septal passage it can be predicted that lung lavage will be at least as efficient at lower doses.

M. LIPPMANN: By what mechanisms can lavage "provoke" clearance?

Dr NOLIBÉ: First, lavage increases particle entry into the interstitium as a result of pneumocytes type 1 lesions and, second, fluid movements push the particles either via the lymphatic ducts to the lymph nodes or beneath the bronchial mucosa through which they can be re-excreted at some specific places.

L. MAGOS: Plutonium dioxide has a wide range of dose–effect relationships ranging from early death from inflammation to neoplasm. Why did you choose such a high dose in your experiments which either caused early death or interstitial pneumonitis? Can you extrapolate the effect of lavage to lower doses? Why did you not use a dose which can cause only neoplasm, as earlier lecturers showed that plutonium dioxide can be measured at this low level?

Dr NOLIBÉ: The experiments were started 5 years ago. This paper describes the lavage procedure and its beneficial effects on acute and subacute lesions. Data cannot be extrapolated to lower doses and neoplasms. We expect to answer the question on the effects of lavage on Pu-induced lung neoplasms in baboons during the next 10 years!

H. SMITH: You have demonstrated that bronchopulmonary lavage is effective in experimental animals. However, one has to persuade the clinician that the procedure is safe. Since the technique involves multiple anaesthesia, would you comment upon the anaesthetic risk?

Dr NOBILÉ: I think, in fact, that is the main risk, as is stated in the paper. We carried out about 100 lavages. There were five mortalities, one due to a rupture of the cuffs of the apparatus and subsequent drowning, one by haemorrhage and three probably due to the anaesthetics. But I must say that I am not competent on a clinical level to discuss the risks of anaesthesia. Obviously this will be studied by the team which is now responsible for applying this therapy in the case of accidents. You obviously have to weigh up which risk is more dangerous—the inhalation or the treatment? All we can say is that the number of accidents was as shown—now it is up to the medical team to decide.

V. PRODI: Do you think that the lavage technique is ready to be applied to humans in the case of serious inhalation accident?

Dr NOLIBÉ: I do think so. We have discussed with clinicians the application of this technique to accidental inhalations. The therapy has already been applied by R. O. McClellan in a case of human accident. The problem is now to bring patients and clinicians to accept repeated lavages which are necessary in serious inhalation accidents.

LUNG RESPONSE TO LOCALIZED IRRADIATION FROM PLUTONIUM MICROSPHERES

E. C. ANDERSON, L. M. HOLLAND, J. R. PRINE and R. G. THOMAS

Los Alamos Scientific Laboratory, University of California, New Mexico, U.S.A.

Abstract—Uniform spherical 10-μm diameter particles of ZrO_2 ceramic, containing various concentrations of PuO_2, have been injected into the jugular vein of Syrian hamsters with subsequent permanent lodgement in the lung capillaries. The number of particles injected has varied from 2000 to 2 000 000 and the specific activity has been from 0.16 to 59 pCi/sphere so that lung burdens range from 0.2 to 700 nCi. To date, approximately 3000 hamsters have been committed to the experiment and two-thirds have died—the expected rate for normal animals. Little biological damage has been observed, and only five primary lung tumours have been found that may be due to radiation delivered to the lung. To provide a comparison to more uniform radiation, soluble polonium has also been instilled intratracheally. Results from the microspheres suggest that localized lung irradiation alone is not sufficient cause for tumour induction and is much less hazardous than diffuse exposure.

INTRODUCTION

The process of tumorigenesis is complicated: the mechanisms involved are not well known and are being pursued vigorously. That irradiation of biological tissues under certain conditions will elicit various forms of cancer has been known for many years. These malignant transformations from normal tissue have been the result of both external radiation and internally deposited radionuclides. Among the latter, plutonium is generally regarded as one of the most hazardous *in vivo* radiation sources, whether deposition is in the lung following inhalation (BAIR and THOMPSON, 1974) or in the skeleton and liver following administration of soluble forms (MAYS and DOUGHERTY, 1972). Their experimental studies used the beagle dog as a test subject and doses far exceeding the current guidelines for ^{239}Pu, both for the occupationally exposed and for the general population. Many humans who were occupationally exposed in the 1940s and who still carry measurable lung burdens are being followed to see if they indicate an increased incidence of lung neoplasia (HEMPLEMANN *et al.*, 1973). To date, even though certain lung burdens exceed the recommended permissible value and have been maintained for 30 years, no primary cancers have been observed that could be attributable to exposure to plutonium. Thus, there is a data gap between large doses which produce lung tumours in dogs and low doses (comparable to current guidelines) which have produced no detectable damage in humans.

The primary purpose of these studies was to administer particulate plutonium sources to the lung using a sufficient number of variables with regard to total dose and dose rate to help define more clearly the relationships between these variables and the incidence of lung cancer. A unique method of lodging radioactive particles in the lung capillaries for the lifetime of the animal was chosen to enable calculation of the localized dose around these particles and to result in a well-defined pattern of dose *vs.* tumour incidence. The use of a few particles would assist immensely in defining the "hot-particle" problem in cancer induction, and the administration of large numbers of particles would give a comparison with the diffuse dose which resembles more closely the pattern following inhalation. The results of these studies have wide and important practical implications regarding the use of nuclear power, particularly where plutonium breeder reactors are involved. Since the experiments involve comparison of particulate *vs.* diffuse irradiation, it is hoped that the pertinent results can be extrapolated to man.

METHODS

The radionuclides of choice (plutonium-238, plutonium-239, promethium-147, cobalt-57) were dispersed in ceramic spheres of ZrO_2 of 10-μm diameter. Both sphere diameter and specific activity were very uniform, the coefficients of variation of these parameters being less than 2%. The spheres were injected into the jugular vein of Syrian hamsters, from which they randomly lodged in the lung capillaries, and served as discrete sources of irradiation to lung tissue. The spheres are plainly visible under the microscope and provide ZrO_2 markers for the regions irradiated, even though the plutonium content corresponds to particles of respirable size. Particle distribution within the lung tissue is extremely uniform (ANDERSON *et al.*, 1974).

The microspheres were prepared by a modification of the sol–gel process developed by the Oak Ridge National Laboratory and others for fuel elements (MCBRIDE, 1967). Very uniform particles were obtained by using equipment such as described by FULWYLER (1971). A 40-μm diameter stream of aqueous ZrO_2 sol was injected into a 1-mm stream of 2-ethyl-l-hexanol in coaxial laminar flow. The 2-ethyl-l-hexanol contained 0.1% NH_4OH and 0.05% Triton X-100, a surfactant. The sphere size was determined by sol concentration, pressure differential between sheath and core streams, and frequency of the sonic oscillator controlling the rate of droplet formation. To prepare 10-μm ceramic spheres, the following conditions typically were used: sol concentration 5.34 g/l., sheath pressure 34 p.s.i.g. (pound/inch^2, gauge) core pressure 55 p.s.i.g. and oscillator frequency 22kH.

Approximately 8×10^7 droplets were produced in about 1 h running time from 40 ml of sol. They were collected in 6 l. of 2-ethyl-l-hexanol and, after 2 h dehydration time with constant gentle stirring, the gelled microspheres were collected on a 47-mm diameter, 14-μm pore nylon Millipore filter. They were then washed repeatedly with heptane to remove the 2-ethyl-l-hexanol and, after brief drying, were transferred to a 50-ml centrifuge cone and suspended three times in absolute methanol. The product was transferred to an alpha-alumina crucible and dried overnight at 200°C. Firing started at 200°C and increased to 1000°C by 200° increments at hourly intervals. Final temperature was maintained for 2 to 3 h. The spheres underwent the following size transformations in the process: freshly gelled 29- to 30-μm diameter; heptane-washed 21- to 22-μm diameter; methanol-washed 18- to 19-μm diameter; and fired 10-μm diameter.

The diameter of the spheres was determined from measurement of the lattices which the spheres often form when a suspending solvent evaporates from a monolayer. The spheres became hexagonally closepacked to a high degree of accuracy, and measurements could be made over as many as 20 sphere diameters with attendant reduction in optical errors of boundary identification. Repeated measurements under these conditions showed coefficients of variation of less than 1% on measurement of the average sphere diameter. The average sphere diameters ranged from 9.90 to 10.87 μm over 11 batches. The mean was 10.28, with a coefficient of variation (CV) of 3.2% among batches, corresponding to a mean volume of 571 μm^3. Although no direct measurement of the particle mass was made, it was calculated from the total mass generated and the frequency of droplet formation (number of droplets formed) to range from 2.62 to 2.98 ng for the 11 batches, with a mean of 2.80 ng and a CV of 4.3% among batches. From the volumes and masses arrived at above, the average sphere density of each batch was calculated to range from 4.25 to 5.60 g/cm^3, similar to the reported density for ZrO_2.

Because cobalt-57 emits a readily detectable gamma ray of approximately 140 keV and has a convenient half-life of approximately 270 days, it was used routinely as a radioactive tracer. It has no beta particle emission, and the radiation dose delivered to the animal from gamma emission is negligible compared to that from the "hot particles" themselves. Using this technique, the body burdens of injected hamsters could be determined readily by NaI (T1) crystal counting. The amount of radionuclide per sphere could be determined from the amount of radioactivity (plutonium-238, plutonium-239, promethium-147, cobalt-57) added to the ZrO_2 sol and the total number of particles generated and independently by direct radiation counts on known numbers of spheres. The amount of cobalt-57 generally used as a tracer was 0.5 pCi/sphere.

The experiments completed to date are defined in Table 1. The number of spheres injected was varied from 2000 to 1 600 000 per hamster, and the specific activity from 0.07 to 59 pCi/sphere. With the number of variables shown, the lung burdens have been as low as 0.14 and as high as 710 nCi/lung; this latter value represents an alpha particle disintegration rate of 1.67×10^6/min. In a few cases, adjunct materials were added intratracheally to the lung to study any possible synergistic effects. These are shown in the last column of Table 1. Using both male and female Syrian hamsters, the injections were performed at approximately 90 days of age. When the animals were moribund and death was imminent, they were sacrificed with chloroform. All animals were examined grossly upon death, and selected tissues were examined for histopathological changes resulting from the radiological insult. The lungs were perfused with 10% formalin *in situ*, and other organs were preserved in formalin for later slide preparation and staining with haematoxylin-eosin.

RESULTS AND DISCUSSION

Mean survival times given in Table 1 were determined from probit plots of fractional survival *vs.* time. Interpretation of microsphere effect on hamster survival is complicated by changes which have occurred during the course of these experiments. This is demonstrated in Fig. 1 in which two distinct survival curves are shown. The upper curve represents earlier experiments (1971–1972 exposures) and shows a possible slight

TABLE 1. SUMMARY OF EXPOSURES OF HAMSTERS TO INTRAVENOUS PLUTONIUM MICROSPHERES

Date of exposure	Number of animals	Spheres per animal	Specific activity (pCi/sphere)	Lung Burden (nCi)	Mean survival time (days of age[a])	Other insults
1971 May	69	2000	0.07	0.14	630	
May	71	2000	0.22	0.44	795	
May	74	2000	0.91	1.82	765	
June	71	2000	0.42	0.84	670	
June	71	2000	4.30[b]	8.60	635	
June	71	2000	13.30[b]	26.00	620	
June	72	2000	59.00[b]	118.00	650	
August	71	2000	2.10[b]	4.20	720	
August	47	10 000	0.22	2.20	830	
November	154	6000	4.30[b]	26.00	720	
December	148	6000	59.00[b]	354.00	615	
1972 February	142	6000	0.22	1.30	695	
July	20	1 600 000	0.07	112.00	715	
July	34	300 000	0.42	126.00	655	
December	30	6000	8.90[b]	53.00	(350)	Cytoxin
1973 April	109	60 000	0.91	55.00	490	
April	107	80 000	8.90[b]	710.00	395	
April	102	80 000	2.10[b]	168.00	515	
May	104	80 000	0.22	18.00	680	
June	37	400 000	0.42	170.00	505	
June	109	150 000	0.06	9.00	455	
July	97	500 000	0.03	15.00	470	
July	44	50 000	0.91	45.00	440[c]	
October	26	900 000	0.016	14.00	480	
October	15	500 000	0.016	8.00	395	
November	53	40 000	0.06	2.40	385	
November	52	20 000	0.06	1.20	450	
1974 January	52	20 000	0.19	3.80	390	
January	51	40 000	0.19	7.60	385	
January	60	60 000	1.60	96.00	455	$C_2F_2Cl_4$
May	76	60 000	2.10[b]	126.00	450	Zymosan
May	71	30 000	0.19	11.00	550	Zymosan

[a] Animals exposed at age 100 days.
[b] Plutonium-238; all others contain plutonium-239.
[c] Weanlings exposed at age 30 days.

decline in survival time with increasing dose, but the effect is not statistically significant. The highest dose of 360 nCi was obtained by exposure to 6000 microspheres of specific activity 59 pCi/sphere. It is estimated that about 2% of the total lung mass was irradiated in this experiment. The median dose to the cells at risk is calculated to be 650 krad/yr; averaging the dose over the entire lung mass gives a yearly dose of about 36 krad. The cluster of four exposures near 100 nCi was obtained by a variety of conditions, ranging from 2000 to 1 600 000 spheres of specific activities 0.07 to 59 pCi/sphere. The fraction of lung irradiated varied from about 1% to nearly 100%, with no detectable effect on survival.

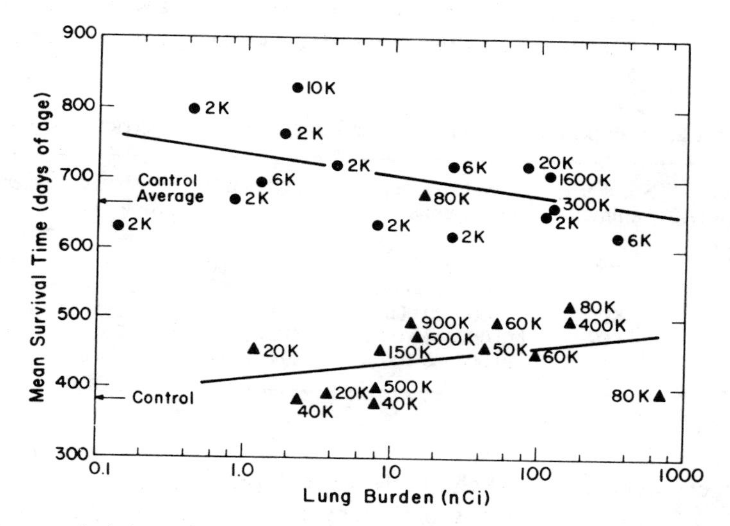

FIG. 1. Mean survival times for experimental hamsters as a function of lung burden (in nCi of plutonium). The two subgroups correspond to different suppliers. The number beside each point is the number of microspheres administered: (—●—) first supplier and (—▲—) second supplier.

Absence of radiation-induced life shortening is also suggested by the 1973–74 exposures (the lower curve of Fig. 1). The apparent increase of survival with dose is not statistically significant. The highest of all exposures, 720 nCi from 80 000 spheres (about 20% of lung irradiated) of activity 8.8 pCi/sphere, may show significant life shortening. The cause of the rather abrupt change in mean survival time in early 1973 has not been identified, and no detectable pathology is associated with the shortened survival. During a transition period, hamsters obtained from both suppliers showed both survival times, making the effect unlikely to be a strain difference.

To date there have been only five primary lung tumours disclosed in a total of 846 experimental hamsters and none in 140 controls (SMITH *et al.*, 1976). Of great importance at this time is the application of these data to some of the current vibrations related to the "hot-particle" controversy over plutonium-239. It has been stated by TAMPLIN and COCHRAN (1974) that a single microscopic particle with alpha activity greater than 0.07 pCi will produce lung tumours with a probability of 5×10^{-4}, independent of particle activity and number of particles. The experiments reported here using the hamster as a test model would definitely rule out such a hypothesis. In fact, if all the data collected to date are summarized as in Table 2, the fallacy in the Tamplin–Cochran prediction can be observed. Only the particles that meet their criteria of hot particles (0.07 pCi) have been included. The animals have been grouped by time since injection, number of spheres per animal, and specific activity per particle. The predicted number of tumours (Tamplin–Cochran model) was calculated by multiplying the total number of spheres by 5×10^{-4}. For the 1565 hamsters reported in Table 2, there were 88 000 000 spheres injected, and the predicted number of tumours would be 44 000 compared to the five that have been observed. This information is concrete evidence that this type of modelling is quite erroneous. The enormous discrepancy between prediction and experimental result appears to render the Tamplin–Cochran model and the GEESAMAN (1968) hypothesis completely untenable.

TABLE 2. TUMOURS PREDICTED BY TAMPLIN–COCHRAN "HOT-PARTICLE" MODEL

Duration of experiment (wk)	Number of animals	Spheres per animal	Total spheres	Predicted tumours[a]	Specific activity (pCi/sphere)
178	570	2000	1 140 000	580	0.07–59.00
173	54	300 000–1 600 000	42 000 000	21 000	0.07–0.42
95–169	527	6000–20 000	3 900 000	1950	0.22–59.00
87	146	150 000–400 000	31 000 000	15 500	0.06–0.42
39–48	268	20 000–60 000	10 000 000	5000	0.06–1.60

[a] By the Tamplin–Cochran model.

These experiments also shed light on the general question of the relative hazards of diffuse *vs.* localized alpha irradiation of the lung. Experiments by LITTLE and co-workers (1970, 1973) confirmed at our Laboratory show that exposure of the hamster lung to instilled solutions of polonium-210 results in very high tumour incidence, approaching 100% for lung burdens of 200 nCi. The results reported here show that localized irradiation by static particles is virtually non-tumorigenic even at burdens up to 700 nCi in the same animal. The reason for this surprising impotence is not known, but presumably it lies in the differences in radiation dose distribution in the two cases. In any event, the results indicate that hazard estimation based on the assumption of uniform exposure is likely to be conservative when applied to "hot spot" exposures of the lung by insoluble PuO_2 particles.

Future experiments will include the continued use of possible synergistic substances to hasten the process of lung carcinogenesis. It is thought that through such experimentation a better idea of the mechanisms involved in tumorigenesis may be uncovered. Localized alpha irradiation alone does not appear to be sufficient to bring about malignant transformation, and by studying additional insults that will mediate such alterations we stand to learn more of the basic processes. The added insults used to date (Table 1) have not served to increase the incidence seen with "hot particles" alone.

Acknowledgement—This work was performed under the auspices of the U.S. Energy Research and Development Administration.

REFERENCES

ANDERSON, E. C., HOLLAND, L. M., PRINE, J. R. and RICHMOND, C. R. (1974) *Experimental Lung Cancer* (edited by KARBE, E. and PARK, J. F.) pp. 430–442. Springer, Berlin.

BAIR, W. J. and THOMPSON, R. C. (1974) *Science, N.Y.* **183,** 715–722.

FULWYLER, M. J. (1971) U.S. Patent Application Serial No. 123362(70).

GEESAMAN, D. P. (1968) *An Analysis of the Carcinogenic Risk from an Insoluble Alpha-Emitting Aerosol Deposited in Deep Respiratory Tissue.* Report UCRL-50387. Lawrence Livermore Laboratory, University of California.

HEMPELMANN, L. H., LANGHAM, W. H., RICHMOND, C. R. and VOELZ, G. L. (1973) *Hlth Phys.* **25,** 461–479.

LITTLE, J. B., GROSSMAN, B. N. and O'TOOLE, W. F. (1970) *Morphology of Experimental Respiratory Carcinogenesis* (edited by NETTESHEIM, P., HANNA, M. G., Jr. and DEATHERAGE, J. W., Jr.). AEC Symposium Series 21, U.S. Atomic Energy Commission report CONF-700501, National Technical Information Service, U.S. Department of Commerce, Springfield, Virginia.

LITTLE, J. B., GROSSMAN, B. N. and O'TOOLE, W. F. (1973) *Radionuclide Carcinogenesis* (edited by SANDERS, C. L. BUSCH, R. H., BALLOU, J. E. and MAHLUM, D. D.) pp. 119–137. AEC Symposium Series 29, U.S. Atomic Energy Commission report CONF-720505, National Technical Information Service, U.S. Department of Commerce, Springfield, Virginia.

MAYS, C. W. and DOUGHERTY, T. F. (1972) *Hlth Phys.* **22,** 793–801.

MCBRIDE, J. P. (1967) *Laboratory Studies of Sol-Gel Processes at the Oak Ridge National Laboratory.* Report ORNL-TM-1980. Oak Ridge National Laboratory.

SMITH, D. M., PRINE, J. R. HOLLAND, L. M. and ANDERSON, E. C. (1976) in *Biological and Environmental Effects of Low-Level Radiation.* Vol. II, pp. 121–129. International Atomic Energy Agency, Vienna.

TAMPLIN, A. R. and COCHRAN, T. B. (1974) *Radiation Standards for Hot Particles. A Report on the Inadequacy of Existing Radiation Exposure of Man to Insoluble Particles of Plutonium and Other Alpha-emitting Hot Particles.* Natural Resources Defense Council, Washington, D.C.

DISCUSSION

D. K. CRAIG: In our ^{239}PuO: exposed dogs at Battelle, we see a very clear dose-related lymphopenia that is persistent, even at doses of the order of 1 nCi/g of dog lung. Have you seen any similar lymphopenia in the hamsters of this study?

Dr THOMAS: As far as lymphopenia is concerned, we just do not have the haematological data to show this. We are now doing some chromosome work on circulating lymphocytes but that is extremely difficult in the hamster.

O. G. RAABE: The Tamplin–Cochran model predicted an induction time of around 10 years before the formation of cancer caused by "hot" particles; do your hamsters normally live that long?

Dr THOMAS: This is important if you are of the school that believes it takes a certain length of time to cause cancer—obviously our hamsters don't live 10 years. If you are of the school that believes that it is a fraction of the life span that is governing, then the 10 years is inconsequential. I don't know the answer to this.

E. A. MARTELL: Is it not possible that, in these Los Alamos experiments using ceramic spheres with a minimum of 0.07 pCi of Pu per sphere, the α intensity is sufficiently high to over-irradiate the cells at risk? It should be noted that the local α intensities are some 10^8 to 10^9 times that of natural alpha radiation levels in the lungs of non-smokers and about 10^5 times that of insoluble radioactive smoke particles. Thus it is suggested that the very low incidence of cancer in these Los Alamos experiments indicates an overkill for such immobile "hot" particles, and that alpha radiation-induced tumours result from much lower alpha particle activities and dose rates. Such considerations may explain the higher tumour incidence for the Battelle Northwest Laboratory Pu inhalation studies.

Dr THOMAS: Yes.

D. K. CRAIG: At Battelle we have exposed rats to a very wide range of inhaled doses of a series of transuranium compounds, including $^{238}PuO_2$, $^{239}PuO_2$, $^{241}AmO_2$ and $^{244}CmO_2$, as well as more soluble compounds. We have observed a clear dose-related carcinogenic response from insoluble $^{239}PuO_2$ particles in the lung. As far as life span is concerned, we have observed an increase over the controls at the lower dose levels, with a progressive decrease in life span relative to the control animals as the dose increased. There is no doubt that it is possible to obtain lung cancers in rats from inhaled alpha-emitting particles, the type of cancer depending upon the dose level and the particular radionuclide involved. Exposures to the other materials are more recent and I am not as familiar with the histopathological results. The $^{238}PuO_2$ was more soluble than the very insoluble $^{239}PuO_2$, even though prepared in identical fashion. $^{244}CmO_2$ was very soluble, being rapidly translocated to the liver and bone of the rats.

E. P. RADFORD: Intravenous injection is clearly different from the inhalation route used in the Hanford experiments, where tumours were consistently observed. I would also draw attention to the recent report of LITTLE *et al.* (1973) who showed bronchial tumours in hamsters given polonium intratracheally at very low doses.

Dr THOMAS: Most of the hamster studies have not been by inhalation but by intratracheal instillation. There is a big difference between the traumatic insults of the two methods on the hamsters.

L. MAGOS: Have you found any difference in the data to show that hamsters are more resistant to chemical carcinogens than rats or mice?

Dr THOMAS: No. I think the reason the hamster was chosen arose from the results of Saffiotis' work with benzopyrene. You would think from chemical carcinogen studies that hamsters would be an ideal animal to study. Comparisons between animals like these that are sensitive to chemical carcinogens in the lung and animals like the dog have not yet been sufficient to yield results.

F. F. HAHN: We are suffering with the Syrian hamster at the Lovelace Foundation, but I think there can be valuable data derived from radiation carcinogenesis studies compared with chemical carcinogenesis studies in the Syrian hamster. If you look at chemical carcinogenesis studies and the studies of Dr Little with polonium there is a high incidence of lung tumours. Both of these instances usually involved repeated intratracheal instillations of material. I think there is something related to the repeated injury or the dose pattern in time or space that results from intratracheal injections that has something to do with development of tumours in the airway of Syrian hamsters.

Were the five tumours you noted in the study not concentrated in any dose level, but randomly scattered through all dose levels?

Dr THOMAS: Yes, that's right.

J. BRAIN: Isn't one of the hallmarks of your experiment the fact that the particles injected have practically no mobility? The normal processes of clearance concentration by macrophages and translocation to the bronchial epithelium are prevented. The particles are trapped in the pulmonary circulation. How does that affect the probability of carcinogenesis in your model?

Dr THOMAS: I think it is highly unusual for people to get 10-μm spheres in the jugular vein so I agree with you. I tried to make it clear that the movement that takes place after inhalation may very well have something to do with the formation of lung tumours. The problem is that the people at Lovelace have exposed hamsters by inhalation to plutonium dioxide and have the same results as we do. Is that not true?

F. F. HAHN: Yes, we have exposed hamsters by inhalation to both ^{238}Pu and ^{239}Pu dioxide using a pattern similar to that at Los Alamos, varying specific activity and the number of particles calculated to irradiate various portions of the lung. These studies are still in progress and tumours may develop in these animals, but to date we have not seen lung tumours in any of the animals, although we have had animals die with radiation pneumonitis. This has been done for one year and this is well past the time when Dr Little reported occurrence of tumours, in a matter of weeks to months. So this is inexplicable at the present time.

L. M. SWINBURNE: By the technique used, the main target tissue would seem to have been vascular endothelium. What were the types of tumours observed?

Dr THOMAS: The length of the alpha trace is approximately 45 μm in unit density tissue; is not that much longer than the endothelial linings of the capillaries? The five tumours were a haemangiosarcoma, an undifferentiated sarcoma, two mucinous adenocarcinomas and a benign adenoma.

M. KUSCHNER: Commenting on Dr Hahn's remarks, may I say that one can produce tumours in hamsters with a single large dose (such as 40 mg) of a chemical carcinogen, methylcholanthrene.

Commenting on Dr Brain's remark, may I say that the tumours in hamsters are often peripheral and that the bronchi are not peculiarly susceptible. The determinant of where tumours develop in these animal systems is where the dose is delivered.

The astonishing feature of Dr Thomas' paper is the apparent total lack of response to levels of radiation which should have produced, at the least, marked radiation fibrosis. Have you considered observing any immunological parameters in these animals?

Dr THOMAS: We are removing the thymus at one day in a series of hamsters. These will be exposed later in the same manner to see if the removal of the thymus cells will by any way allow them to develop lung tumours.

L. MAGOS: What is your further plan? Have you any hope to have some positive results from this work?

Dr THOMAS: The people who started working on these experiments had things very nicely predicted as to how many tumours would arise under a set of circumstances. They became very discouraged. I feel that the negative results in these experiments are extremely important, far more important than if we had 200 lung tumours. They are stimulating us to do immunological studies and allowing us to get at some of the mechanisms.

COMPARATIVE PULMONARY CARCINOGENICITY OF INHALED BETA-EMITTING RADIONUCLIDES IN BEAGLE DOGS*

F. F. HAHN, S. A. BENJAMIN, B. B. BOECKER, C. H. HOBBS, R. K. JONES, R. O. MCCLELLAN and M. B. SNIPES

Inhalation Toxicology Research Institute, Lovelace Foundation, Albuquerque, N.M., U.S.A.

Abstract—Beta-emitting radionuclides are important constituents of isotope inventories in light water reactors and may pose an inhalation hazard to industrial workers or the general population if they are released. To study the biological effects of such potential exposures, a series of life span studies was initiated in which beagle dogs were exposed to aerosols of relatively insoluble fused clay particles containing ^{90}Y, ^{91}Y, ^{144}Ce or ^{90}Sr. Groups of dogs exposed to each radionuclide received graded initial lung burdens of radioactivity. When combined with the varied physical half-lives of the four radionuclides, this resulted in a wide variety of radiation doses and dose patterns to the lung. Deaths (> 640 days after exposure) were generally associated with pulmonary neoplasia in dogs that inhaled ^{91}Y, ^{144}Ce or ^{90}Sr. These dogs had cumulative lung doses to death >20 000 rads. Exposure to ^{144}Ce or ^{90}Sr with dose rates that decreased slowly induced pulmonary haemangiosarcomas. Pulmonary irradiation from ^{91}Y, with a rapidly decreasing dose rate, resulted in pulmonary epithelial tumours. No malignant lung tumours have been seen within 1540 days after exposure to ^{90}Y. The animals in the main studies have been observed for 1342 to 2756 days after exposure.

INTRODUCTION

The use of radioactive materials for scientific and industrial purposes has created a need for better understanding of the biological effects of ionizing radiations. Accidents involving nuclear power reactors and fuel reprocessing plants could result in the release of fission product radionuclides. These beta-emitting radionuclides would enter the body primarily by inhalation and deposition of small particles in the lung and would result in irradiation of the lung and adjacent organs.

The biological effects of inhaled beta-emitting radionuclides are important considerations in the risk–benefit analysis of nuclear power reactor systems. Human epidemiological studies have shown that external or internal irradiation of the lung may have late-occurring sequelae, including pulmonary neoplasms. These studies, however, have dealt with external irradiation from X-rays, gamma rays or neutrons, or with internal

* Research performed under United States Energy Research and Development Administration Contract No. E(29-2)-1013 and conducted in animal-care facilities fully accredited by the American Association for Accreditation of Laboratory Animal Care.

irradiation from radon and radon daughters (N.R.C. Advisory Committee, 1972; UNSCEAR, 1972). No comparable data exist for man exposed by inhalation to beta-emitting radionuclides.

Experimental animal studies have confirmed the limited data from human epidemiological studies documenting the pulmonary carcinogenicity of external irradiation and internal alpha-emitting radionuclides (SANDERS *et al.*, 1970). Animal studies with beta-emitting radionuclides in the lung have shown that they are carcinogenic; however, the dose response patterns and tumour incidences are not well enough understood to make meaningful quantitative predictions of man's response to inhaled beta-emitters. (CEMBER, 1964).

A group of studies has been initiated at the Inhalation Toxicology Research Institute to establish the dose–response relationships resulting from the inhalation of different quantities of beta-emitting radionuclides with varied physical half-lives. Beagle dogs have been exposed to relatively insoluble forms of ^{90}Y, ^{91}Y, ^{144}Ce or ^{90}Sr and are being observed for their life span. This report summarizes the current state of the studies and emphasizes dose–response relationships for the production of lung tumours.

MATERIALS AND METHODS

The experimental approach and design of these studies have been described by McCLELLAN *et al.* (1970). Equal numbers of male and female beagle dogs, born and raised in this colony, were given single, brief (2–48 min) nose-only exposures to aerosols of fused clay particles containing ^{90}Y, ^{91}Y, ^{144}Ce or ^{90}Sr in different activity levels to achieve graded initial lung burdens of radioactivity. Aerosols were prepared by cation exchange of the radionuclide into montmorillonite clay, generated with a Lovelace nebulizer and heat-treated by passing through a heating column operated at 1100°C. The aerosols were characterized by examination of samples collected by an electrostatic precipitator, a cascade impactor, and by radioanalysis of air-filter samples. The particle size distributions were polydisperse and could be described by log normal functions with activity median aerodynamic diameters ranging from 0.8 to 2.7 μm and with geometric standard deviations of 1.4 to 2.7. Control dogs inhaled similar heat-treated particles containing a stable form of the elements being studied and deposited an amount of fused clay (100–400 μg in the lung) approximately equal to the amount inhaled and deposited by dogs exposed to the radionuclides in fused clay particles.

Whole-body counting was performed on each dog immediately after exposure and at intervals thereafter to determine the total amount of aerosol deposited in the body during exposure, and its subsequent retention. The amount of aerosol initially deposited in the pulmonary region, the initial lung burden (ILB), was also determined from the whole-body counting data. This was accomplished by fitting multicomponent exponential functions to the data and considering the ILB to be the fraction of the initial body burden associated with all but the first, rapidly clearing, component associated with clearance of the upper respiratory tract and tracheobronchial region (BOECKER and CUDDIHY, in press).

The mean organ absorbed dose rates and cumulative doses were calculated for each dog using its own whole-body retention data and the relationships between lung burden and total burden determined in various parallel studies (BOECKER and CUDDIHY, in press). The equation for cumulative absorbed beta radiation dose is

$$\text{cumulative rad} = \frac{0.0512\ \bar{E}(AF)A_0}{W(TF)} \int_0^t LuB(t)\mathrm{d}t$$

$\bar{E}$ = average β energy in MEV,
AF = fractional absorption of β energy = 1.0 for lung,
A_0 = ILB in μCi,
W = body weight at exposure in kg,
TF = lung weight with blood as fraction of body weight = 0.011,
$LuB(t)$ = lung burden at time t as a fraction of the ILB.

The dogs were 12–14 months old at exposure and were subsequently maintained for life span observation. Each dog was given a physical examination annually and observed daily until death occurred spontaneously or the animal was euthanized in a moribund condition. Complete gross and histopathological examinations were performed at death. Pertinent organs were radioanalysed to document radionuclide retention patterns whenever possible.

RESULTS

Numbers of dogs, range of ILBs achieved and the time since the last dog was exposed in each study are shown in Table 1. Although a series of discrete activity levels was used for planning the inhalation exposures, variability among dogs and exposure conditions produced a spread in initial body and lung burdens at each level such that each entire experiment can be considered a continuous spectrum of ILB values within the range listed.

TABLE 1. REPRESENTATIVE PARAMETERS FOR THE FOUR STUDIES WITH DOGS EXPOSED BY INHALATION TO BETA-EMITTING RADIONUCLIDES IN RELATIVELY INSOLUBLE FORMS

Radionuclide	Approximate effective half-life in lung (days)	Number of dogs	Range of ILB (μCi/kg body weight)	Days since last surviving dog exposed (as of 7/1/75)
^{90}Y	2.6	89	0, 80–5200	1540
^{91}Y	50	96	0, 11–360	1375
^{144}Ce	180	111	0, 0.0024–210	1418
^{90}Sr	400	72	0, 3.7–94	1342

The four radionuclides in these studies provide a wide range in radiation dose patterns to lung. Fused clay particles are relatively insoluble, having a biological half-time in the lung of $\simeq$ 700 days, thus the effective half-life (Table 1) in the lung was greatly influenced by the physical half-life of the radionuclide. The wide variation among isotopes in effective half-life in the lung delivered virtually completed doses to the lung in different times. The percentage of potential infinite dose to the lung at various times after exposure is shown in Fig. 1. Doses resulting from these relatively insoluble beta-emitting radionuclides have been compared to the dose accumulation from inhaled $^{239}PuO_2$ (PARK *et al.*, 1972). The wide range of ILBs achieved with these four radionuclides provides the opportunity to study the relationship between pulmonary carcinogenesis and total radiation dose, dose rate and dose protraction.

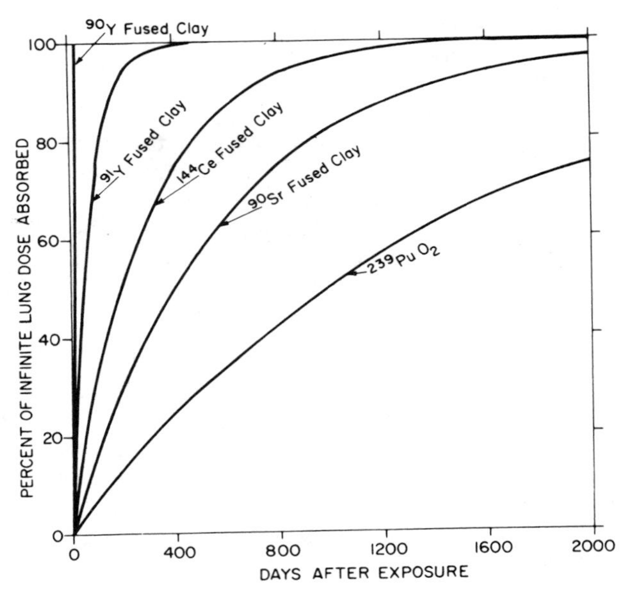

FIG. 1. Percent of the potential infinite dose to the lung as a function of time after exposure to ^{90}Y, ^{91}Y, ^{144}Ce or ^{90}Sr in fused clay particles. These are compared to the dose from $^{239}PuO_2$.

Within the lung, the radiation dose resulting from beta-emitting radionuclides is much more uniform than that from alpha-emitting radionuclides because of the greater penetration of the beta particles. However, SNIPES *et al.* (1975) have shown that the dose from ^{90}Sr in fused clay particles to various structures in the thorax may vary from nearly zero to four times the calculated average dose to the lung.

All dogs that died or were euthanized within 600 days after inhalation exposure in all four studies had various degrees of radiation pneumonitis, pulmonary fibrosis and pulmonary vasculitis. In this time period, dogs exposed to ^{144}Ce or ^{90}Sr generally had more active inflammation and pulmonary fibrosis than dogs exposed to ^{90}Y or ^{91}Y perhaps due to their longer average survival time after inhalation exposure and the influence of continuing irradiation. Some of these early effects have been reported by MCCLELLAN *et al.* (1970) and HOBBS *et al.* (1972).

Forty dogs, twenty-eight with primary malignant lung tumours, have died at times ranging from 644 to 2396 days after inhalation exposure. The number of dogs dead with tumours, times after exposure and lung doses are summarized in Table 2. Several dogs died with primary haemangiosarcomas of the heart or mediastinum and several died with primary bone tumours or epithelial tumours associated with the nasal cavity, but have not been included in these data.

The numbers and types of malignant pulmonary tumours seen to date vary from study to study. None of the dogs exposed to ^{90}Y has died yet with a malignant pulmonary tumour; however, a small benign pulmonary adenoma was an incidental finding in one dog that died of pulmonary fibrosis at 903 days after exposure. All dogs in the ^{91}Y study that died at later times had bronchiolo-alveolar carcinomas. Several also had other types of pulmonary carcinomas. All dogs in the ^{144}Ce and ^{90}Sr studies that died with tumours had widely disseminated primary pulmonary haemangiosarcomas. In addition to these tumours, several dogs had other malignant pulmonary tumours including bronchiolo-alveolar carcinoma, bronchogenic adenocarcinoma, epidermoid carcinoma or fibrosarcoma.

TABLE 2. PRIMARY MALIGNANT PULMONARY TUMOURS OBSERVED TO DATE (7/1/75) IN DOGS EXPOSED TO BETA-EMITTING RADIONUCLIDES INHALED IN A RELATIVELY INSOLUBLE FORM

Radionuclide	Number dead with malignant lung tumour	Days after exposure to death (range)	Dose to lung to death (rads)
^{90}Y	0	—	—
^{91}Y	5	1116–1613	16 000–25 000
^{144}Ce	9	750–2396	22 000–61 000
^{90}Sr	14	644–1213	34 000–68 000

The most frequently found tumour, haemangiosarcoma, was clinically aggressive and usually killed the dog within 3 months from the time of initial radiographical or clinicial diagnosis. At necropsy, haemangiosarcomas were characterized by irregularly shaped, dark red, blood-filled pulmonary nodules measuring from one mm to about 10 cm in diameter. They numbered from a few to several hundred nodules per lung. The larger nodules were more often found in the parenchyma of the anterior lobes in dogs exposed to ^{144}Ce. In dogs exposed to ^{90}Sr, distribution of nodules was more random and the number of nodules per lung greater. Distant metastases were common and most frequently involved brain, heart, kidneys and adrenals. The histological appearance varied from dog to dog, but was similar in lung and distant metastases. They consisted of poorly circumscribed masses composed of capillary or cavernous vascular sinusoids lined by plump pleomorphic endothelial cells (Fig. 2). Acute and chronic haemorrhage was frequent in and around tumour nodules. Bronchi, bronchioles, blood and lymph vessels and the pulmonary parenchyma were frequently compressed or destroyed by invading tumour nodules. Case histories of several of these dogs have been reported (HAHN *et al.*, 1973a; BENJAMIN *et al.*, 1975).

The fibrosarcoma seen in one dog exposed to ^{144}Ce was distinct from the haemangiosarcoma found in the same lung and metastasized to different sites. Histologically, it

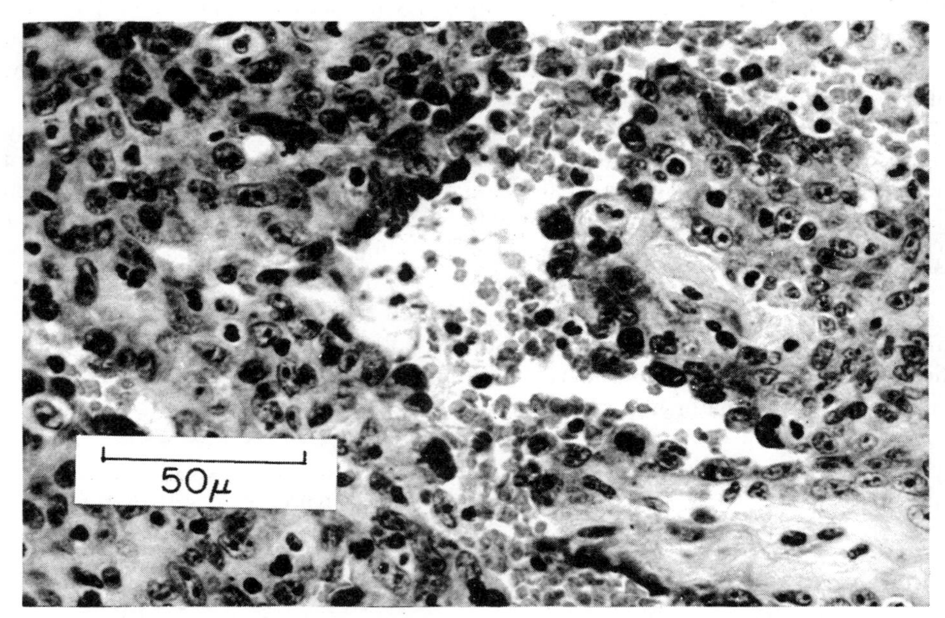

FIG. 2. Photomicrograph of a pulmonary haemangiosarcoma showing neoplastic cells in mitosis. H and E stain.

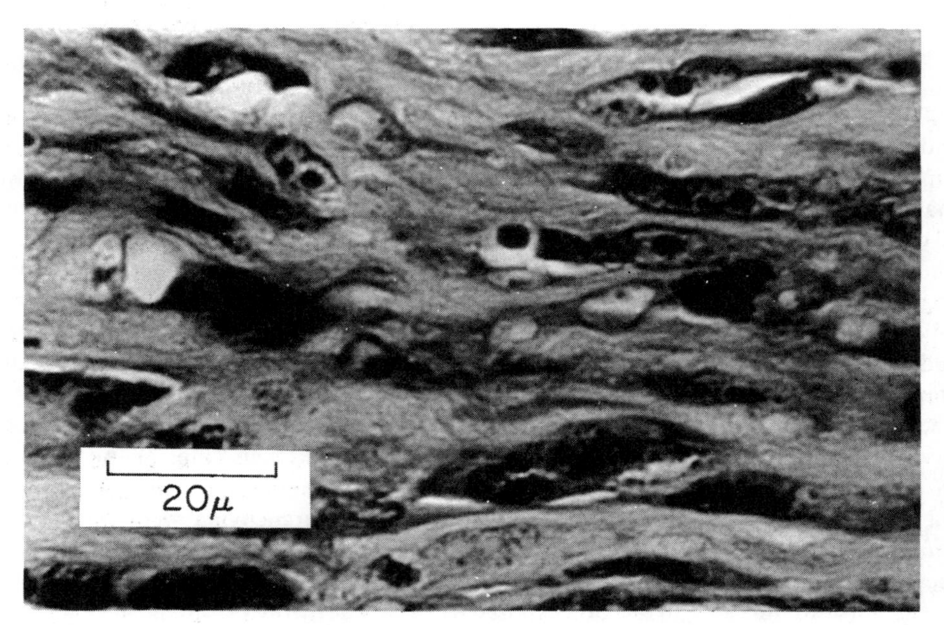

FIG. 3. Photomicrograph of a pulmonary fibrosarcoma showing anaplastic fibroblasts. H and E stain.

contained large swirled masses of mature connective tissue interspersed with well-differentiated fibroblasts and surrounded by anaplastic fibroblasts with frequent mitotic figures, Fig. 3.

The bronchiolo-alveolar carcinomas had a more prolonged clinical course than the haemangiosarcomas. One dog lived as long as 867 days from initial diagnosis to death. The gross appearance at necropsy also differed. Yellowish ill-defined tumour masses were found in much or all of one or several lung lobes but did not distort the normal contour of the lung. Distant metastases were found only in the lymph nodes of the thorax. Histologically, medium-sized, round or cuboidal cells in clumps or ribbons filled the alveoli, but did not greatly alter the alveolar architecture (Fig. 4). The cells dilated and filled many pulmonary lymphatics. Several dogs also had pulmonary carcinomas of other types intimately combined with the bronchiolo-alveolar carcinomas. These were mucin producing adenocarcinomas and epidermoid carcinomas (Fig. 5).

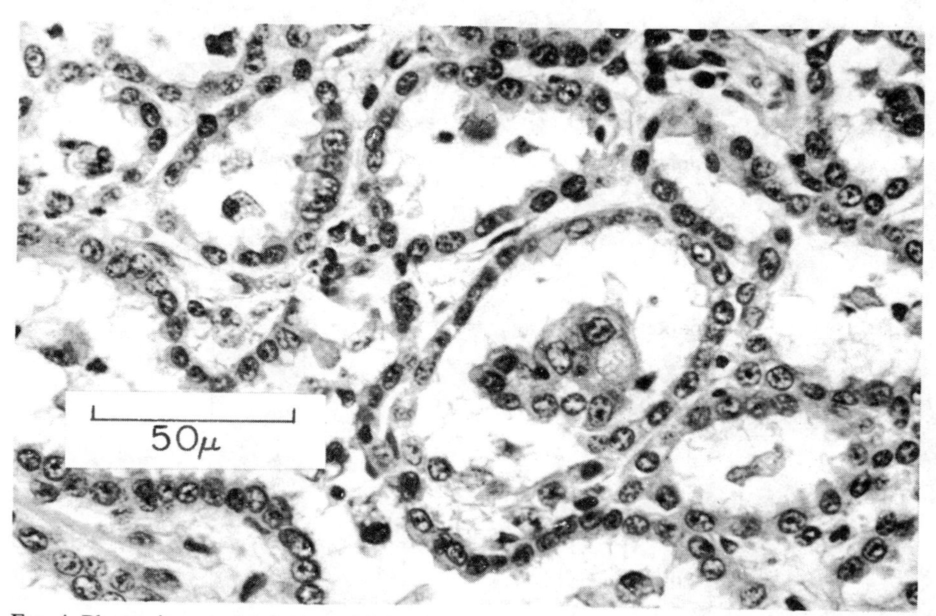

FIG. 4. Photomicrograph of a bronchiolo-alveolar carcinoma showing the characteristic growth pattern along alveolar walls. H and E stain.

The relationship of radiation dose to lung and survival time for dogs dying with malignant pulmonary tumours after inhalation of beta-emitting radionuclides is shown in Fig. 6. Five dogs in the ^{91}Y study have died with lung tumours 1342 to 1613 days after inhalation with radiation doses to lung of from 16 000 to 25 000 rads. Nine dogs in the ^{144}Ce study have died with lung tumours 750 to 2396 days after inhalation exposure with radiation dose to lung of from 23 000 to 61 000 rads. Fourteen dogs in the ^{90}Sr study have died with lung tumours 644 to 1213 days after inhalation exposure with radiation doses to lung of 34 000–68 000 rads.

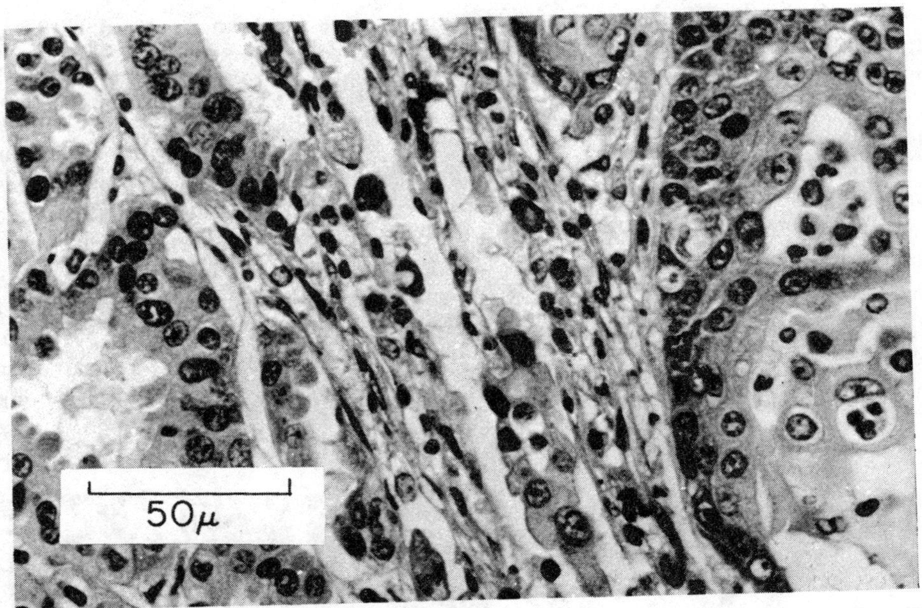

FIG. 5. Photomicrograph of an epidermoid carcinoma showing intimate growth with bronchiolo-alveolar carcinoma.

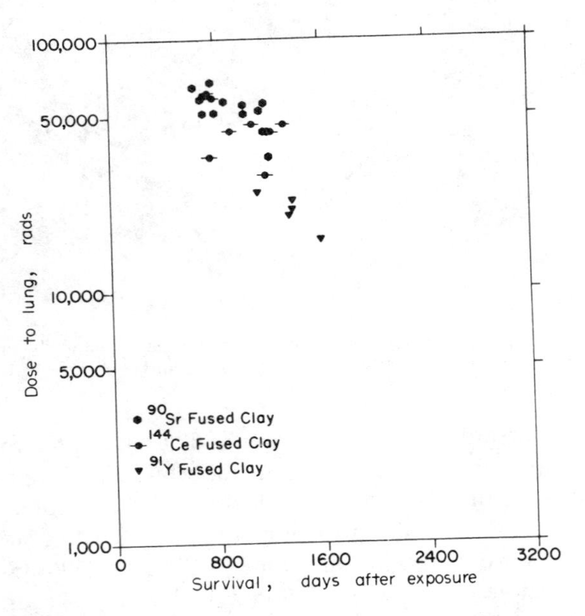

FIG. 6. Survival times and radiation dose to lung for dogs dying with malignant pulmonary tumours after inhalation of beta-emitting radionuclides.

DISCUSSION

Although these studies with inhaled, relatively insoluble, beta-emitting radionuclides are still in progress, some comparisons of dose-response relationships can be made. The shortest observation period from time of inhalation exposure for dogs still alive is 1342 days. Thus, comparisons have been made only through this period and deal with dogs exposed to ^{144}Ce and ^{90}Sr in fused clay particles since these are studies with sufficient numbers of tumours for analysis. The cumulative incidence of malignant pulmonary tumours in dogs that inhaled ^{144}Ce or ^{90}Sr in fused clay particles is shown in Fig. 7. Incidence rates were calculated using a procedure of ROSENBLATT *et al.* (1971)

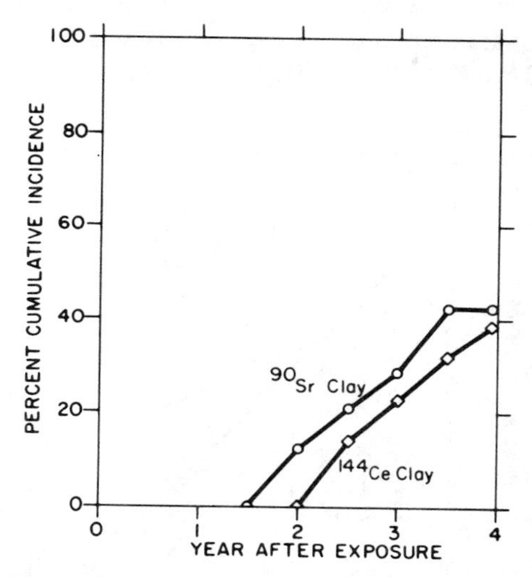

FIG. 7. Cumulative incidence of malignant pulmonary tumours in dogs that inhaled ^{144}Ce or ^{90}Sr in fused clay particles and died within 1350 days after exposure.

based on life table methods of incidence calculation. The groups chosen for comparison are all dogs in each study which survived at least 600 days after exposure and had potential infinite dose to lung of 22 000 rads, the lowest dose which has resulted in a primary lung tumour in these two studies, as of 7/1/75. Using the potential infinite dose in the group selection disregards dose rate or dose protraction as a factor. However, when the two cumulative incidences are compared, it is seen that the total incidence to 1350 days after exposure and the slopes of the two curves are essentially the same. This indicates that, for this time period after exposure and at these doses and dose rates to lung, the total dose must be a major factor in the cumulative incidence of lung tumours. The incidence curve for dogs exposed to ^{90}Sr is shifted to the left which indicates that dose protraction in these dose and dose-rate ranges results in fatal lung tumours at slightly earlier times after exposure.

Average dose rates for the dogs with lung tumours in these two studies are shown in Fig. 8. The dose rate in the dogs with ^{144}Ce is initially higher but decreases much faster than the dose rate in the dogs with ^{90}Sr. It should be recognized that comparison of these two studies over this time period deals essentially with induction of one tumour type, pulmonary haemangiosarcoma.

Epithelial tumours of the lung, mainly bronchiolo-alveolar carcinomas, have been induced after the inhalation of ^{91}Y in fused clay particles. Five dogs with doses to the lung of 16 000–25 000 rads died 1115 to 1613 days after inhalation of ^{91}Y in fused clay particles. Epithelial tumours are comparable to the tumour types usually seen after the inhalation of $^{239}PuO_2$ by dogs (PARK *et al.*, 1972). In these latter studies, four dogs died within 1613 days after inhalation exposure and had an average radiation dose of 4800 rads to the lung; doses were calculated with uniform dose distribution and a lung weight to body weight ratio of 0.011. The relative biological effect for induction of bronchioloalveolar tumours by inhaled alpha- and beta-emitting particles appears to be 4–5. This is in contrast to the relative biological effect for induction of bronchiolo-alveolar tumours by inhaled alpha emitters and haemangiosarcomas by inhaled beta emitters of about 10 (HAHN *et al.*, 1973a).

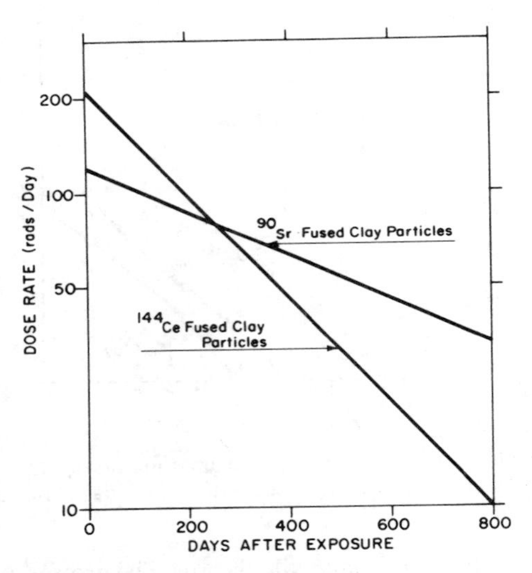

FIG. 8. Average dose rates to lung for dogs that inhaled ^{144}Ce or ^{90}Sr in fused clay particles and died with malignant pulmonary tumours within 1350 days after exposure.

The propensity for the protracted pulmonary irradiation from inhaled beta-emitting radionuclides to produce haemangiosarcomas as opposed to the epithelial tumours induced by inhaled $^{239}PuO_2$ has been commented on by HAHN *et al.* (1973b) and JONES *et al.* (1974). Speculations on the reasons for the differences relate to the differences in linear energy transfer between alpha and beta emitters, differences in penetration of the particles and differences in dose patterns at the cellular level. Since ^{91}Y in fused clay particles has, to date, been shown to induce epithelial tumours of the lung and not sarcomas, other factors must also be involved in these differences. In these studies, the pulmonary irradiation from ^{91}Y is quite different from that of $^{239}PuO_2$; the emission is different (beta *vs.* alpha), the dose rate is different (relatively high *vs.* low) and the dose protraction is different (short *vs.* long). Both types of irradiation do cause pulmonary fibrosis which may play a role in the induction of pulmonary carcinomas, especially bronchiolo-alveolar carcinomas.

REFERENCES

BENJAMIN, S. A., HAHN, F. F., CHIFFELLE, T. L., BOECKER, B. B., HOBBS, C. H., JONES, R. K. and McCLELLAN, R. O. (1975) *Cancer Res.* **35,** 1745–1755.

BOECKER, B. B. and CUDDIHY, R. G. (in press) *Hlth Phys.*

CEMBER, H. (1964) *Prog. exp. Tumor Res.* **4,** 251–303.

HAHN, F. F., BENJAMIN, S. A., BOECKER, B. B., CHIFFELLE, T. L., HOBBS, C. H., JONES, R. K., McCLELLAN, R. O., PICKRELL, J. A. and REDMAN, H. C. (1973a) *J. natn. Cancer Inst.* **50,** 675–698.

HAHN, F. F., BENJAMIN, S. A., BOECKER, B. B., CHIFFELLE, T. L., HOBBS, C. H., JONES, R. K., McCLELLAN, R. O. and REDMAN, H. C. (1973b) *Radionuclide Carcinogenesis* (edited by SANDERS, C. L., BUSCH, R. H., BALLOU, J. E. and MAHLUM, D. D.) AEC Symposium Series No. 29, pp. 201–214, U.S. Department of Commerce, Springfield, Virginia.

HOBBS, C. H., BARNES, J. E., McCLELLAN, R. O., CHIFFELLE, T. L., JONES, R. K., LUNDGREN, D. L., MAUDERLY, J. L., PICKRELL, J. A. and RYPKA, E. W. (1972) *Radiat. Res.* **49.** 430–460.

JONES, R. K., HAHN, F. F., HOBBS, C. H., BENJAMIN, S. A., BOECKER, B. B., McCLELLAN, R. O. and SLAUSON, D. O. (1974) *Experimental Lung Cancer, Carcinogenesis and Bioassays* (edited by KARBE, E. and PARK, J. F.) Springer, Heidelberg, New York.

McCLELLAN, R. O., BARNES, J. E., BOECKER, B. B., CHIFFELLE, T. L., HOBBS, C. H., JONES, R. K., MAUDERLY, J. L., PICKRELL, J. A. and REDMAN, H. C. (1970) *Morphology of Experimental Respiratory Carcinogenesis* (edited by NETTESHEIM, P., HANNA, M. G. and DEATHERAGE, J. W.) pp. 395–415. A.E.C. Symposium Series No. 21, U.S. Department of Commerce, Springfield, Virginia.

NATIONAL RESEARCH COUNCIL ADVISORY COMMITTEE ON THE BIOLOGICAL EFFECTS OF IONIZING RADIATION (1972) *The Effects on Populations of Exposure to Low Levels of Ionizing Radiation*, pp. 145–156. National Academy of Sciences, National Research Council, Washington, D.C.

PARK, J. F., BAIR, W. J. and BUSCH, R. H. (1972) *Hlth Phys.* **22,** 803–810.

ROSENBLATT, L. S., HETHERINGTON, N. H., GOLDMAN, M. and BUSTAD, L. K. (1971) *Hlth Phys.* **21,** 869–875.

SANDERS, C. L., THOMPSON, R. C. and BAIR, W. J. (1970) *Inhalation Carcinogenesis* (edited by HANNA, M. G., NETTESHEIM, P. and GILBERT, J. R.) pp. 285–303. A.E.C. Symposium Series No. 18, U.S. Department of Commerce, Springfield, Virginia.

SNIPES, M. B., HULBERT, A. J. and RUNKLE, G. E. (1975) in: *Biomedical Dosimetry. Proceedings of an International Symposium, Vienna, Austria, March 1975.* pp. 683–694. International Atomic Energy Agency, Vienna.

UNITED NATIONS SCIENTIFIC COMMITTEE ON THE EFFECTS OF ATOMIC RADIATION (1972) *Ionizing Radiation: Levels and Effects*, vol. 2, pp. 417–420. United Nations, New York.

DISCUSSION

G. W. DOLPHIN: Have you looked at changes in the blood count?

Dr HAHN: Yes, extensive clinical evaluation has been carried out on all the dogs. There is a lymphopenia following the exposures and it is dose related. The length of the depression relates to the prolongation of the radiation dose to the lung. The acute irradiation from ^{90}Y causes an abrupt drop and a relatively fast recovery of the peripheral leucocyte numbers as opposed to ^{90}Sr which has a protracted irradiation and gives a drop and a slower recovery to normal levels—in fact they may not reach normal levels for a number of years.

E. P. RADFORD: A comment concerning the differential sensitivity of bronchial and peripheral lung tissues. The tumours observed in irradiated animals are more likely to be peripheral. There is evidence in man that the bronchial epithelium is more radiosensitive than the peripheral tissues. The Hiroshima survivors had whole-body irradiation with neutrons, and the lung cancers observed are primarily bronchial in origin. In the uranium miners inhaling radon daughters, the lung parenchyma secured a radiation dose of about the same level as the bronchial epithelium, yet only one alveolar cell tumour has been observed by Dr Saccomanno compared with about 200 bronchial tumours.

Dr HAHN: I have one comment; with the protracted irradiation we see with exposure to ^{90}Sr and ^{144}Ce we get tumours essentially of lung blood vessels. On the other hand, we see carcinomas of various types with the more acute radiation exposure with ^{91}Y. In coming years it will be interesting to see if we have a shift to more carcinomas with this briefer radiation dose to the lungs.

R. E. ALBERT: Was the earlier tumour induction by ^{90}Sr compared to ^{144}Ce due to a higher dose? If not, why not?

Dr HAHN: Generally those dogs dying earlier with lung tumours had higher radiation doses. The first dog to die with a lung tumour after inhalation of ^{90}Sr died 116 days before the first dog to die with a lung tumour after inhalation of ^{144}Ce.

G. W. DOLPHIN: The doses quoted in the paper are calculated for the lung, but the dose to the immune system throughout the body is of importance. This dose could possibly be measured by chromosome aberration studies in lymphocytes.

Dr HAHN: Yes, we have to remember that all the structures in the thorax are being irradiated to some degree after inhalation of beta-emitting particles. In fact, lesions may be seen in these other structures, for example we have seen primary tumours of the heart and mediastinum. Obviously lymphocytes passing through the lung are being irradiated. We are conducting lymphocyte function studies on many of these dogs.

M. KUSCHNER: I think you would agree that the appearance of these particular tumours is unexplained and unexpected. Tumours in man are very often multifactorial—tumours in uranium miners occur exclusively in cigarette smokers, for example. There are combinations of factors involved in the production of the tumour, and the animal models can be manipulated just as man is manipulated by the multiple things to which he is exposed. When an angiosarcoma develops one begins to wonder about specific sensitivity; there may be some genetic basis for instability in that particular tissue.

Dr HAHN: You are certainly right in your comments. Haemangiosarcomas are rare in people. They are relatively common in dogs in many sites but not as a primary tumour of lung. It may be correct that haemangiosarcoma is one of the tumour types which are induced readily in dogs by carcinogens. There have been reports, however, of haemangiosarcomas induced in other tissues, such as skin and bone, and in other species, such as rat and mouse, by beta-emitting radionuclides. These instances may relate to protracted beta irradiation and may not be species specific.

R. G. THOMAS: The tumours found at Battelle in the plutonium-exposed dogs were not angiosarcomas. This suggests a difference in the α and β radiation effect on the lung.

Dr HAHN: Yes, the difference may be the dose distribution in the lung and the resulting lesions. I did mention that in the ^{91}Y studies we have seen epithelial tumours, mainly bronchiolo-alveolar carcinomas, that are similar to those seen in dogs exposed to PuO_2. The occurrence of these tumours may be related to the pulmonary scars that are seen in both studies.

E. P. RADFORD: The results in these experiments do not necessarily show a high radio-sensitivity of the blood-vessel epithelium, since the doses at which the haemangiosarcomas appeared were very high indeed. In response to Dr Kuschner I quite agree with his comment about the multifactorial nature of carcinogenesis in man. But I should correct one misconception—the non-smoking uranium miners *are* developing bronchial tumours, the latent period appears to be prolonged compared to the smokers. The dose–response data are now much closer for the non-smokers than for the smokers.

SESSION 8*

Thursday, 25th September

TALC

* The papers on Gases and Vapours given in this Session have been published in *The Annals of Occupational Hygiene*, Vol. 19, no. 1 (1976).

CHEMICAL AND PHYSICAL PROPERTIES OF BRITISH TALC POWDERS

F. D. POOLEY and N. ROWLANDS

Department of Mineral Exploitation, University College, Cardiff, Wales

Abstract—An examination of bulk talc samples imported into Great Britain has shown that they are extremely variable in their talc mineral content. Major contaminating minerals present with the talc are chlorite, carbonates and quartz. The chemistry of samples examined varied with their mineralogical content which also accounted for observed differences in particle morphology. Tremolite fibres were found in three samples, one of which contained the mineral as a major phase. No other varieties of asbestos were detected.

INTRODUCTION

There is only one indigenous source of talc in the British Isles, which supplies only a minor part of the British talc market, and this is in the Shetlands on the Island of Unst.

The majority of material used in Britain and referred to as talc is imported either in a powder form or as a rock which is crushed and ground as required. The name "talc powder" refers commercially to a material which contains talc as one of its principal ingredients and commercial samples vary in their actual talc mineral content from 95% to less than 40% by weight. The major sources of British talc by country are

TABLE 1. UNITED KINGDOM: IMPORTS OF TALC BY COUNTRIES, 1969–1972*

Country	Tonnes			
	1969	*1970*	*1971*	*1972*
Norway	18 321	16 666	19 025	17 973
France	10 493	14 195	13 168	11 056
Italy	9018	8475	7877	7737
China	8062	9804	9802	11 332
India	2029	3696	1943	1499
Belgium	1596	2448	2448	2415
U.S.A.	984	1043	1301	1000
Netherlands	841	959	650	1231
West Germany	266	566	589	988
Other countries	441	526	494	364
Total	52 051	58 378	57 297	55 595

* Source: H.M. Customs and Excise.

listed in Table 1. These countries often supply material of different grades and also material from several sources within that country. There are many countries which supply small amounts and also some who re-export material from other countries to Britain. Most talc mineral imported into Britain is raw material which is used by a wide variety of industries. Some talc, however, is imported in the form of finished articles and this is very difficult to trace and quantify but probably represents only a small proportion of imported talc. The estimated consumption of talc on the basis of industrial use in Britain is listed in Table 2. This list represents only major usage; minor uses of talc are very extensive.

TABLE 2. ESTIMATED CONSUMPTION OF TALC BY USER IN U.K. 1970

	1000 tonnes	*Per cent*
Roofing felt	22	33
Paint and plastics	20	30
Cosmetics	10	15
Rubber	9	13
Fertilizers	3	4
Ceramics	2	3
Paper	1	1
Miscellaneous	1	1
	68	100

GEOLOGY AND MINERALOGY OF TALC

Talc is a phyllosilicate consisting of a tri-octahedral brucite-like sheet sandwiched between two sheets of linked SiO_4 tetrahedra. The talc crystal is made up of stacks of these composite layers held together by the weakest of chemical bonds—the Van der Waal's forces. This stacking can be disturbed by the slightest forces causing slipping of composite layers and the development of a perfect cleavage parallel to the basal plane, accounting for the important soft lubricating texture of talc.

The chemical composition of pure talc, $Mg_3Si_4O_{10}(OH)_2$, on the basis of oxide weight percentages is: MgO—31.7%; SiO_2—63.5%; H_2O—4.8%. Naturally occurring talc, however, contains many elemental substitutions, aluminium or titanium may substitute for silicon while iron, nickel, manganese, chromium and aluminium may substitute for magnesium. Iron and nickel seem to substitute most commonly for magnesium and talc with a complete iron substitution for magnesium has been recorded. Nickel substitution in talcs associated with serpentine bodies have also been recorded and can be as large as 0.5% by weight.

The crystalline structure of the talc has been demonstrated to be mainly triclinic although earlier data suggest a monoclinic structure. Optical properties of talc particles vary depending upon the presence of small amounts of elemental substitutions in the talc. In polarized light talc is colourless and under crossed-nicols shows high-order birefringence colours with an extinction angle close to 0°.

Commercial deposits of talc are commonly derived from altered serpentinized ultra-mafic rocks or low-grade metamorphosed carbonate rocks such as dolomite. The alteration of serpentinite rocks is accomplished by the metasomatism of serpentine by the introduction of CO_2 to produce a talc–carbonate rock. The metamorphism of dolomite rocks involves a reaction with SiO_2 also to form a talc–carbonate rock. During the formation of talc many minor mineral phases may be formed in the talc ore, depending upon the elemental impurities in the rock; the changes themselves may also involve formation of intermediate mineral phases before talc is finally formed. The mineralogical composition of a talc ore may therefore vary considerably depending upon location but is usually fairly consistent in composition from any one source.

The composition of a talc ore may be further complicated by the presence of intrusions of the surrounding waste rock into the talc ore (lithological inclusions) which may be mined and processed with the talc for sale. A listing of some of the major and minor minerals that may be found in association with commercial talc samples is given in Table 3. As far as the minor minerals are concerned the list is certainly not complete there being many other trace minerals which can be found in talc samples.

TABLE 3. COMMON MINERAL IMPURITIES ASSOCIATED WITH TALC

Major	Magnesite	$MgCO_3$
	Dolomite	$CaMgCO_3$
	Chlorite	$Mg_5Al_2Si_3O_{10}(OH)_8$
	Tremolite	$Ca_2Mg_5Si_8O_{22}(OH)_2$
	Anthophyllite	$(Mg, Fe)_7Si_8O_{22}(OH)_2$
	Quartz	SiO_2
Minor	Calcite	$CaCO_3$
	Actinolite	$Ca_2(Mg,Fe)_5Si_8O_{22}(OH)_2$
	Muscovite	$KAl_2(Si_3Al)\ O_{10}(OH, F)_2$
	Rutile	TiO_2
	Serpentine	$Mg_6Si_4O_{10}(OH)_8$
	Pyrite	$Fe\ S_2$
	Enstatite	$MgSiO_3$
	Olivine	$(Mg,Fe,Mn)_2SiO_4$
	Magnetite	Fe_3O_4

Together with chlorite, the carbonate minerals magnesite and dolomite are by far the most common of the minerals associated with talc; chlorite may be present in any one of several forms depending upon its chemical composition.

EXAMINATION OF BRITISH TALC

Samples of talc mainly in a powdered form representing the majority of talc materials imported into Great Britain have been examined by a variety of mineralogical, chemical and physical techniques to obtain a better description of their composition. The samples were obtained from the major importers of talc before they had been subjected to further treatment, i.e. grinding or blending, and were assumed to be typical of the material imported from the various world sources. Talc is brought into

Great Britain in batch shipments often in large amounts and to obtain representative samples of every shipment would be a monumental task.

MINERALOGICAL COMPOSITION

The mineralogy of the samples was investigated using a variety of techniques including X-ray diffraction, thermal gravimetric analysis, differential thermal analysis, optical microscopy and electron microprobe analysis. The mineralogy of the samples was found to be extremely variable, the talc content being 42—96% by weight. The most common accessory minerals were carbonates, mainly magnesite, a little dolomite and calcite. The carbonate mineral content of the samples ranged from 0.5 to 44% by weight. Chlorite minerals were found to be almost as common in the samples as the carbonate minerals. In several cases, however, chlorite was not detected and the range of chlorite content varied from 0% to 55%. Quartz was established as the next most common ingredient and was found to occur in eleven out of the twenty-seven samples; it was usually found in only minor amounts, i.e. 1–2% with the exception of one sample where it exceeded 5%. Other minor mineral phases detected included rutile magnetite and tremolite. Tremolite was found in one sample to be over 30% by weight and detectable in two other samples.

The wide range in mineralogical composition between the talc samples is best illustrated by the analysis of several powders in Table 4. Quantitative mineralogical

TABLE 4. TYPICAL QUANTITATIVE MINERALOGICAL DATA OBTAINED FROM SEVERAL SAMPLES BY DTA, TGA, AND X-RAY DIFFRACTION ANALYSIS (% by weight)

Talc	Chlorite minerals	Carbonate minerals	Other minerals detected
92%	N.D.	5.5%	None
98%	1%	0.5%	None
46%	51%	1%	Quartz
88%	11%	2.5%	Quartz
84%	13%	N.D.	None
92%	3%	0.5%	Quartz
56%	N.D.	37%	5% Quartz
49%	N.D.	6%	>30% Tremolite

analyses by DTA, TGA and X-ray diffraction techniques are sensitive to approximately 1–2% by weight. They are also comparative techniques and require a mineral standard for calibration purposes. Mineralogical standards are very difficult to produce with identical characteristics to the minerals contained in the samples being analysed, and estimates of the mineral content of a sample may therefore often vary by several per cent. The relatively high detection levels of the techniques, i.e. 1–2%, also means that trace mineral fractions are often not detected in powder samples although they may be observed with the optical or electron microscope.

The talc samples were also examined with an electron microscope microprobe analyser to establish the presence of any asbestos minerals. Using this technique three samples were found to contain tremolite fibres; in two of these the fibres were not detected by other means. None of the samples were found to contain chrysotile asbestos although in several samples, fibres similar in morphology to chrysotile were observed. When analysed they were found to have a chemistry comparable to sepiolite (meerschaum).

PHYSICAL CHARACTERISTICS OF BRITISH TALC SAMPLES

The majority of British imported talc samples are marketed in a powder form and vary from very coarse to extremely fine powders. Powders are ground to varying degrees of fineness to suit individual industrial applications. Many of the powders which were examined with a Quantimet 720 image analysis system consisted of particles finer than 53 μm while a number of special preparations of certain grades which were micronized (finely ground) samples consisted of particles finer than 20 μm. For the majority of samples a median diameter of 25 μm was obtained from sizing data, with an average upper particle size of approximately 65 μm. The size distribution of the powders on a particle number basis was found to be very unstable and to be dependent upon the energy employed in the dispersion of the samples, in preparation for size analysis. The instability is due mainly to the very soft and fragile nature of talc.

The morphology of the particles in the samples varied considerably and was found

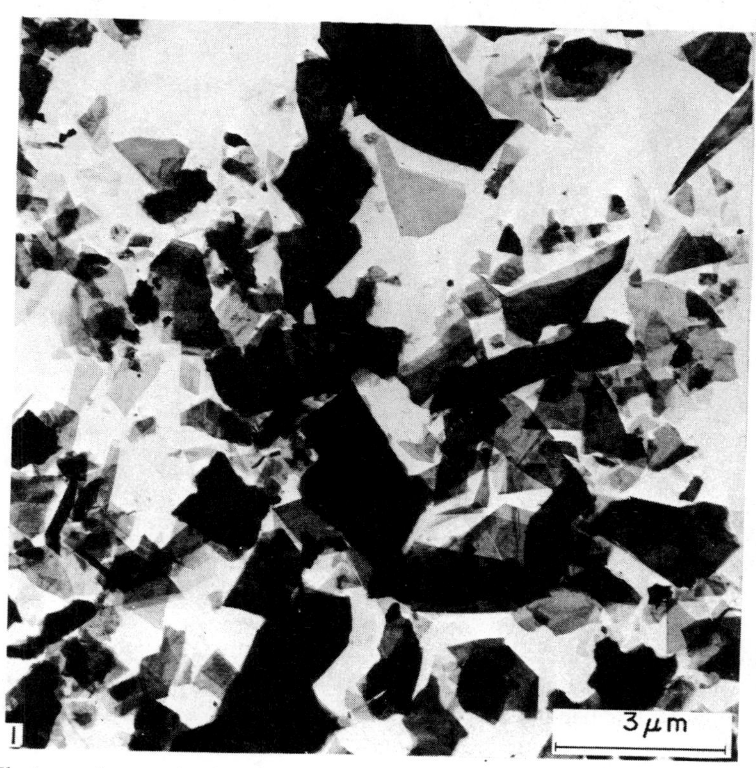

FIG. 1. Electron micrograph of pure talc particles illustrating their thin plate-like morphology.

to be mainly dependent upon mineralogical composition. Those samples consisting mainly of talc were composed of flat, angular, flaky particles often extremely thin. With an increase in carbonate mineral content the flaky particles were reduced in number and more compact and rounded particles were observed. The one sample containing major tremolite was found to be extremely fibrous. The three distinct morphological appearances are illustrated by Figs. 1–3. Those samples with major chlorite content were also found to be fairly flaky in appearance, the flakes being not as angular or as thin as the purer talc samples, however.

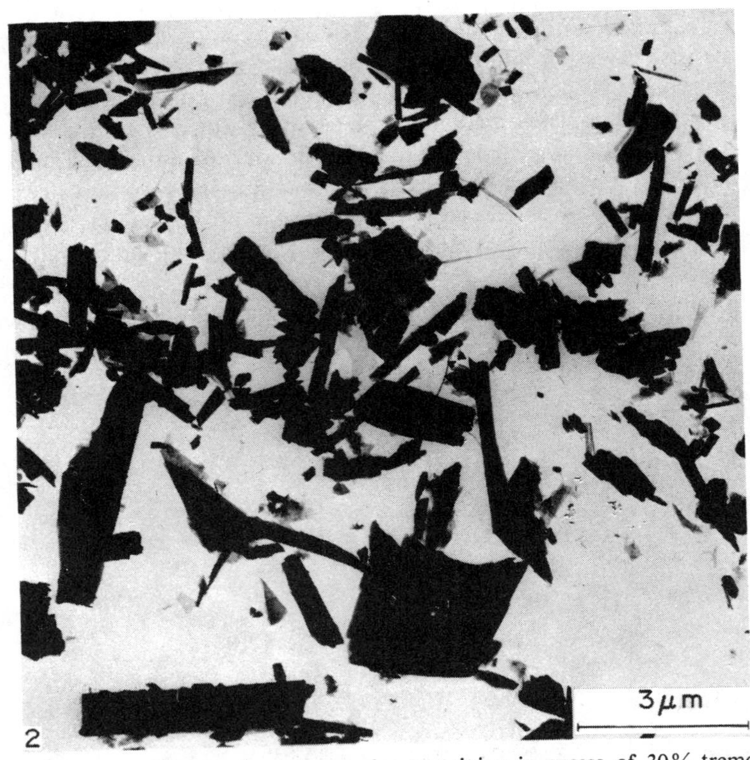

FIG. 2. Electron micrograph of a talc powder containing in excess of 30% tremolite. The majority of the fibrous particles are tremolite.

Fibrous mineral particles, i.e. with an axial ratio greater than 3 : 1 could be found in all of the samples examined and appeared to increase in frequency with the fineness of the powder. These fibrous particles were often flat laths or rolled sheets of talc although fibrous particles of chlorite were also observed.

Sepiolite fibres which were found in several of the samples when examined with the electron microscope, have a very similar appearance to chrysotile asbestos fibre. They were only identified as being sepiolite by microprobe analysis and also their difference in morphology to chrysotile as they do not have the tubular structure visible at high magnification on the electron microscope that the latter possesses.

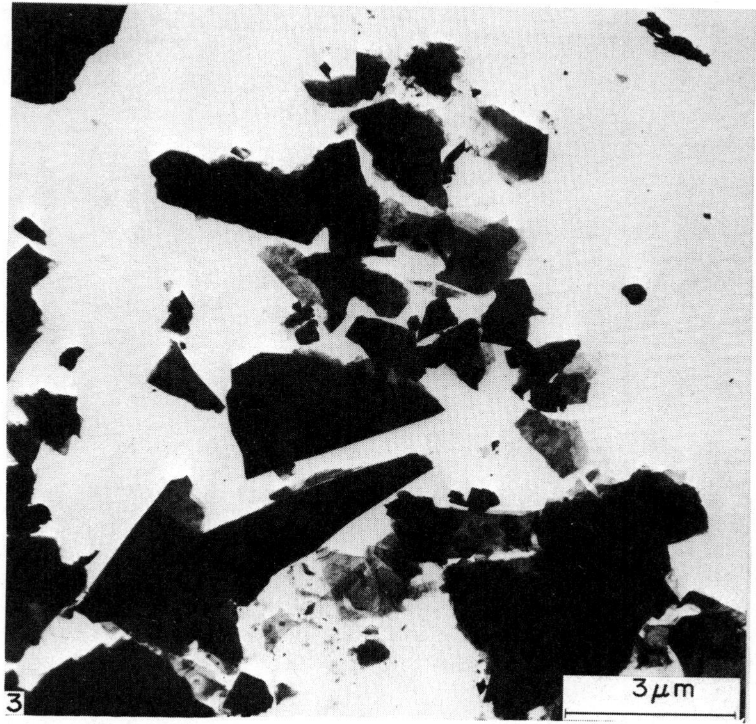

FIG. 3. Electron micrograph of a talc powder containing carbonate and chlorite minerals.

CHEMICAL COMPOSITION OF BRITISH TALCS

The chemical analysis of talc samples was found to be most easily performed using X-ray fluorescence analysis. Wet chemical analysis of talc samples is extremely difficult due to the inability to dissolve talc readily even in the strongest of acid or alkaline solutions. The purity of the various powders can be related almost directly to the mineralogical composition of the powders, the level of impurities being related to the amount of elements other than magnesium and silicon present in the sample. Analyses of samples representing some of the extremes of mineralogical composition are illustrated by Table 5. Generally it can be stated that an increase in aluminium content reflects chlorite mineral content and a drop in silica content and increase in CO_2 reflects carbonate content.

An examination of the trace element content of the samples revealed that potassium and manganese were fairly common in all samples. A number of the powders also contained small quantities of the transition metals nickel, cobalt and chromium, while others did not. The samples containing the transition metals were found to be related directly to ultramafic talc deposits while the talcs derived from metamorphosed dolomites were deficient in these elements.

TABLE 5. VARIATION IN MAJOR ELEMENTAL CHEMISTRY OF TALC POWDERS WITH CHANGE IN MINERAL COMPOSITION

Mineralogical description of sample	Major oxide weight percentage composition						
	MgO	SiO_2	CaO	Fe_2O_3	TiO_2	Al_2O_3	CO_2*
(a) High-grade talc	30.40	62.10	0.20	0.28	0.05	0.03	0.2
(b) Chlorite-rich talc	31.00	41.90	0.70	1.70	0.14	10.80	1.0
(c) Carbonate-rich talc with high quartz content	29.73	52.05	2.00	0.98	0.05	0.50	18.00
(d) Tremolite-rich talc	24.75	59.70	5.50	0.20	0.05	1.00	0.60
(e) Carbonate-rich talc with high magnetite content	28.90	38.90	0.80	6.23	0.05	1.00	18.80

* CO_2 obtained by thermal gravimetric analysis.

The bulk analysis reflects only the combined mineral content of the sample and not the actual chemistry of the talc it contains.

Analysis of talc particles in each of the samples with a microprobe analysis system revealed that the only element other than magnesium and silicon detectable in most of the specimens was iron. The iron content varied from an undetectable level to almost 5% of the mineral by weight as Fe_2O_3. The samples containing talc with a high iron content were again directly related to ultramafic talc deposits, talc derived from altered limestone deposits being very low in iron.

CONCLUSIONS

Mineral powders which are used in Great Britain and which are commonly referred to as "talc powders" vary a great deal in their actual talc mineral content. The major contaminants found in the powders were carbonate and chlorite minerals together with quartz and tremolite. Only three of the twenty-seven samples examined were found to contain tremolite asbestos fibres and none of the samples were found to contain chrysotile asbestos fibres. The mineralogy of the powders examined was found to influence their particle morphology and chemistry. It was found that the powders could be divided into two groups mainly on the basis of their chemistry: those derived from altered serpentine rocks and those from altered dolomite deposits. The former contain measurable quantities of the transition elements nickel, chromium and cobalt.

ANIMAL EXPERIMENTS WITH TALC

J. C. WAGNER,* G. BERRY,* T. J. COOKE,† R. J. HILL,*
F. D. POOLEY‡ and J. W. SKIDMORE*

Abstract—Italian talc has been tested on rats using three routes, intra-pleural inoculation, inhalation and ingestion. Groups exposed to superfine chrysotile asbestos and untreated controls were included for comparison. In all the experiments animals were allowed to live out their lives. The intra-pleural inoculation of talc produced no mesotheliomas in contrast to eighteen produced by the chrysotile asbestos. After ingestion, one leiomyosarcoma occurred with Italian talc and one with chrysotile asbestos. Whether these tumours are a consequence of the feeding is uncertain. The inhalation studies demonstrated that with equal dosage, talc can produce a similar amount of fibrosis as asbestos. However, the chrysotile exposed rats developed lung adenomas, adenomatosis and an adenocarcinoma, whereas the only lung tumour seen in animals exposed to talc was a small adenoma, which may have been an incidental finding.

INTRODUCTION

In these studies we have investigated the biological properties of a single type of talc, using the same methods as we have applied to various types of asbestos. Talc was introduced into rats by three routes—intra-pleural, inhalation and ingestion. We had facilities for testing a single talc dust, and decided to use the Italian talc which is a major source of cosmetic talc used in Great Britain. The literature on the biological effects of cosmetic and consumable (used in confectionery) talc is confusing and some of the results unjustifiably alarming. The more sensational findings have naturally attracted a lot of publicity. Therefore, we have been forced to devote a large amount of experimental resources in an attempt to put the possible hazards resulting from the inhalation of cosmetic and consumable talc into perspective. The inhalation study has not been completed and this is a preliminary communication, as far as this route is concerned.

MATERIALS AND METHODS

The main experimental material was Italian talc. The mineral sample used in this study was obtained from a shipment of talc material imported from a mine in Northern Italy where talc has been produced for over 70 years. Talc from this particular mine was chosen for two reasons. First, because it has been used in Great Britain for over 50 years and secondly, because over 40% of the cosmetic grade talc used in Great Britain is obtained from this source.

* Medical Research Council Pneumoconiosis Unit, Penarth, Wales.
† Department of Paediatric Pathology, Welsh National School of Medicine, Cardiff, Wales.
‡ Department of Mineral Exploitation, University College, Cardiff, Wales.

This particular talc is referred to in the talc trade as Italian 00000 grade. It is imported in a ready-milled form, with an upper particle size of 70 μm and a mean particle size of 25 μm. The talc sample was found to contain 92% talc mineral by weight together with 3% chlorite and 1% carbonate minerals; quartz was also found in the powder at approximately the 0.5–1% level.

Extensive investigation of this particular grade of talc had been performed for a 2-year period prior to the start of the animal experimentation, and samples which were over 30 years old had been examined as well as more recent imports. Virtually no change in the mineralogical composition of the material has been detected. No asbestos minerals of either the tremolite or chrysotile varieties have been detected in the many samples of this powder examined. A mineralogical study of the talc mine itself has shown that tremolite can be found in isolated sections of the mine but this could not be traced into the final product. This is probably due to the selective mining procedures adopted in the mine where the talc is mined by hand.

For comparison the sample of super-fine chrysotile asbestos (SFA chrysotile) which we have previously shown to give a high mesothelioma rate after intra-pleural inoculation (WAGNER *et al.*, 1973) was included and there were also controls exposed to neither material.

The experimental animals were barrier-protected caesarian-derived rats of the Wistar strain bred at the Unit from a stock given to us by Imperial Chemical Industries, Pharmaceutical Division, Alderley Edge, Cheshire.

In each group of animals there were equal numbers of males and females and allocation to the treatment groups was at random. The rats were caged in fours except when in the inhalation chambers when they were caged in sixes. The inhalation chambers were in a separate room. The rats were fed on a proprietary brand of autoclaved cubes and water *ad libitum*. The animal house was supplied with filtered air. Except for the scheduled killings, each rat was allowed to live until it died naturally or appeared to be distressed; full necropsy examinations were carried out.

INTRA-PLEURAL INOCULATION EXPERIMENT

The dose was 20 mg per rat made up as a suspension in physiological saline, with a concentration of 50 mg/ml. Injection was into the right pleural cavity using the method described by WAGNER and BERRY (1969). There were 48 rats injected with the talc, 48 with SFA chrysotile and 48 controls injected with saline. Injection was in January 1973 when the rats were between 8 and 14 weeks old, and the last animal died in September 1975.

The results are given in Table 1 which includes the mean survivals after injection and the numbers with a mesothelioma. As expected, mesotheliomas occurred in a proportion of the rats injected with SFA chrysotile. In fact, fewer occurred than was expected since in our previous experiments (WAGNER and BERRY, 1969; WAGNER *et al.*, 1973) this material produced mesotheliomas in 65% of the animals. However, in these previous experiments there was longer survival and after allowing for this the present mesothelioma rate was similar to that in our first experiment. The shorter survival in

TABLE 1. INTRAPLEURAL INOCULATION EXPERIMENT

Material injected	No. injected	Mean survival (days)	Number with mesothelioma
Italian talc	48	655	0
SFA chrysotile	48	598	18
Saline controls	48	691	0

the present experiment was probably due to the rats having lost their SPF status. Also, as expected, the mean survival of the SFA-injected rats was reduced in comparison with the controls. No mesotheliomas were observed in the talc-injected animals. Howevei, injection site granulomas were common and a small pulmonary adenoma was found in one rat which died 25 months after injection. There was no other relevant pathology of the lungs in these animals. The mean survival was about a month less than the controls, but this difference could have been due to chance ($P > 0.25$).

INHALATION EXPERIMENT

Rats were exposed in 1.4 m^3 chambers which could hold up to 48 rats; caged in sixes. The dust clouds were generated for $7\frac{1}{2}$ h a day and 5 days per week. The respirable dust concentrations were measured daily using a Casella Type 113A size-selective gravimetric dust sampler, and variations were allowed for by adjusting the concentrations on the following days, so that the required dosage, calculated as the product of concentration and time, was achieved uniformly in a specific time. The SFA cloud was generated using the generator designed for the U.I.C.C. standard reference samples of asbestos (TIMBRELL *et al.*, 1968) and in the cabinets about 80% by weight of the cloud was respirable. The talc cloud was generated using a Wright dust feed mechanism and about 40% was respirable. Exposure started in February 1973, with 48 rats exposed to talc and 48 to SFA chrysotile. After 6 months' exposure half of the rats were removed and transferred to ordinary cages, and were replaced by another 24 per dust. These rats were in turn removed and replaced after 3 months' exposure, and all exposure ceased after another 3 months. Thus there were 96 rats exposed to each dust, 48 for 3 months, 24 for 6 months, and 24 for 12 months. There were also the same numbers of controls which were kept in ordinary cages in racks. At the start of each exposure period the majority of the rats were between 6 and 8 weeks old. The mean respirable dust concentration was 10.8 mg/m^3 for each dust and the cumulative doses, i.e. the products of concentration and time, were approximately 4100, 8200 and 16 400 mg/m^3 h for the 3-month, 6-month and 12-month exposures. Ten days after the end of each exposure period some rats were sacrificed and there were also sacrifices 1 year later.

For the sacrificed rats an assessment was made of the severity of fibrosis in the lungs. Sections of both lungs were examined in random order without knowledge of the dust or length of exposure. The sections were observed on a viewing screen of a Projectina microscope 4013 BK at a magnification of $\times 85$. The fibrosis in each lung was assessed on a seven-point scale: 1: nil, 2: minimal, 4: slight, 6: moderate and 8: severe. Illustrative examples can be seen in WAGNER *et al.* (1974).

The mean fibrosis scores of the rats sacrificed at the end of exposure and one year later are shown in Table 2. The main features are that both Italian talc and SFA chrysotile produced fibrosis to a similar extent, and that there was some evidence of progression after exposure had discontinued in the longer exposed animals.

TABLE 2. INHALATION EXPERIMENT—MEAN FIBROSIS AT END OF EXPOSURE AND 1 YEAR LATER (number of rats)

Material	Time	Length of exposure		
		3 months	6 months	12 months
Italian talc	End of exposure	2.2 (8)	2.7 (6)	3.4 (6)
	1 year later	2.4 (8)	3.4 (4)	4.6 (4)
SFA chrysotile	End of exposure	2.8 (8)	3.0 (6)	3.2 (6)
	1 year later	2.2 (8)	3.2 (4)	4.2 (4)
Controls	End of exposure	1.8 (8)	1.9 (6)	1.3 (6)
	1 year later	1.6 (8)	1.5 (3)	1.9 (3)

Most of the animals in the 6- and 12-month exposure groups had died by 6th June 1975, but over half of those in the 3-month groups were still living. Therefore, the 3-month groups will not be considered further in this paper.

The numbers of rats with lung tumours are shown in Table 3. None occurred in the control rats, there was one adenoma in the rats exposed to talc and there were seven

TABLE 3. INHALATION EXPERIMENT—LUNG TUMOURS

Material	Exposure	Number exposed	Sacrificed	Died	Number of lung tumours		
					Adenomas	Adenomatosis	Adenocarcinoma
Italian talc	6 months	24	10	12	0	0	0
	12 months	24	10	12	1	0	0
SFA chrysotile	6 months	24	10	8	0	1	0
	12 months	24	10	11	3	2	1
Controls		48	18	27	0	0	0

lung tumours, including one adenocarcinoma in the SFA groups. In addition, one rat in the SFA 1-year group had a widespread lymphosarcoma. However, as we showed previously (WAGNER *et al.*, 1974) tumours of this type (lymphomas and leukaemias) are an occasional finding in our rats independent of treatment.

INGESTION EXPERIMENT

Rats were fed the test materials with a dose of 100 mg per day per rat. The food mixture was prepared in batches sufficient for 5 days. The basic mixture consisted of equal amounts by weight of coarsely powdered Spillers small-animal diet and Horlicks malted milk. This mixture was chosen because the rats liked it and could be easily trained to eat it quickly and completely. 244 g of the basic mixtures was added to 16 g of the test material in a 20 × 30 cm polythene bag. The bag was sealed and the contents mixed by rubbing between the hands. The contents were then weighed into 5 equal parts and sealed in 5 × 13 cm polythene bags. On the day before a bag was required 5 cm^3 of deionized water were injected with a hypodermic syringe and the contents kneaded into a uniform stiff dough. This was rolled in the palms, still sealed in the bag, and then shaken out on a polythene rolling sheet. The cylinder of dough was then rolled out to the length of a dose-cutter on which it was then laid and divided into 32 portions by drawing a scalpel through the slots in the cutter. The doses were stored in the polythene bag until the next day. This improved the consistency, making them drier and firmer. The doses were administered by dividing the rectangular cages into four compartments. The mesh floor was covered with aluminium and the rats introduced. A daily record was kept for each rat of how much of the dose was consumed. In fact after the first 2 weeks, it was rare for the whole pellet not to be consumed and overall over 98% of the planned dose was consumed, the minimum consumption of one rat being 85%. There were 32 rats fed talc, 32 SFA chrysotile and 16 controls fed with the basic mixture only. Feeding started in February 1973, when the rats were between 21 and 26 weeks old, and was carried out on 101 days in the next 5 months. Except when the doses were being administered the rats had access to the normal diet.

At post-mortem the abdominal organs were examined and the entire alimentary canal removed and fixed *en bloc* in 10% neutral formalin, together with the liver, spleen, kidneys, heart, lungs and any suspected pathological lesion. Tissue for histological examination was taken from the liver, spleen, stomach, ileum, caecum, rectum, omentum, lesser omentum, mesentery and parietal peritoneum and any other site of pathology. Tissues were processed on a tissue processor, embedded in paraffin wax, sectioned at 5 μm bulk stained in haematoxylin and eosin and mounted in DPX. Care was taken during the post-mortem and while handling wet tissues not to introduce possible contamination particularly from glove powder. No steps were taken to eliminate possible contamination via chemical reagents such as the fixatives. Further tissue blocks will be taken for electron microscopical and electron probe identification of minerals.

Two animals from each treatment were sacrificed 3 months after the feeding had finished, and the last animal died in September 1975. The mean survivals from the start of feeding were 614 days for talc, 619 for SFA chrysotile and 641 days for the controls, ignoring the sacrificed animals.

Abnormalities of the gut were found in only two rats. A rat fed talc had a leiomyosarcoma of the stomach. A tumour of this type may have occurred in a rat fed SFA chrysotile although the diagnosis is not certain (possibly it is a reticulum celled sarcoma). Other findings were an adrenal adenoma in a control rat, sarcomas of the uterus in two rats fed talc, and in one fed SFA and a lymphosarcoma in a rat fed SFA. These latter findings are not considered as consequences of the feeding because of their location; also we have previously observed three sarcomas of the uterus out of 126 control rats (WAGNER *et al.*, 1974). The two leiomyosarcomas of the stomach could possibly be a consequence of the feeding although malignant tumours of the digestive organs and peritoneum do occur in our rats in the absence of treatment, and we found three in the group of controls referred to above, although none was a leiomyosarcoma.

REFERENCES

TIMBRELL, V., HYETT, A. W. and SKIDMORE, J. W. (1968) *Ann. occup. Hyg.* **11**, 273–281.
WAGNER, J. C. and BERRY, G. (1969) *Br. J. Cancer* **23**, 567–581
WAGNER, J. C., BERRY, G and TIMBRELL, V. (1973) *Br. J. Cancer* **28**, 173–185.
WAGNER, J. C., BERRY, G., SKIDMORE, J. W. and TIMBRELL, V. (1974) *Br. J. Cancer* **29**, 252–269.

DISCUSSION

S. J. ROTHENBURG: Were the particle size distributions similar for the samples of talc and chrysotile?

J. C. MARTIN: In the inhalation experiments, how much dust was retained in the lungs at the end of exposure? Do you think that retention and clearance are the same for each dust tested; if not, can one really say that the fibrogenic potential is the same?

MR SKIDMORE: Whilst continuous sampling was used to determine respirable mass concentrations only occasional samples were obtained for microscopical examination. These indicated that the respirable fraction of the talc cloud contained approximately 1300 particles/ml larger than 1 μm. Between 1 and 2% of these were fibrous with lengths up to about 20 μm and diameters between 1 and 2 μm. The SFA cloud contained approximately 500 fibres/ml longer than 5 μm plus a substantial number of shorter fibres and non-fibrous particles of similar chemical composition.

Retention and clearance were certainly not the same for the two dusts. For talc, in those rats sacrificed at the end of exposure, there were 2.5, 4.7 and 12.2 mg talc per rat in the lungs after 3, 6 and 12 months' exposure. With the chrysotile much smaller amounts were found and even after 12 months, the mean was only 0.8 mg. One reason for using the inhalation route is to allow these differences to play their part; that is, the actual rather than the potential effect is determined.

E. K. CUNDY: You say that your mineral is free of fibrous particles of the tremolite type. Was any electron microscopy carried out on this sample to check the absence or otherwise of fibrous particles?

W. SMITHER: You said that you found no tremolite or asbestos in this talc. Have you found any fibres at all? This conference has learned that fibre morphology is the important factor. Would you care to characterize the fibres you found in talc? Would you say that they conform to the classical description of asbestos—that is a hydrated fibrous silicate? If so, must we change the classical description of asbestos or must we accept that there are asbestos fibres in cosmetic talc?

DR POOLEY: The examinations performed on the talc included X-ray diffraction analysis, differential thermal and thermal gravimetric analysis on the bulk material while the transmission electron microscope fitted with an energy-dispersive X-ray analyser was used to study single fibres in the samples in an effort to detect asbestos. The many fibrous particles analysed in the samples, i.e. those particles with a $> 3:1$ axial ratio, were found to be laths of talc or chlorite mineral.

Dr Smither poses a very interesting question concerning the definition of asbestos. If we look very closely at industrial silicate materials imported into Great Britain for use by the various manufacturing industries, we find that these materials contain numerous fibrous particles. One example is the mineral sepiolite which is a magnesium silicate which forms very fine fibre very similar to chrysotile but yet is not called asbestos. If you ask me whether or not the fibres found in talc look like commercial asbestos then I would say "no". The diameters of the fibres found in the talc samples were generally in excess of 1 μm whereas the majority of commercial asbestos minerals have fibre diameters which are below 1 μm.

W. SMITHER: Were there any ferruginous bodies in the pathological sections?

DR WAGNER: No.

J. R. LYNCH: Since most of what we know about the biological effect of asbestos indicates that the fibre shape may be the most important factor, it seems that we should regard all respirable mineral fibres, regardless of how they may be described industrially or mineralogically, as presenting a potential hazard similar to asbestos in the absence of evidence to the contrary.

MR SKIDMORE: The talc sample we tested was mainly non-fibrous, i.e. less than 2% of the particles were fibres. Also these fibres were coarser than typical asbestos fibres. Our experiments have surely provided evidence that this talc has an actual and potential carcinogenic hazard at least an order of magnitude less than asbestos, but provide no evidence on the possible effects of non-asbestos *fibrous* material.

D. K. CRAIG: At Battelle, we have exposed groups of 100 hamsters to talcum powder in various exposure regimens, the maximum cumulative exposure being 6000 mg h/m^3, delivered over a year at a respirable concentration (as measured by the MRE horizontal elutriator) of 8 mg/m^3. This talcum powder came from Vermont. We observed no significant difference in the lung pathology of the control and the exposed animals, we saw no significant fibrosis in animals, we saw no ferruginous bodies in their lungs and we saw no fibres in any of the samples we took of the talcum powder aerosols.

G. W. WRIGHT: Since fibrous as well as non-fibrous respirable particles are reported in the air to which these animals were exposed, one cannot be certain which, or perhaps both, may be the fibrogenic agent. Which do the authors believe is the effective agent?

A similar situation has recently come to my attention in humans exposed to flux-calcined diatomaceous earth. The chest roentgenogram of persons thus exposed often shows a diffuse non-nodular pattern similar to asbestosis.

The dust examined by electron microscopy shows the presence of long thin fibres said to be quartz. This observation raises the possibility that it is these fibres that may account for the non-nodular component in these roentgenograms.

R. J. RICHARDS: Mineral particles do adsorb organic materials on to their surface; perhaps this effect should receive some consideration in relation to the biological potential of the "mineral".

A. MORGAN: Why did you select the SFA chrysotile for comparison? Electron micrographs of this material show that it is inhomogeneous and contains both very fine fibres and "chunks" of material which may consist of chrysotile compacted during milling. Tests such as protein adsorption and haemolysis show that it does not behave as a typical chrysotile. Would you hazard a guess as to whether it is the fibrous phase or the "chunks" which is responsible for the reported biological effects?

Dr WAGNER: The SFA chrysotile has produced a higher mesothelioma rate after intrapleural injection than any of the asbestos samples we have used, and as we were looking for gastrointestinal tumours after feeding for the first time we decided to include it for this reason. Actually in the injection and inhalation experiments other chrysotile samples, including one of the U.I.C.C. samples, were also used, but they are not reported in this paper which is primarily concerned with talc.

J. C. McDONALD: Have you any information on the frequency of mesothelial tumours in animals exposed to talc containing tremolite?

G. W. GIBBS: Did you see pleural calcification in your animals?

Dr WAGNER: We have no experience of talc or tremolite in our previous experiments but we have an injection experiment in progress involving tremolite. I saw no pleural calcification in the talc experiments, in contrast to one of our previous experiments with samples of Canadian chrysotile.

M. KUSCHNER: Was the *pattern* of fibrosis in the lung produced by talc similar to that produced by asbestos? Secondly, did the *amount* of fibrosis in the pleura on intra-pleural instillation differ with each of these materials?

Dr WAGNER: In the lung the patterns were very similar but previously I have observed a slight difference between chrysotile and crocidolite. The pattern with chrysotile is similar to that described by Professor Heppleston with a focal alveolar lipoproteinosis around the respiratory bronchioles. The talc produced the same type of reaction. As far as the pleura is concerned the fibrosis was much more marked with the talc than the chrysotile.

V. TIMBRELL: Fibrous and flaky materials such as talc have in common the ability to produce large particles of small aerodynamic size, the aerodynamic size of a fibre being related to the diameter and that of a flake to its thickness. Thus thin flakes of talc can have diameters 25 μm or greater and yet be respirable. Like long fibres, such large flakes may not be cleared by macrophages, etc., and may thus remain in contact with the same cells indefinitely and produce fibrosis.

It is necessary to differentiate between fibrogenicity and carcinogenicity which may not be directly related. STANTON and WRENCH (*J. natn. Cancer Inst.*, 1972, **48**, 797) and ourselves have shown that the *carcinogenic* potential of fibrous materials is related to the particle shape and not that *fibrogenicity* is dependent on the particles being fibrous. It is thus understandable how inhaled talc particles may be fibrogenic without being carcinogenic.

TALC—RECENT EPIDEMIOLOGICAL STUDIES

GAVIN HILDICK-SMITH

Rutgers Medical School and Johnson & Johnson,
New Brunswick, N.J., U.S.A.

Abstract—Talc dusts are categorized into cosmetic grades consisting predominantly of talc mineral free of asbestos, and industrial grades containing varying amounts of mineral talc combined with other mineral dusts.

Concern has been expressed on the hazard to health of talc dusts encountered in the environments of talc-mine employees and of consumers. Data obtained from recent epidemiological studies of mine employees exposed to cosmetic-grade talc dusts are reviewed to assess the health hazard of talc mineral dust.

Study of the respiratory system of talc-mine employees exposed to cosmetic grade talc dusts shows that the pulmonary function and chest X-ray findings were similar to those observed in control subjects, but an increase in symptoms was noted in smoking talc miners.

Review of the cause of death of talc-mine millers exposed to 20 mppcf cosmetic talc dust for as long as 40 years showed no difference in the incidence of the causes of death from data obtained from a control cohort; miners exposed to 600 mppcf of talc mineral dust (containing 5% quartz) showed a higher incidence of respiratory deaths than the controls.

The incidence of deaths from pulmonary tumours and all tumours was numerically lower for the talc millers and statistically lower for talc miners than recorded for the control cohort, indicating that cosmetic-grade talc is not a carcinogen.

The short exposure to small amounts of cosmetic-grade talc in the normal use of talc-containing cosmetic products indicates that cosmetic-grade talc as used in such products is not a hazard to health.

RECENTLY attention has been focused on the health hazard of industrial and cosmetic-grade talc dusts used by industry and in consumer products, on which there are limited epidemiological data by which to assess their precise effect on health.

Talc, which is hydrated magnesium silicate $Mg_3Si_4O_{10}(OH)_2$ (PAULING, 1930), was known to the ancient Egyptians, Assyrians and Chinese and has been used ever since. The current largest use of talc is in such industrial products as ceramics, paint and paper and industrial processes like the manufacture of rubber goods. The talc used in such products and industries is referred to as industrial talc (THOMPSON, 1974) as it is usually composed of talc combined with a variety of mineral dusts to provide the desired physical properties. Industrial talcs can have a low mineral talc content and may contain free silica and other minerals and can contain asbestos.

Due to the possible health hazard of industrial talc dusts, government regulations control the amount and type of dust to which workers are exposed. At this time the maximum talc dust exposure is defined as a Threshold Limit Value (TLV) of 20 mppcf nonfibrous particles and five fibres per ml in a working environment based on an 8-h day for a 5-day working week (A.C.G.I.H., 1973). The grade of talc that is used in cosmetic and toiletry products is called cosmetic talc which is mined from selected talc deposits and can be defined as containing at least 90% mineral talc that is free of detectable amounts of asbestos, but associated with limited amounts of other minerals.

Talc was mined and used industrially for many decades until THOREL (1896) published the first report of talc pneumoconiosis. Talc pneumoconiosis was subsequently reported in workers exposed to industrial-grade talcs, usually before industrial environments were improved (DEVILLIERS, 1961; DREESSEN, 1933; GREENBERG, 1947; MILLMAN, 1947; PORRO *et al.*, 1942). Unfortunately most published medical reports on talc dusts relate to the use of industrial-grade talc and provide no precise data on the composition or the amount of talc dust to which workers were exposed. The exact factors responsible for any ill effects reported cannot, therefore, be accurately assessed. In order to determine the effect of talc dusts on health, it is important to identify the amount and composition of talc dusts in the working environment.

Epidemiological studies have been initiated with cosmetic-grade talc dusts in an attempt to assess the effect of talc mineral dust on the respiratory system and the result of prolonged exposure to such dust.

A review of recent epidemiological studies is submitted to assist in evaluating the effect of exposure to cosmetic-grade talc dusts on mine employees and assess whether the normal use of cosmetic-talc products is a hazard to the health of the consumer.

PULMONARY MORBIDITY STUDIES

KLEINFELD *et al.* (1965) reported that talc millers exposed for an average of 19 years to 62.3 mppcf of an industrial talc containing tremolite, anthophyllite and free silica had a significantly higher incidence of respiratory symptoms, abnormal pulmonary function tests and chest X-ray findings than recorded for a control group.

GREEN and SYLWESTER (unpublished) initiated a prospective study of talc-mine employees designed to monitor respiratory system function in relation to a cosmetic talc dust environment. Data obtained on seventy mine employees were compared with similar data obtained from a control group of subjects employed in non-dusty industries.

The British Medical Research Council questionnaire was used to obtain health data, and pulmonary function information was gathered by use of a Stead–Wells spirometer. AP and lateral chest X-rays were taken under controlled conditions and read by trained personnel.

The main employees had worked for an average duration of 4.6 years and were exposed to an average dust count of 7.6 mppcf. The cosmetic grade talc produced by the mine undergoes a purification procedure in the mill so that the final product consists of more than 90% platy talc, free of asbestos and free silica.

The seventy talc-mine employee population contained eight non-smoking subjects and sixty-two who smoked or had smoked. The eight non-smokers were symptom-free and showed no difference in pulmonary function tests or chest X-ray findings from the control subjects. The data on miners who smoked were compared with data from a control group matched for age and duration of employment drawn from non-dusty industries and consisted of 247 subjects who smoked.

Review of the pulmonary function data obtained on the smoking miners and smoking and non-smoking control subjects showed no statistically significant difference in the measurements of FVC or FEV_1 (when assessed as per cent predicted values using predictions derived from Vermont non-mineral industries, taking into account the person's age, sex, height, and smoking habits) or in the FEV_1/FVC ratios (Table 1a).

TABLE 1. COMPARISON OF PULMONARY MORBIDITY IN TALC MINERS (SMOKERS) AND CONTROLS (after GREEN and SYLWESTER, unpublished)

	Talc miner smokers	Smoking controls	Non-smoking controls
Sample size	62	247	122
(a) *Lung Function Variables*			
No. cigarettes/day	24.8	20.5	0
FEV_1/FVC (%)	81.4	81.0	82.5
FVC (% of predicted)	103.5	100.2	102.1
FEV_1 (% of predicted)	101.9	100.0	103.1
Lung X-ray localized opacities (no. of cases)	2	9	8
Lung X-ray diffuse opacities (no. of cases)	4	15	10
(b) *Other Variables*			
Cough (no. of cases)	14 (23%)	49 (20%)	5 (4%)†
Phlegm (no. of cases)	14 (23%)	23 (9%)†	5 (4%)†
Wheeze (no. of cases)	20 (32%)	51 (21%)*	15 (12%)†
Wheeze + shortness of breath (no. of cases)	7 (11%)	30 (12%)	8 (7%)
No symptoms (no. of cases)	7 (11%)	94 (38%)	89 (73%)
Cough for 3 months of year/subjects with cough	9/14 = 64%	41/49 = 84%	2/5 = 40%
Phlegm for 3 months of year/subjects with phlegm	10/14 = 71%	19/23 = 83%	3/5 = 60%

* = $P < 0.10$. † = $P < 0.01$.

Review of the chest X-ray findings shows fewer localized and diffuse opacities were seen in the smoking talc workers than the smoking or non-smoking control subjects (Table 1a).

The data obtained on pulmonary symptoms show that smoking workers reported an incidence of cough and wheezing similar to that of smoking non-talc workers but higher than non-talc working non-smokers. A higher incidence of phlegm was reported for the smoking miners than smoking and non-smoking control. There was no difference in incidence in the three groups studied when assessed for cough or phlegm production over a period of 3 months for each year or wheeze combined with shortness of breath for a similar period (Table 1b).

CAUSE OF DEATH OF TALC-MINE EMPLOYEES

The long-term follow-up of workers exposed to mineral dusts has revealed that the critical environmental factors which determine the nature and rate of onset of disease, are dust count, length of exposure and specific type of dusts. Enterline *et al.* (1973) showed that there was a critical level (125 mppcf-years) of exposure to chrysotile asbestos dust and duration of employment of chrysotile mine workers below which pulmonary cancer did not occur.

Epidemiological studies on the cause of death of talc-mine employees can be valuable in assessing the rate of onset and type of disease produced by specific talc dusts encountered in an industrial environment. Epidemiological studies of the cause of death of talc miners were initially conducted on workers exposed to industrial grade talc containing asbestos minerals and later on those exposed to cosmetic-grade talc dust free of asbestos.

Kleinfeld *et al.*, (1967) published data on the cause of death of miners exposed for more than 15 years to industrial talc dust containing tremolite and anthophyllite and reported an incidence of malignancy that was four times greater in the older miners (60–79 years) than the general public in contrast to miners in the age group 45 to 59 years.

In a subsequent follow-up publication Kleinfeld *et al.*, (1974) reported on the cause of death of workers from the same mine and showed that the incidence of deaths due to malignancy in the miners was not statistically different from the expected incidence in the general population.

Kleinfeld attributed the drop in incidence of malignancy to the reduction in dust counts, a median dust range of 413 to 30 mppcf before 1945, to 63 to 3 mppcf in 1945 to 1965.

Rubino *et al.* (unpublished) conducted a study on the cause of death of Italian talc-mine employees to establish whether the mining of cosmetic-grade talc free of asbestos was associated with causes of death different from those observed in a control population. The study consisted of reviewing the cause of death obtained from death certificates of employees who began mine work between 1921 and 1950, and who had worked for a minimum of 1 year. The control data were obtained from the records of subjects who lived in a non-industrial rural community 38 miles from the mine by randomly selecting data on male subjects who matched the birth date of individuals in the mine employee cohort and recording the cause of death of those who had died after 1921.

The data on a total population of 1784 mine employees consisting of 1346 miners (88.9% of the total miner census) and 438 millers (91.6% of total miller census) were compared with the data obtained from the control cohort (Table 2A).

Table 2B presents an analysis of the years of exposure of 1325 miners (mean 14.9 years) and 428 millers (mean 15.8 years). Four hundred and fifty-seven (34%) miners and 170 (39%) of the millers had 20 years' exposure and 206 (15%) miners and 57 (13%) millers had more than 30 years' exposure to talc dust.

The air dust content was determined by reviewing records obtained from 1948 until today, with the air dust concentration being constant from 1921 to 1949.

Records of dust counts show that miners were exposed to 600 mppcf of talc dust

TABLE 2. DEATH STATISTICS OF TALC-MINE EMPLOYEES COMPARED WITH CONTROLS (after RUBINO *et al.*, unpublished)

A. *Vital status of 1346 miners and 438 millers with completed follow up compared with respective controls*

		Dead	Alive	Death certificates obtained
Miners	Number	704	642	667
	Per cent	52.3	47.7	94.7
Controls	Number	851	495	813
	Per cent	63.2	36.8	95.5
Millers	Number	227	211	218
	Per cent	51.8	48.2	96
Controls	Number	275	163	254
	Per cent	62.8	37.2	92.4

B. *Length of exposure to talc of 1325 miners and 428 millers*

Years of exposure	Miners		Millers	
	Number	Per cent	Number	Per cent
1–9	652	49.2	190	44.4
10–19	216	16.3	68	15.9
20–29	251	18.9	113	26.4
30–39	200	15.1	50	11.7
40–49	6	0.5	7	1.6
Total	1325	100	428	100

C. *Miners—observed* vs. *expected deaths and ratios*

Latency	Exposed *vs.* controls comparison			
	Total exposed		Controls	
	Obs./Exp.	Ratio	Obs./Exp.	Ratio
0–1	68/84.2	0.81†	100/83.8	1.19†
11–20	110/119.6	0.92	127/117.2	1.08
21–30	203/208.8	0.97	206/200.2	1.03
31–40	188/207	0.91	220/200.9	1.10
41–50	126/157.5	0.80†	184/152.4	1.21†
50+	9/14.1	0.64*	14/8.9	1.57*
Total	704/791.2	0.89†	851/763.3	1.11†

* Statistically significant at 5% level.
† Statistically significant at 1% level.

TABLE 2—*continued.*

D. *Millers—observed* vs. *expected deaths and ratios*

	Exposed *vs.* controls comparison			
	Total exposed		Controls	
Latency	Obs./Exp.	Ratio	Obs./Exp.	Ratio
0–10	16/29.6	0.54†	43/29.4	1.46†
11–20	46/41.7	1.10	36/40.2	0.90
21–30	66/67.9	0.97	69/67.1	1.03
31–40	57/72.5	0.79†	87/71.5	1.22†
41–50	38/42.2	0.90	37/32.8	1.13
50+	4/4.5	0.89	3/2.5	1.20
Total	227/258.4	0.88†	275/243.5	1.13†

† Statistically significant at 1% level

E. *Miners—observed/expected deaths and ratio by cause*

	Total exposed		Controls	
Cause of death	Obs./Exp.	Ratio	Obs./Exp.	Ratio
Infectious diseases	56/66	0.85	75/64.5	1.16
All tumours	100/129.5	0.77†	155/125.1	1.24†
Lung cancer	9/20.2	0.45†	31/19.5	1.59†
Gastrointestinal cancer	46/49.9	0.92	54/49	1.10
Nervous system diseases	9/9.9	0.91	10/9.8	1.02
Cardiovascular diseases	208/276.1	0.75†	334/265.5	1.26†
Respiratory diseases	142/102	1.39†	58/97.5	0.59†
Gastrointestinal diseases	49/59.1	0.83*	68/57.2	1.19*
Senility	12/11	1.09	10/10.8	0.93
Accidents	68/64.7	1.05	60/62.6	0.96
All other causes	23/33.5	0.69†	43/32	1.34†

* Statistically significant at 5% level.
† Statistically significant at 1% level.

F. *Millers—observed/expected deaths and ratio by cause*

	Total exposed		Controls	
Cause of death	Obs./Exp.	Ratio	Obs./Exp.	Ratio
Infectious diseases	14/17.6	0.80	21/17.2	1.22
All tumours	42/46.2	0.91	48/43.5	1.10
Lung cancer	4/7.6	0.53	11/7.3	1.51
Gastrointestinal cancer	16/19	0.84	21/17.9	1.17
Nervous system diseases	4/2.5	1.60	1/2.5	0.40
Cardiovascular diseases	72/92	0.78†	106/85.9	1.23†
Respiratory diseases	25/21.5	1.16	17/20.3	0.84
Gastrointestinal diseases	20/21.8	0.92	22/20.1	1.09
Senility	4/4.6	0.87	5/4.4	1.14
Accidents	28/26.7	1.05	24/25.2	0.95
All other causes	9/9.8	0.92	10/9.2	1.09

* Statistically significant at 5% level.
† Statistically significant at 1% level.

from 1920 to 1950, at which time the dust level was progressively reduced to a level of 2 mppcf by 1965, where it has remained. The millers were exposed to a dust level of 30 mppcf in 1920 when this level was gradually lowered to 10 mppcf by 1975.

The cosmetic-grade talc to which the miners were exposed consists of platy talc free of asbestos minerals but containing 5% of silica dust which arises from the footwall rock in the mine. The talc dust to which the millers were exposed was not less than 90% pure talc, free of asbestos but containing 0.5% by weight of free silica and 3–4% by weight of chlorite and 1–2% by weight of carbonate (WAGNER *et al.*, this Symposium; pp. 647–652).

A review of the overall data on total deaths in the control groups and those of the miners and millers shows that for the miners there were 704 deaths as opposed to 851 deaths in the control group, with 227 deaths in the miller group as opposed to 275 deaths in the control group. The data for the miners (Table 2C) show no relationship exists between the ratio of observed to expected deaths among miners except in those with 41–50 years' exposure in which there is a significantly lower number of deaths than the expected values.

The total number of deaths observed in the miners is significantly less than those for the control cohort. Review of the observed and expected deaths in the miller cohort shows a significantly lower number of deaths in the millers of the age group with 31–40 years of exposure and a significantly lower overall incidence of death for the millers (Table 2D).

Review of death in miners in the major categories analysed (Table 2E) shows a significantly higher incidence of deaths from respiratory disease. In contrast, in the case of deaths due to all tumours as well as lung cancer and cardiovascular disease, the observed deaths are statistically lower than those noted in the control group.

Review of the cause of death in the miller cohort shows no difference between observed and expected deaths except in cardiovascular deaths which showed an observed number of deaths below expected values (Table 2F).

The data obtained from this study show the miners exposed to 600 mppcf cosmetic talc mineral dusts containing 5% silica have a higher incidence of deaths from respiratory disease than the control group or the millers exposed to 20 mppcf cosmetic talc dust containing less than 0.5% free silica. In addition, the lower incidence of overall tumours and lung cancer reported in the mine employees in contrast to the control group indicates that dust encountered in the mine or cosmetic-grade talc dust encountered in the mill is not a carcinogen in the population studied.

DISCUSSION

In recent years interest has been focused on the potential hazard of talc dusts present in industrial and consumer environments. As industrial and consumer talcs can be significantly different in their mineral composition, a review of recent epidemiological studies has been undertaken to identify the potential hazard to health of mine workers and consumers exposed to cosmetic-grade talc dusts. The effect of industrial grade talcs on the health of those exposed to them will be determined by appropriate epidemiological studies.

Initial data obtained from an ongoing epidemiological study of pulmonary function in talc-mine workers exposed to cosmetic-grade talc have been submitted.

The data show that non-smoking talc miners showed no difference in incidence of pulmonary symptoms, chest X-ray and pulmonary function findings from the control population studied. The workers who smoked also showed no difference in pulmonary function tests and chest X-ray findings from the control subjects. The smoking talc workers had a similar incidence of cough and wheeze but a higher incidence of phlegm as compared to the smoking and non-smoking control subjects.

These data indicate that workers exposed to the cosmetic-grade talc dust environment described did not show evidence of pulmonary disease. The significance of increased incidence of phlegm in miners who smoke, in the absence of abnormal pulmonary function and chest X-ray findings, has yet to be determined.

It is of interest to note that talc dust is not an allergen and that available data show that talc dust is readily ingested by pulmonary macrophages, which does not alter the viability of the cells or their phagocytosis of colloidal particles (DI LUZIO, unpublished).

In college-age subjects, smoking has been shown to induce a significant increase in incidence of cough, phlegm and wheezing as opposed to the incidence noted in a non-smoking control group (PETERS and FERRIS, 1967). In addition, in a survey of respiratory symptoms reported among employees working in a chrysotile asbestos mine (MCDONALD *et al.*, 1972), it was shown that smoking was a determinant in producing bronchitic symptoms. ROSSITER and WEILL (1974) have indicated that smoking in a dust environment produces an adverse synergistic effect which is demonstrated by pulmonary lung function tests. These data suggest that workers exposed to a dust environment who smoke may run a higher risk of developing pulmonary disease than non-smokers. Prospective study of workers who smoke in dusty environments will, however, determine whether or not pulmonary disease develops.

As long-term exposure to dusts may produce pulmonary fibrosis or pulmonary cancer, the evaluation of the cause of death of workers who have had prolonged exposure to cosmetic-grade talc dust is important. RUBINO *et al.* (unpublished) showed that miners exposed to 600 mppcf talc dust containing *circa* 5% of free silica arising from the rock wall in the mine had a higher incidence of death from respiratory disease as compared to the controls. Millers exposed to cosmetic grade talc dusts at an average level of 20 mppcf for periods up to 40 years showed an incidence of respiratory disease similar to that for the control cohort, which suggests that this level of cosmetic talc dust exposure does not induce a degree of pulmonary disease that is responsible for death.

Kleinfeld reported that miners exposed to levels as high as 413 mppcf of industrial-grade talc containing tremolite had a higher incidence of pulmonary cancer in the older age group than control subjects and later reported that the difference was not noted when the dust level was lowered.

MERLISS (1971), BLEJER and ARLON (1973), HENDERSON *et al.* (1971) and PELFRENE and SHUBIK (1975) suggested that talc containing chrysotile or talc alone might be carcinogenic.

The study conducted by RUBINO *et al.* (unpublished) showed that total tumours and pulmonary tumours reported were numerically lower for millers and statistically lower for miners compared with the incidence in the control cohort. These data would indicate that talc is not a carcinogen. This observation is supported by a study conducted in hamsters by WEHNER (unpublished) and those reported by SMITH (1965, 1973), POTT and FRIEDRICHS (1972) and GROSS *et al.* (1970) where animals which had talc given intrathoracically or inhaled it for prolonged periods and followed to natural death did not develop cancer.

Review of exposure time and dust concentration encountered by the consumer, in contrast to that of the talc-mine employees exposed to cosmetic talc dust, gives an indication of the difference in exposure to talc dust. A consumer exposed to cosmetic talc dust for one minute a day would be exposed to talc dust for one 480th the daily 8-h exposure time of a talc miner or miller.

The normal usage of a commercially available cosmetic talc dusting product exposes the consumer to a total weekly exposure of talc of 0.102 mppcf-hours (SIVERTSON, unpublished). The talc millers in the study reported by RUBINO *et al.* (unpublished) were exposed to an average dust count of 20 mppcf (the TLV foı talc) which provides a weekly time weighted average of 800 mppcf-hours per week of talc dust which is 7800 times greater than the weekly time weighted dust count exposure to which a consumer is exposed.

The data submitted indicate that the normal use of cosmetic products containing cosmetic-grade talc is not a hazard to health.

REFERENCES

AMERICAN CONFERENCE OF GOVERNMENTAL INDUSTRIAL HYGIENISTS (1973). *Threshold Limit Values for Chemical Substances and Physical Agents in Workroom Environments.* A.C.G.I.H., Cincinnati, OH.

BLEJER, H. P. and ARLON, R. (1973) *J. occup. Med.* **15**, 92–97.

DEVILLIERS, A. J. (1961) *Occup. Hlth Rev.* **13**, 3–14.

DI LUZIO, N. (unpublished) Personal communication, 1975.

DREESSEN, W. C. (1933) *J. ind. Hyg. Toxicol.* **15**, 66–78.

ENTERLINE, P., DE COUFLE, P. and HENDERSON, V. (1973) *Br. J. ind. Med.* **30**, 162–166.

GREEN, G. and SYLWESTER, D. (unpublished) Personal communication, 1975.

GREENBERG, L. (1947) *Yale J. biol. Med.* **19**, 481–501.

GROSS, P., DE TREVILLE, R. T. P. and CRALLEY, L. J. (1970) *Pneumoconiosis, Proceedings International Conference, Johannesburg, 1969* (edited by SHAPIRO, H. A.) pp. 220–224. Oxford Univ. Press, Cape Town.

HENDERSON, W. J., JOSLIN, C. A. F., TURNBULL, A. C. and GRIFFITHS, K. (1971) *J. Obstet. Gynaec. Br. Commonw.* **78**, 266–272.

KLEINFELD, M., MESSITE, J., SHAPIRO, J. and SWENCICKI, R. (1965) *Archs envir. Hlth* **10**, 431–43.

KLEINFELD, M., MESSITE, J., KOOYMAN, O. and ZAKI, M. (1967) *Archs envir. Hlth* **14**, 663–667.

KLEINFELD, M., MESSITE, J. and ZAKI, M. H. (1974) *J. occup. Med.* **16**, 345–349.

MCDONALD, J. C., BECKLAKE, M. R., FOURNIER-MASSEY, G. and ROSSITER, C. E. (1972) *Archs envir. Hlth* **24**, 358–363.

MERLISS, R. R. (1971) *Science, N.Y.* **173**, 1141–1142.

MILLMAN, N. (1947) *Occup. Med.* **4**, 391–394.

PAULING, L. (1930) *Proc. Nat. Acad. Sci. U.S.A.* **16**, 123–129.

PELFRENE, A. and SHUBIK, P. (1975). *Nouv. Presse méd.* **4**, 801–803.

PETERS, J. M. and FERRIS, B. G. (1967) *Am. Rev. resp. Dis.* **95**, 774–782.

PORRO, F. W., PATTON, J. R. and HOBBS, A. A. JR. (1942) *Am. J. Roentg.* **47**, 507–524.

POTT, F. and FRIEDRICHS, K. H. (1972) *Naturwissenschaften* **59**, 318.

ROSSITER, C. E. and WEILL, H. (1974) *Bull. Physiopath. resp.* **10**, 717–725.

RUBINO, G. F., SCANSETTI, G., PIOLATTO, G. and ROMANO, C. (unpublished) Meeting of American Occupational Medical Association, San Francisco, April 1975.

SIVERTSON, J. N. (unpublished) Personal Communication, 1974.

SMITH, W. E., MILLER, L., ELSASSER, R. E. and HUBERT, D. D. (1965) *Ann. N.Y. Acad. Sci.* **132**, 456–488.

SMITH, W. E. (1973). *Am. ind. Hyg. Ass. J.* **34**, 227–228.

THOMPSON, C. S. (1974) International Circular, IC-863, pp. 22–44. U.S. Bureau of Mines, Washington.

THOREL, C. (1896) *Beitr. path. Anat.* **20**, 85–101.

WEHNER, A. P. (unpublished) XVIII International Congress on Occupational Health, Brighton, England, September, 1975.

DISCUSSION

D. MALCOLM: Was the method of estimating talc dust the same from 1921 to 1975?

Dr HILDICK-SMITH: No.

D. MALCOLM: In 1948, when talc was used as a mould lubricant for casting battery grids, some fifty casters were X-rayed, and some showed early nodulation. Six have since died of pneumoconiosis. The type of talc and concentration were not known. Some men may have been ex-miners.

G. W. WRIGHT: Did you find any X-ray abnormalities in the men about whom you are reporting?

Dr HILDICK-SMITH: No.

J. C. MCDONALD: I am unclear and concerned about the choice of controls in the mortality study and their comparability with the study population. It is stated only that they were a random sample of persons of the same birth date from a neighbouring community. Miners are a self-selected group who survive long enough to be employed in heavy work. Were the controls similarly selected from survivors to the same point in time?

Dr HILDICK-SMITH: The controls were selected from agricultural workers living 40 miles from the mine. Each control had a birth date of a mine employee and had to be alive in 1921.

SESSION 9

Friday, 26th September

EPIDEMIOLOGICAL STUDIES (1)

THE EFFECT OF QUARTZ AND OTHER NON-COAL DUSTS IN COALWORKERS' PNEUMOCONIOSIS

PART I: EPIDEMIOLOGICAL STUDIES

W. H. WALTON, J. DODGSON, G. G. HADDEN and M. JACOBSEN

Institute of Occupational Medicine, Edinburgh, Scotland

Abstract—The 10-year attack rate of pneumoconiosis among 3154 faceworkers (initially of category 0/– or 0/0) at twenty collieries has been examined as a function of the individual exposures to respirable dust and its various mineral constituents. The overall mass of respirable dust was found to be the most significant variable, confirming the earlier findings based on colliery mean data. The probability of radiological progression also increased with age. The inclusion of non-coal or quartz in addition to "dust" improved the correlation, the effect being that the probability of progression appeared to fall with increasing mineral content. However, since there is a negative correlation between coal rank and the mineral content of the dust at collieries, an alternative interpretation might be that coals of lower rank are less harmful. In either case, the inclusion of an interaction term between quartz and the clay minerals, kaolin and mica, further improved the correlation; an apparent increase in the hazard with increasing quartz exposure being reversed in the presence of high clay mineral exposure. No generalization concerning the effect of quartz as such is possible from our data. When models derived from the combined data were used to estimate pneumoconiosis progression at individual collieries, substantial variations between observed and expected values were found, indicating the existence of factor(s) not reflected in the environmental data available. Until the reasons for these differences have been further elucidated, the simple mass concentration of respirable dust, unadjusted for composition, remains, in our opinion, the most suitable index of the dust hazard for places in British coal mines when the quartz content does not exceed 7.5% (the limit of the present data).

INTRODUCTION

Although quartz and other crystalline forms of silica have long been recognized as a health hazard in industries and mines where silicosis occurs, its importance in the development of coalworkers' pneumoconiosis remains a controversial topic. Many investigations of the effect of quartz and other non-coal minerals in coalworkers' pneumoconiosis have been carried out in an attempt to resolve this problem: these include major epidemiological studies in British (JACOBSEN *et al.*, 1971) and German coalfields (REISNER, 1971; LEITERITZ *et al.*, 1971); post-mortem examinations of coal-miners' lungs (CASSWELL *et al.*, 1971); animal experiments (SCHLIPKOTER *et al.*, 1971; LE BOUFFANT *et al.*, 1973) and measurements of the cytotoxicity of mine dusts (ROBOCK and KLOSTERKÖTTER, 1971).

Results from the first phase of the National Coal Board's epidemiological research into the relationship between pneumoconiosis and dust exposure, leading to the introduction of new gravimetric dust standards for British coal mines, were reported by JACOBSEN *et al.* (1971) at the 1970 B.O.H.S. International Symposium on Inhaled Particles. These authors demonstrated a strong correlation between the progression of simple pneumoconiosis among coal-face workers at twenty collieries over a 10-year period and the colliery mean (coal-face) mass concentration of respirable dust. A similar finding was reported by REISNER (1971). Additional effects due to quartz were noted by both JACOBSEN *et al.* (1971) and LEITERITZ *et al.* (1971) but could not be quantified. JACOBSEN *et al.* (1971) anticipated that more useful information on the effects of dust composition might emerge when the detailed dust exposures of individual workmen were examined. (Mean values of the individual dust exposures were quoted by Jacobsen *et al.*, but the data were not available in time for use in the statistical analysis.) Further information on the composition and other characteristics of the airborne dust at the pneumoconiosis field research (PFR) collieries was given by DODGSON *et al.* (1971).

MCLINTOCK *et al.* (1971) discussed the attack rate of progressive massive fibrosis (PMF) in British coal mines as a whole, and, at the PFR collieries, they examined its relationship to the dust exposure of the individuals concerned. They found that, although the PMF-attacked men were associated with a higher mean dust exposure than the men without PMF, they were not exposed to higher concentrations of quartz dust during the period studied.

The autopsy studies of CASSWELL *et al.* (1971) indicated that the coal and mineral contents of the lung were the main contributors to radiological appearance with the mineral content contributing about four times as much as an equal weight of coal but inclusion of the quartz content in the statistical analysis did not improve the correlation. A possible explanation of the absence of evidence for a quartz effect in coalworkers' pneumoconiosis may be found in the results of the cytotoxicity and animal experiments (ROBOCK and KLOSTERKÖTTER, 1971; SCHLIPKÖTER *et al.*, 1971; LE BOUFFANT *et al.*, 1973). These suggest that quartz itself may vary in toxicity and that the presence of other minerals, including coal and clay minerals, may inhibit its activity.

Investigations into the effects of dust composition in coalworkers' pneumoconiosis have continued at the PFR collieries, and further analyses based on the dust exposures of the individual members of the populations studied by JACOBSEN *et al.* (1971) are reported here. It was discovered that small errors arising from the use of too few decimal places in the original computation of the individual exposures to quartz and other minerals were cumulatively significant, and hence the exposures had to be recalculated. We take the opportunity to correct the mean exposure data quoted in the earlier paper. It has to be remembered also that the gravimetric data used to calculate the exposures were derived indirectly from particle concentrations measured by thermal precipitator. More reliable data are expected from the second phase of the research which has been continued at ten of the original PFR collieries using gravimetric sampling methods with compositional analysis. The fifth cycle of (approx. 5-yearly) radiological surveys, marking the end of a second 10-year period of study, is currently in progress, and the further data obtained will be analysed when this has been completed.

Parallel with these field studies this Institute is carrying out autopsy studies on deceased coalminers from the PFR collieries whose detailed work and medical histories are known. The first results of this work are given by DAVIS *et al.* (p. 691). Follow-up studies on men who have left these collieries either for retirement or for other reasons are in progress. In addition, investigations of the cytotoxicity of the air-borne dusts collected at the PFR collieries have been started.

This paper aims to review the earlier PFR data supplemented by the later information on individual exposures referred to above. Various mathematical models are examined to explore those factors which should be included in further studies to clarify the effect of quartz and other non-coal minerals in coalworkers' pneumoconiosis.

ENVIRONMENTAL AND RADIOLOGICAL DATA

Details of the population studied, the methods used for the environmental and radiological measurements together with the data obtained during the first 10 years of the PFR at twenty collieries were described by JACOBSEN *et al.* (1971).

Population

The present study relates mainly to the same survivor population of 4122 face workers at twenty PFR collieries as studied by JACOBSEN *et al.* (1971). These were coal-face workers at the times of the first and second 5-yearly radiological surveys and either working at the face or elsewhere underground at the third surveys; their chest X-ray films had been specially read. Particular attention has been given to the sub-population of 3154 men whose chest X-rays showed no evidence of change at the first surveys, as these were considered to be least affected by previous industrial history.

An additional study has been made of men at the same PFR collieries who worked in stone and to whom the lower stone dust standards applied for some part of the time. No men were wholly engaged in such work over the 10-year period.

The first surveys took place between 1953 and 1958, and the third surveys between 1963 and 1968. The periods of observation at the different collieries were therefore staggered by some 5 years overall.

Environmental Data

The methods of dust measurement and of deriving personal cumulative exposures were described by JACOBSEN *et al.* (1971), who also gave references to earlier publications.

Each colliery population was divided into occupational groups based on place of work and occupation. The shift-average (portal to portal) dust concentration was determined for each group. Personal dust exposures were calculated from the numbers of shifts worked in different groups, the shift time and the corresponding dust concentrations. On the other hand, the colliery mean dust concentrations used by JACOBSEN *et al.* (1971) in the earlier analysis were simply obtained by averaging all the shift concentrations measured for coal-face workers.

During most of the period, the dust measurements were made with the thermal precipitator (T.P.). The particle counts were subsequently converted to mass concentrations by the application of mass number indices (MNIs) determined experimentally by side-by-side sampling with thermal precipitators and MRE gravimetric dust samplers. It is not known whether the colliery MNIs remained constant during the 10-year study, but microscopical determinations of particle size made during the period of T.P. sampling suggest that any changes were relatively small.

No compositional measurements were made during the period of T.P. sampling other than microscopical counts of the proportion of non-coal particles. Compositional analyses were made on the gravimetric samples taken during the side-by-side sampling mentioned above and during the later regular gravimetric sampling. These measurements demonstrated good agreement between the gravimetric "ash" determinations and the microscopical measurements of "non-coal". Mean non-coal percentages were quoted by JACOBSEN *et al.* (1971) together with quartz percentages estimated on the assumption that the quartz contents of the gravimetric ashes were the same as those of the non-coal fractions of the earlier T.P. samples.

Subsequently, determinations of the proportions of quartz and kaolin plus mica particles in the original T.P. samples, selected and bulked by occupational group or combined groups, were completed using an interference microscope technique (DODGSON, 1963; DODGSON *et al.*, 1971). The relationship of these measurements to those obtained by gravimetric techniques was examined and appropriate correction factors applied. The resulting data enabled computation of individual exposures to non-coal (ash), quartz and kaolin/mica as well as total respirable dust. The quartz exposures given by JACOBSEN *et al.* were obtained in this way, but contained the computational errors referred to above and corrected in Table 1 of the present paper. This table reproduces the colliery data given by JACOBSEN *et al.* (1971), with minor corrections and additions.

There are some variations in the relationships (Table 1) between the exposure and environmental data. This is to be expected because of the movement of men between occupational groups and their varying times at work. The average number of hours worked by an individual in the 10-year span was 17 400. A few of the quartz data show differences (quartz exposure/dust exposure as compared with the percentage of quartz in the dust) that cannot wholly by explained in this way and suggest abnormalities either in the interference microscope estimations or in the constancy of the quartz-in-ash ratios.

Further estimations of the composition of the phase 1 T.P. dust samples are currently being made using a micro-analysis technique based on infrared absorption, recently developed by DODGSON and WHITTAKER (1974). These should yield more accurate data.

Radiological Data

The X-ray films taken in the early PFR surveys were first "read" for pneumoconiosis at the times of the surveys but temporal changes in reading standards became apparent and so the first survey films were re-read using standardized procedures (RAE, 1967) near the times when the second survey films were assessed. These "definitive" readings were reported by ROGAN *et al.* (1967). The third survey films were read by the same procedure but again apparent changes in reading levels caused concern. Further special film readings were therefore carried out on the first and third survey films of the face-workers present at both surveys. The film-pairs for each man were viewed together and

TABLE 1. PROGRESSION, ENVIRONMENTAL AND EXPOSURE DATA FOR COHORT OF 4122 FACE WORKERS OVER APPROXIMATELY 10 YEARS BETWEEN FIRST AND THIRD MEDICAL SURVEYS

Coalfield	Colliery	Coal rank, % carbon	Number of men	No. in category at 1st survey and % progressing: 0/– or 0/0		0/1		1/0		Mean environmental data			Mean exposures		Time 1st to 3rd survey
				No.	%	No.	%	No.	%	Dust conc. (mg/m^3)	% Non-coal	% Quartz	Dust, gh/m^3	Quartz gh/m^3	Years
	P	84.1	234	229	0.0	2	0.0	2	0.0	1.60	36	4.3	28.2	1.02	10.0
Scottish ..	O	85.4	319	290	1.0	18	5.6	6	33.3	1.60	42	5.5	32.1	1.07	9.9
..	S	82.0	129	118	0.8	6	0.0	2	0.0	1.20	62	5.8	20.0	1.16	10.1
..	J	82.6	254	241	1.7	8	12.5	4	100.0	3.40	43	3.0	43.8	3.52	10.7
Northumberland	D	84.0	113	106	0.0	5	20.0	1	0.0	1.60	43	3.0	31.7	0.62	11.0
Cumberland	M	86.9	261	195	8.2	22	40.9	19	31.6	4.40	44	6.8	69.3	2.32	10.5
Durham ..	Y	86.3	293	189	4.2	36	25.0	20	30.0	5.00	35	3.4	89.6	1.72	10.5
..	T	89.7	281	175	18.9	37	48.6	19	57.9	4.80	33	5.9	83.6	2.43	10.9
Yorkshire ..	G	85.3	268	235	3.8	19	36.8	11	45.5	2.60	43	6.2	47.8	2.47	10.2
..	X	85.2	160	121	19.8	20	60.0	12	75.0	4.50	51	7.8	72.9	3.57	11.5
Lancashire	A	87.8	80	54	25.9	13	61.5	4	75.0	7.20	19	1.2	166.1	2.18	11.0
North Wales	L	84.9	196	127	14.2	28	17.9	20	35.0	5.90	39	6.9	92.9	4.17	11.1
Notts	Q	81.1	291	264	10.2	19	36.8	6	66.7	5.90	51	5.1	137.3	7.20	10.9
Warwick	C	81.8	215	188	3.2	16	37.5	7	42.9	2.50	42	4.2	40.4	1.71	10.2
South Wales ..	W	94.0	99	66	19.7	17	64.7	6	50.0	5.00	31	3.2	75.1	1.81	11.0
(anthracite) ..	E	92.7	76	37	2.7	13	30.8	9	22.2	4.45	19	0.8	58.0	1.84	10.2
South Wales ..	I	91.2	161	70	14.3	26	46.2	17	76.5	3.60	18	2.2	59.1	1.23	10.8
(steam coal) ..	F	91.9	146	65	26.2	35	65.7	10	60.0	8.20	20	2.3	151.7	2.24	11.0
South Wales (bituminous)	V	90.6	335	211	11.4	36	44.4	26	46.2	5.10	28	2.8	99.7	2.72	10.3
Kent	B	88.6	211	187	4.3	15	20.0	3	33.3	4.20	32	2.0	70.9	2.37	11.0
All collieries		86.8	4122	3168	7.4	391	39.1	204	47.5	4.14	36	4.1	72.4	2.53	

TABLE 2. EXPOSURES BETWEEN FIRST AND THIRD SURVEYS OF MEN OF CATEGORY 0/– OR 0/0 AT FIRST SURVEY. BY COLLIERY, 3154 MEN*

Colliery	Number	Mean age at 1st survey	Dust exposure gh/m³			Non-coal exposure gh/m³			Quartz exposure gh/m³			Mean exposures			% Prog.
			Range	Mean	s.d.	Range	Mean	s.d.	Range	Mean	s.d.	Kaolin and mica. gh/m³	$E_Q \times E_K$	$\frac{E_Q \times E_K}{E_D}$	
A	53	27.8	54.6–304.8	156.8	65.9	12.9– 45.6	27.6	8.0	1.17– 3.26	2.20	0.55	11.51	26.8	0.17	26.4
B	187	33.8	38.3– 110.1	70.8	12.9	14.0– 29.0	20.6	2.8	1.44– 3.82	2.38	0.42	11.54	27.0	0.38	4.3
C	188	39.4	19.9—68.2	40.4	8.8	10.1– 30.6	18.8	4.0	0.85– 3.04	1.73	0.42	3.75	6.7	0.16	3.2
D	106	38.1	9.4– 71.6	32.0	13.1	4.9– 26.0	13.6	4.4	0.22– 1.21	0.62	0.24	3.99	2.7	0.08	0
E	36	34.3	26.3– 95.7	59.3	20.8	6.7– 19.2	13.5	3.0	0.58– 3.21	1.86	0.86	6.74	14.4	0.21	2.8
F	65	33.0	42.5–309.2	156.9	54.3	12.1– 64.7	30.6	9.3	1.07– 4.33	2.31	0.65	13.24	33.2	0.21	26.2
G	235	34.4	19.6– 76.3	48.0	10.3	7.2– 27.3	18.5	3.1	1.14– 3.80	2.47	0.42	6.83	17.2	0.36	3.8
I	70	33.2	31.0– 89.2	56.3	15.8	8.6– 16.6	11.6	1.5	0.46– 1.70	1.20	0.29	11.91	14.4	0.26	14.3
J	241	36.4	16.7– 81.0	43.9	13.4	7.1– 42.2	20.6	7.7	1.24– 7.22	3.54	1.28	7.50	30.3	0.62	1.7
L	127	35.4	44.6–151.5	92.4	19.7	15.8– 57.4	36.0	8.3	1.76– 6.54	4.11	0.99	13.92	59.5	0.62	14.2
M	194	36.4	24.1–134.2	69.4	21.8	9.1– 54.8	30.0	8.4	0.64– 4.18	2.34	0.64	7.97	20.0	0.27	8.2
O	289	37.2	11.5– 50.3	32.0	6.7	4.9– 28.7	14.0	3.3	0.26– 2.26	1.07	0.39	3.91	4.6	0.13	1.0
P	228	37.1	12.8– 54.7	28.2	7.6	4.7– 18.3	9.9	2.2	0.52– 1.89	1.02	0.25	4.43	4.8	0.16	0
Q	264	34.5	42.5–260.4	137.7	43.5	24.6–149.9	79.9	24.7	3.11–14.04	7.21	2.06	45.23	354.7	2.36	10.2
S	118	37.3	8.7 –35.8	20.1	6.2	6.7– 25.7	14.4	4.1	0.49– 2.04	1.16	0.34	4.62	5.7	0.27	0.8
T	170	34.6	18.8–141.0	82.8	26.4	6.9– 41.0	27.1	5.7	0.47– 4.14	2.43	0.55	7.10	17.9	0.23	17.1
V	210	34.3	25.4–173.2	98.7	26.9	9.3– 45.2	24.8	7.0	0.84– 6.52	2.79	1.18	6.75	19.9	0.19	11.0
W	65	32.2	22.4–167.2	71.2	29.9	7.6– 31.1	21.0	5.0	0.88– 3.90	1.77	0.52	6.25	11.3	0.17	18.5
X	120	34.7	43.4–103.2	72.6	11.9	23.4– 58.0	41.3	6.1	1.90– 5.00	3.62	0.60	12.71	46.9	0.64	19.2
Y	188	35.4	42.0–133.5	88.1	21.6	16.6– 49.5	32.5	5.9	0.69– 3.93	1.64	0.50	11.08	18.3	0.20	4.3

* Excluding 14 category 0/– or 0/0 men from Table 1 who developed lesions other than of simple pneumoconiosis.

classified by eight radiologists working independently and using the 12-point elaboration of the I.L.O. 1959 classification (LIDDELL and LINDARS, 1969). Each film was assigned to a category on the 12-point scale based on the mean of the eight readings and progression was considered to have occurred if the classifications of the two films differed by one or more categories (JACOBSEN *et al.*, 1971). The results are summarized by colliery in Table 1.

Our studies of the face-worker group have been concentrated on the men whose films were classified 0/– or 0/0 at the first survey. Fourteen of the men so classified in Table 1 were excluded because they developed lesions other than of simple pneumoconiosis, leaving a total of 3154 men. Table 2 gives the dust exposures and other details of this sub-group. The numbers of men starting in other categories are small for statistical purposes: nevertheless it is notable that the order of ranking of collieries by per cent progression from category 0/1 is very similar to that for the 0/- or 0/0 group (Table 3). The ranking order is either the same or different by only one place for eleven of the twenty collieries. Only three collieries show ranking order differences of more than three places. The changes are greater for the 1/0 group, probably because of the very small numbers involved.

For our studies of men other than the selected face-worker group, we have used either the "definitive" readings or "clinical" readings made at the time of survey.

TABLE 3. RANKING ORDER OF COLLIERIES BY % PROGRESSION FROM DIFFERENT INITIAL CATEGORIES

Order	Initial Category		
	0/– or 0/0	0/1	1/0
1	F	F	J
2	A	W	I
3	X	A	A
4	W	X	X
5	T	T	Q
6	I	I	F
7	L	V	T
8	V	M	W
9	Q	C	V
10	M	Q	G
11	B	G	C
12	Y	E	L
13	G	Y	B
14	C	B	O
15	E	D	M
16	J	L	Y
17	O	J	E
18	S	O	D
19	D	S	S
20	P	P	P

The X-ray voltages used in the first surveys were all "normal" (60–65 kV) but higher voltages (*ca.* 100 kV) were used at some collieries in the third surveys. Assessments of film quality (definition, density, contrast) have been made. We have considered the possible disturbing effects of such factors, but have not been able to detect their influence in the present study.

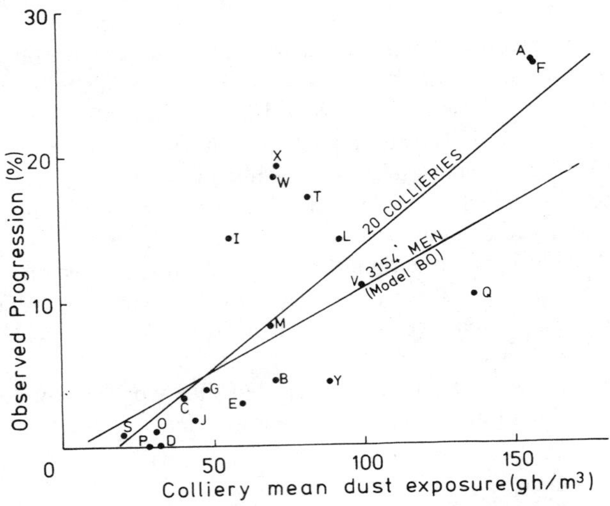

FIG. 1. Progression *vs.* dust exposure, by colliery.

PROGRESSION *VS.* DUST EXPOSURE

Faceworkers

Only 7.3% of the 3154 faceworkers with 0/– or 0/0 X-rays at the first survey showed progression. This fact determines that any analysis of the results must be in terms of probabilities. We have therefore used the probability of progression, or the fraction of men who progressed within a group, as the response variable.

Figure 1 gives a plot of per cent progressions *vs.* mean dust exposure for the twenty collieries. The correlation coefficient is 0.79. Use of (mean dust concentration) × (years between surveys) instead of mean exposures gives a correlation coefficient of 0.84. These are similar to the data given by JACOBSEN *et al.* (1971) using slightly different indices. Also shown for comparison is the regression line for the probability of progression *vs.* dust exposure obtained by statistical analysis of individual responses to individual dust exposures for the 3154 men.

In Table 4 the population of 3154 men has been subdivided by dust exposure. The percentage of men who showed progression of pneumoconiosis within each exposure range is plotted against the exposure in Fig. 2. A closely linear relationship is seen, the correlation coefficient based on the mean values for the nine ranges being 0.96. The slope and intercept of the regression line differ from that for the twenty collieries in Fig. 1. At least three factors will have contributed to the difference. Firstly, different numbers of men were employed at the various collieries; secondly, collieries with

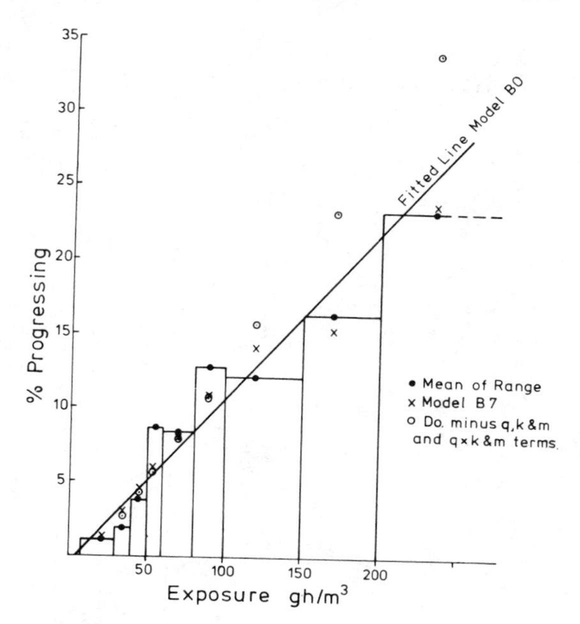

FIG. 2. Histogram of percentage of men progressing within different exposure ranges, based on 3154 individual exposures. The linear regression curve is that computed from the 3154 exposures, with dust and progression as the only variables (Model B0).

higher pneumoconiosis prevalence contributed relatively less data for analysis of progression from category 0/– or 0/0; and thirdly, there were substantial variations in exposures experienced by individuals who had worked in the same colliery. Some of these effects have been discussed by JACOBSEN (1972; 1975).

Extensive statistical analyses have been made of results using various mathematical models and individual values of all the measured parameters summarized by exposure range in Table 4A.

The models examined were of the form:

$$P_C = f(y)$$

where $y = a_0 + \Sigma a_X E_X + a_{XY} E_{XY} + a_T T$,

a_0, a_X, etc. = constants,

E_X = exposure to constituent "X" of the dust, e.g. all dust (D), non-coal (N), quartz (Q), kaolin and mica (K),

E_{XY} = an interaction term comprising the product or quotient of the exposures to two or more constituents, e.g. $E_Q \times E_K$,

T = age at first survey (A), or years of previous work at the coal face (H).

(P_C, per cent progression, is used instead of the fractional progression, P, in order to reduce the number of zeros in the numerical values of the constants).

Also used as an exposure parameter was the exposure to coal dust alone, (D – N), multiplied by a coal-rank weighting factor.

Various forms of functional relationship between P and y were tried including

TABLE 4

A. DISTRIBUTION OF PROGRESSION AND OF MINERAL EXPOSURE BY DUST EXPOSURE, FIRST TO THIRD SURVEY, FOR ALL MEN OF CATEGORY 0/– OR 0/0 AT FIRST SURVEY

Dust exposure, gh/m³		9–30	30–40	40–50	50–60	60–80	80–100	100–150	150–200	200–309	Overall
	Range	9–30	30–40	40–50	50–60	60–80	80–100	100–150	150–200	200–309	Overall
	Mean	22.9	34.8	44.8	54.9	70.4	89.5	119.2	170.5	235.2	68.2
Number of men		471	495	398	288	536	384	405	134	43	3154
Mean age at 1st survey yr.		38.5	36.6	37.2	35.6	34.8	34.2	33.6	30.4	30.6	35.5
Progressors %		1.1	1.8	3.8	8.7	8.4	12.8	12.1	16.4	23.3	7.3
Non-coal exposure gh/m³	Range	4.7–20.3	8.8–25.7	9.0–29.0	9.2–39.3	8.6–49.6	10.1–62.3	18.3–89.1	20.7–117.0	24.3–149.9	4.7–149.9
	Mean	11.0	14.7	18.8	23.3	27.1	32.2	43.9	75.1	75.6	26.8
	s.d.	3.1	2.5	3.5	5.3	8.6	10.7	19.3	32.9	47.3	20.0
Kaolin + mica exposure gh/m³	Range	1.5–7.3	1.5–16.4	2.2–17.1	2.1–19.4	3.1–32.2	2.5–37.9	1.8–56.9	8.5–74.7	12.3–88.9	1.5–88.9
	Mean	3.6	4.8	6.6	8.0	10.0	11.8	18.5	41.8	42.7	10.7
	s.d.	1.0	1.9	2.8	3.0	4.0	6.3	13.9	22.1	31.0	12.1
Quartz exposure gh/m³	Range	0.2–2.6	0.5–3.7	0.5–4.8	0.8–5.7	0.9–7.2	1.0–6.6	1.2–8.8	1.5–11.3	2.0–14.0	0.2–14.0
	Mean	0.9	1.5	2.3	2.6	2.6	3.0	3.9	6.4	6.6	2.6
	s.d.	0.4	0.7	0.9	1.0	1.1	1.2	1.9	3.0	4.5	1.9
Quartz exp. × kaolin + mica exp.	Mean	3.65	7.53	15.63	21.64	28.17	38.84	94.91	329.9	411.21	47.00
Quartz %	Range	1.4–9.8	1.3–10.0	1.2–10.5	1.4–10.1	1.2–10.3	1.1–7.3	0.9–6.7	0.9–6.4	1.0–5.9	0.9–10.5
	Mean	4.2	4.3	5.1	4.7	3.7	3.3	3.3	3.8	2.9	4.0
	s.d.	1.7	1.8	2.0	1.9	1.7	1.3	1.6	1.7	2.1	1.8

B. DISTRIBUTION OF PROGRESSION BY DUST SUBDIVIDED BY % QUARTZ

Quartz %	No.	% Prog.	No.	% Prog.	No.	% Prog.	No.	% Prog.	No.	% Prog.	No.	% Prog.	No.	% Prog.	No.	% Prog.	No.	% Prog.	No.	% Prog.
0–2.5	74	0	58	1.7	31	3.2	26	19.2	119	4.2	122	9.8	178	14.0	45	33.3	24	29.2	677	10.5
2.5–5.0	262	1.1	311	1.6	197	5.1	183	8.7	325	8.0	214	14.5	143	9.8	49	6.1	9	22.2	1693	6.5
5.0–7.5	115	1.7	87	3.4	116	2.6	50	6.0	70	17.1	48	12.5	84	11.9	40	10.0	10	10.0	620	7.1
7.5 +	20	0	39	0	54	1.9	29	3.4	22	9.1	0	—	0	—	0	—	0	—	164	2.4

$P = \sin^2 y$ and the logistic function $y = \ln [P/(1 - P)]$, the direct linear relationship $P = y$, however, proved to be the most successful as might perhaps be expected from Fig. 2. Further details of the methods of analysis together with the equations of the most significant fitted curves are given in the Appendix.

The linear models permit calculation of the expected progression in any sub-group of the population very simply from the mean values of the measured variables, age and exposures to different constituents of the dust, and indeed the contributions of the different quantities to the total expected progression are readily seen.

All the models identify age as a significant factor, with similar coefficients a_T averaging about 0.185, corresponding to an increase of *ca.* 1.8 in the percentage probability of progression for each 10 years increase in age. Age and past years of work at the coal face are highly correlated ($r = 0.75$) and other statistical analyses showed no advantage in using the latter rather than age which is more easily defined.

Table 5 illustrates the effect of age and of past years by dust exposure for rather coarse groupings of the population. The changes in the proportions of progressors are

TABLE 5. PROGRESSION BY AGE AT FIRST SURVEY, PAST YEARS AT COAL FACE AND DUST EXPOSURE

	Dust exposure, gh/m³						
A. Age at first survey years	8.7 – 50		50–100		100–309		Mean of groups
	No.	% Prog.	No.	% Prog.	No.	% Prog.	% Prog.
−30	262	0.8	330	7.3	220	10.9	6.3
30 – 45	776	2.2	691	10.4	301	17.3	10.0
+45	326	3.1	187	12.3	61	8.2	7.9
Mean of groups		2.0		10.0		12.1	
B. Past years at face							
0 – 10	579	1.2	620	7.6	338	12.1	7.0
10 – 20	380	1.8	383	10.4	165	18.8	10.3
20 – 30	292	4.1	168	14.9	67	11.9	10.6
+30	113	2.7	37	18.9	12	8.3	10.0
Mean of groups		2.7		12.9		12.8	

uneven but the variations with age (or years) become greater as the dust exposure increases except in the extreme high age (years) high exposure groups where there are relatively few men. This suggests that a model in which age (or years of past exposure) interacts with the dust level might better fit the observed data. The age terms a_T and the constants a_0 in the model equations are of approximately equal magnitude and opposite sign at the average age of the population (35.5 years at the first survey) so that for groups unbiased by age the plot of expected progression against exposure passes near to the origin.

Models B0 to B7 (see Appendix) include various combinations of exposure parameters. "Dust" (D) embraces all the mineral constituents of the airborne dust so the other terms non-coal, quartz, etc., represent additional weightings, positive or negative, for these materials.

If, firstly, we consider only a single measure of exposure, a strong correlation is found between the percentage progression of pneumoconiosis, P_C, and dust, the slope a_D of the regression line being 0.1127 (% prog)/(gh/m^3 respirable dust) (Model B0). This line is plotted in Figs. 1 and 2. Other single variables, e.g. non-coal exposure or quartz exposure, correlate much less strongly with pneumoconiosis progression confirming the earlier findings of JACOBSEN et al. (1971). The addition of "age" to the model improves the correlation and gives a slightly higher slope, $a_D = 0.120$ (Model B1).

The introduction of non-coal as an additional variable is striking (Model B2). The dust coefficient a_D is increased to 0.175, but is offset by a strong negative coefficient, $a_N = -0.149$, for non-coal, so that the hazard appears to diminish with increasing non-coal content of the dust. If quartz is introduced into the model instead of non-coal, it also appears to have a negative effect, but the correlation is inferior to that with non-coal (Model B3). These relationships are modified when further constituents are taken into account, as shown later.

The relationship to the quartz content of the dust can also be seen in Table 4B, where the population has been sub-divided by dust exposure and per cent quartz in the dust. For "all exposures", the per cent progression is strikingly less for the +7.5% quartz group than for the −2.5% quartz group (2.4% as compared with 10.5%), but this is distorted by the absence of men with high dust exposures in the former group. However, in the two highest separate exposure ranges, there is also a three-fold reduction in progression between the 0–2.5% and 5–7.5% quartz groups. It may be relevant that 64 out of the 69 men and all but 1 of the 22 progressors in the former group were at the two collieries A and F, whereas all the 50 men of the latter (5–7.5% quartz) group were at colliery Q.

If both non-coal and quartz, as well as dust, are included in the analysis (Model B4) quartz has little effect and the correlation coefficient is no better than for non-coal and dust alone. A further improvement in the correlation coefficient is obtained by the use of quartz, kaolin plus mica and an interaction term quartz — (kaolin plus mica), Model B7. "Non-coal" has not been examined in association with these latter variables.

The "expected progressions" using Models B0, B2 and B7 have been calculated for the populations in each of the exposure ranges used in Table 4 and Fig. 2 and the standard deviations of the differences between the observed and expected progressions were 2.15, 2.47 and 1.51 %, respectively. The estimates provided by the best model, B7, are indicated in Fig. 2.

With Model B7 the combined effects of the quartz, kaolin and mica, and interaction terms are insignificant for exposures less than 100 gh/m^3. In the three higher ranges, however, inclusion of these variables yields "expected progressions" markedly closer to the observed results. This is illustrated graphically in Fig. 2. Overall, for the whole population these terms add -0.02 % to the expected progression.

The models have also been used to estimate the probabilities of progression at the twenty collieries. Table 6 shows the contributions of different terms in the models, the total probabilities, the differences from the observed values, and the standard errors of these differences. The estimated probabilities are plotted against the observed values in Fig. 3. Model B2, as compared with B0, substantially reduces the differences between the observed and the estimated progression at collieries A, F and Q, but makes little impact elsewhere. Model B7 gives predictions very similar to those of B2, the estimated percentage probabilities differing by less than 1 in most cases. It is of interest to note the influence of the quartz, kaolin and mica and product terms in Model B7 (Table 6). Only at colliery Q do these terms have any substantial effect. The negative non-coal term of Model B2 also has greatest effect at colliery Q. The range of exposures at Q is from 42 to 260 gh/m^3 (mean 137.7) and it seems likely that much of the effect previously noted in the high exposure ranges of Fig. 2 arises from this colliery.

The strongly negative effect of the non-coal minerals in the previous models led us to consider a further variable, coal rank (as measured by the % carbon in the coal), since it is known that the percent ash (or non-coal) in the airborne dust shows a negative correlation with coal rank (DODGSON *et al.*, 1971). This relationship applies, of course, only between collieries, the rank of coal mined at a colliery being a constant characteristic of the coal seam(s) worked except occasionally where there have been geological intrusions. It is illustrated by the data in Table 1, which give the relationship: % non-coal = 2.5 (100 − % carbon), $r = 0.80$. The coal rank term tested in the models was of the form:

$$a_C \times (\text{coal exposure}) \times (\%\ \text{carbon} - k).$$

The values of a_C and k determine the weighting given to the coal exposure and its rate of change with coal rank (% carbon). "Coal" is, of course, equal to "dust" minus "non-coal". This term was used in combination with other variables included in the previous models and gave the results detailed in the Appendix, see Models R1 and R3. The correlation coefficients from the binary analyses using the 3154 men were somewhat higher than from any of the models that did not contain a rank factor. The value obtained for k was about 83.6. Generally speaking, the effect of the rank term is to give high rank anthracite coals approximately the same weighting as "non-coal" but to give the lowest rank coals zero weighting.

The results from models R1 and R3 are detailed in Table 6 and those from R1 in Fig. 3. It can be seen from Fig. 3 that Model R1 gives estimated progressions appreciably nearer to the observed values than other models for collieries F, W, T, I, J, C and G, but is less effective at A, L, V and E. The mean of differences between observed and

TABLE 6. COMPONENTS OF ESTIMATED PROBABILITY OF PROGRESSION × 100, BY COLLIERY
(observed mean progression = 9.36%)

Colliery	Model B0		Model B2					Model B7				
	Total = const. & dust	Obs. −Est.	Const. & age	Dust	Non-coal	Total	Obs. −Est.	Const. & age	Dust	Quartz + k & m + q × k & m	Total	Obs. −Est.
A	17.25	9.15	−2.11	27.38	−4.11	21.16	5.24	−4.72	25.48	−0.19	20.56	5.84
B	7.56	−3.26	−0.98	12.36	−3.07	8.32	−4.02	−3.61	11.50	−0.11	7.79	−3.49
C	4.13	−0.93	0.08	7.05	−2.80	4.33	−1.13	−2.57	6.56	0.54	4.52	−1.32
D	3.19	−3.19	−0.16	5.59	−2.02	3.40	−3.40	−2.81	5.20	0.04	2.43	−2.43
E	6.26	−3.46	−0.88	10.35	−2.01	7.46	−4.66	−3.51	9.64	0.23	6.34	−3.54
F	17.26	8.94	−1.13	27.39	−4.55	21.71	4.49	−3.76	25.50	−0.41	21.32	4.88
G	4.99	−1.19	−0.86	8.38	−2.75	4.76	−0.96	−3.50	7.80	0.46	4.77	−0.97
I	5.92	8.38	−1.09	9.83	−1.73	7.01	7.29	−3.72	9.15	−0.39	5.03	9.27
J	4.53	−2.83	−0.49	7.66	−3.07	4.11	−2.41	−3.12	7.13	0.63	4.63	−2.93
L	9.99	4.21	−0.67	16.13	−5.36	10.10	4.10	−3.31	15.01	−0.23	11.47	2.73
M	7.40	0.80	−0.49	12.12	−4.46	7.17	1.03	−3.12	11.28	0.26	8.41	−0.21
0	3.19	−2.19	−0.33	5.59	−2.08	3.17	−2.17	−2.98	5.20	0.24	2.45	−1.45
P	2.76	−2.76	−0.35	4.92	−1.47	3.09	−3.09	−2.99	4.58	0.17	1.76	−1.76
Q	15.10	−4.90	−0.84	24.04	−11.89	11.31	−1.11	−3.48	22.38	−8.60	10.29	−0.09
S	1.85	−1.05	−0.32	3.51	−2.14	1.05	−0.25	−2.96	3.27	0.22	0.52	0.28
T	8.91	8.19	−0.83	14.46	−4.03	9.60	7.50	−3.46	13.45	0.41	10.40	6.70
V	10.70	0.30	−0.88	17.23	−3.69	12.66	−1.66	−3.51	16.04	0.56	13.08	−2.08
W	7.60	10.90	−1.28	12.43	−3.12	8.03	10.47	−3.90	11.57	0.30	7.95	10.55
X	7.75	11.44	−0.81	12.68	−6.15	5.72	13.48	−3.44	11.80	−0.07	8.28	10.92
Y	9.51	−5.21	−0.67	15.38	−4.84	9.87	−5.57	−3.31	14.32	−0.23	10.78	−6.48
Mean	7.79	1.57				8.20	1.16				8.14	1.21
standard error		1.29					1.20					1.14

Colliery	Model R1: Const. & age	Model R1: Coal (rank weighted)	Model R1: Non-coal	Model R1: Total	Model R1: Obs. − Est.	Model R3: Const. & age	Model R3: Coal (rank weighted)	Model R3: Non-coal	Model R3: Quartz + k & m + q × k & m	Model R3: Total	Model R3: Obs. − Est.
A	−1.97	11.57	5.05	14.65	11.77	−4.33	11.20	7.33	0.61	14.81	11.61
B	−0.84	5.34	3.77	8.27	−3.99	−3.21	5.14	5.47	0.72	8.13	−3.85
C	0.21	−0.80	3.43	2.84	0.35	2.17	−0.68	4.99	0.91	3.04	0.15
D	−0.04	0.17	2.49	2.63	−2.63	−2.41	0.22	3.62	0.29	1.71	−1.71
E	−0.76	8.83	2.48	10.55	−7.77	−3.13	8.38	3.60	0.77	9.62	−6.84
F	−1.01	22.23	5.61	26.83	−0.68	−3.37	21.14	8.14	0.49	26.40	−0.25
G	−0.74	1.08	3.39	3.73	0.10	−3.11	1.10	4.92	1.09	4.00	−0.17
I	−0.95	7.21	2.12	8.38	5.91	−3.32	6.86	3.08	0.28	6.91	7.38
J	−0.36	−0.47	3.77	2.94	−1.28	−2.73	−0.37	5.47	1.44	3.81	−2.15
L	−0.55	1.60	6.59	7.64	6.53	−2.93	1.67	9.57	0.97	9.29	4.89
M	−0.36	2.78	5.49	7.92	0.33	−2.73	2.72	7.98	0.92	8.88	−0.63
O	−0.20	0.70	2.56	3.06	−2.02	−2.58	0.71	3.72	0.54	2.39	−1.35
P	−0.23	0.21	1.82	1.80	−1.80	−2.60	0.25	2.64	0.50	0.79	−0.79
Q	−0.71	−2.99	14.62	10.92	−0.70	−3.08	−2.62	21.24	−5.12	10.42	−0.20
S	−0.19	−0.19	2.63	2.25	−1.40	−2.57	−0.16	3.82	0.56	1.65	−0.80
T	−0.70	7.23	4.96	11.49	5.57	−3.06	6.92	7.20	1.05	12.10	4.96
V	−0.75	10.97	4.55	14.78	−3.82	−3.12	10.47	6.61	1.23	15.19	−4.24
W	−1.15	11.06	3.85	13.76	4.71	−3.52	10.48	5.59	0.80	13.35	5.12
X	−0.67	1.09	7.56	7.97	11.19	−3.04	1.11	10.98	1.00	10.04	9.12
Y	−0.54	3.22	5.95	8.63	−4.37	−2.91	3.17	8.64	0.48	9.38	−5.12
Mean				8.55	0.80					8.60	0.76
standard error					1.16						1.09

k & m = kaolin and mica q × k & m = quartz, kaolin and mica interaction term.

predicted progression for each colliery, and the standard errors of these means, are shown in Table 6 for various models.

The suggestion that coal rank is a factor in pneumoconiosis is, of course, not new. There has long been evidence of higher risk in anthracite mines for equal dust counts, but to a very large extent this was accounted for by the higher mass-number indices of the dust at the high rank collieries, as shown by JACOBSEN *et al.* (1971), who could not detect any further effect of rank in the cruder colliery data available at that time.

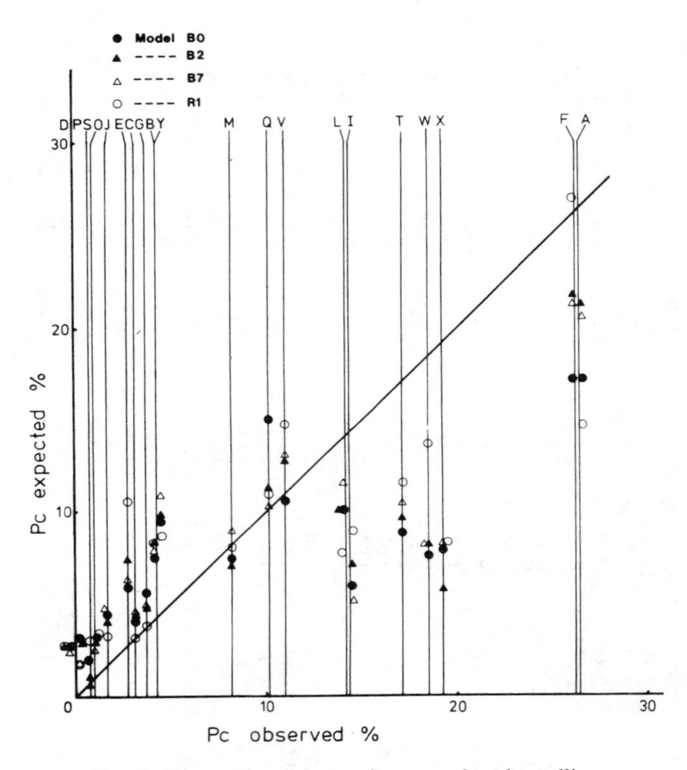

FIG. 3. Expected *vs.* observed progression, by colliery.

Although the models containing coal-rank appear to give the nearest approach overall to the observed progression at the collieries the residual differences between the observed and estimated values remain large in relation to the differences between the models (see Fig. 3), so it would be rash to assert that any of the models examined is "correct." The differences between the models are most pronounced for the low rank collieries and a more detailed study of the data within such collieries should show whether the hazard is predominantly related to the non-coal exposure as indicated by the models with coal rank included or to the coal exposure with a negative component from the non-coal minerals as indicated by the other models. This and other further studies of the data will be undertaken, supplemented by the more accurate micro-analytical data that will shortly be available.

It is noticeable from Fig. 3 and Tables 1, 2 and 6 that major residual differences between observed and expected progressions, of opposite sign, occur between some pairs of collieries from the same coalfields with dust of generally similar character, e.g. collieries W and E in S. Wales, or T and Y in Durham. It seems unlikely that such differences can be explained in terms of our recorded data. There appear to be colliery factors other than coal rank (as measured by % carbon in the coal) that have not yet been identified. Such paired differences are hidden when the colliery populations are considered together as in Fig. 2 and Table 4. (The PFR collieries were selected for their differences, successfully it appears!) The further research in progress, as mentioned in the introduction, is intended to shed light on these unknowns. Meanwhile the present work supports the conclusion of JACOBSEN *et al.* (1971), that the mass concentration of respirable dust provides the best single index of the pneumoconiosis hazard, at least within the range of concentrations and compositions seen in this report.

An example of an unexpected factor of possible significance is provided by colliery T, where a vein of "witherite" (barium carbonate) was exploited in one district of the colliery. Some of the men's X-ray films show heavy lung shadows that may perhaps be attributable to this radio-opaque material. This mineral will be looked for in the further compositional analyses now being made of the old T.P. dust samples, and in the post-mortem lung dust studies described in Part II of this paper (DAVIS *et al.*, p. 691).

Workers in Stone

More stringent dust standards have been prescribed for stone drivages than elsewhere in British coal mines (CHAMBERLAIN *et al.*, 1971), and so the present study was extended to workers in such places. The occupational groupings used at the PFR collieries did not precisely identify all such men, but men classified as "hard headers" can be taken to be closely equivalent. These "hard headers" or stone drivage workers were relatively few in number and none were solely engaged in this work over the 10-year period, their usual alternative occupations being coal drivage or roadway repair work. DODGSON *et al.* (1971) were able to report data for "stonework" based on only twenty-seven bulked samples from seven of the twenty PFR collieries. The ash and quartz contents of these dusts were proportionately 30% and 40% higher than for face work. Mostly, the stoneworkers were not among the population of face workers studied by JACOBSEN *et al.* (1971) and their X-ray films had not been specially read for progression, only the "definitive" or "clinical" readings were available.

Among the total 10-year survivor population of some 12000 men at the twenty collieries, 640 spent some part of the time in hard-heading work, the average being only about 3%. Only twenty men worked for more than 25% of the time as hard headers. The mean dust and quartz exposures of the 640 men (67.3 and 2.5 gh/m^3 respectively) differed little from those of face workers among the population studied by JACOBSEN *et al.* (1971) who had not worked in stone (71.9 and 2.5 gh/m^3), and no differences were seen in the prevalence or attack rate of either simple pneumoconiosis or PMF. All the twenty workers were of category 0 and none showed progression (on the I.L.O. 4-point scale) in the 10-year period. These sparse data provided no evidence of a greater attack of pneumoconiosis among the stoneworkers and do not advance our knowledge of the effect of dust composition.

DISCUSSION AND CONCLUSIONS

Cumulative exposures to respirable dust as a whole and to various mineral components have been calculated for individual members of the 4122 face workers at twenty collieries previously studied by JACOBSEN *et al.* (1971), and the attack rate of pneumoconiosis among the 3154 members of this population who were of category 0/– or 0/0 at the beginning of the period has been examined as a function of dust exposure.

Various functional relationships between the probability of progression and a compound dust exposure parameter were examined; a simple linear relationship fitted the data best for the population who showed no pneumoconiosis at the start of the research. This dust-exposure parameter was the sum of terms comprising the exposures to different mineral constituents multiplied by appropriate coefficients or weighting factors. Interaction terms between minerals were also included, and also the effects of age or years of past exposure.

For the 3154 men, dust exposure (overall mass of respirable dust) was the most significant variable. This confirms the earlier findings of JACOBSEN *et al.* (1971). Probability of progression also increased with age at the beginning of the 10-year exposure. The inclusion of non-coal or individual mineral exposures into the model, additional to dust, improved the correlation; the effect being that the probability of progression appeared to fall with increasing mineral content. This applied to both non-coal and quartz taken individually. When quartz, kaolin and mica, and an interaction term between the minerals were all included, quartz appeared to increase the hazard. At relatively high exposures to kaolin and mica this was offset by the negative coefficients of the other two terms.

When the overall population was sub-divided by dust-exposure range and by % quartz in the dust, the % progression was seen to increase with quartz percentage in some dust ranges and to diminish in others, the overall effect of % quartz being negative as indicated by the statistical analysis. The maximum quartz level was 10.5%; there were few data for concentrations greater than 7.5%.

Some further models were examined in which coal rank (% carbon) was included as a variable. (It is known that the % non-coal in the dust at collieries tends to rise with diminishing rank.) The results indicated that the apparent fall in toxicity of the dust with increasing mineral content might alternatively be explained as a diminishing effect of coal with decreasing rank (% carbon), the non-coal component now having a strong positive effect. Once again the inclusion of an interaction term between quartz and the clay minerals appeared to strengthen the correlation. Further work is needed to distinguish between these alternatives.

When the various models derived from analysis of the pooled data for 3154 men were used to estimate the progression at individual collieries, considerable variations between the observed and estimated values were found. This indicates the existence of a factor (or factors) varying between collieries, but not reflected in any of the environmental data available. Until the reasons for these colliery differences have been further elucidated, the simple mass concentration of respirable dust, unadjusted for composition, remains in our opinion the most suitable index of the dust hazard for places in British coal mines where the quartz content does not exceed 7.5% (the limit of our data). We indicated in the introduction to this paper the further research that is in progress into these matters.

Acknowledgements—We are indebted to many of our colleagues for help, especially to Dr J. Burns for consultation on the medical data and to Mr M. D. Attfield, Mr K.D. Isles and Mr R.C Steele for discussion of the models used, calculation of the best fits and the general processing of the data.

REFERENCES

CASSWELL, C., BERGMAN, I. and ROSSITER, C. E. (1971) *Inhaled Particles III* (edited by WALTON, W. H.) vol. II, pp. 713–726. Unwin Bros., Old Woking. Surrey.

CHAMBERLAIN, E. A. C., MAKOWER, A. D. and WALTON, W. H. (1971) *Inhaled Particles III* (edited by WALTON, W. H.) vol. II, pp. 1015–1030. Unwin Bros., Old Woking, Surrey.

DODGSON, J. (1963) *Nature, Lond.* **199**, 245–277.

DODGSON, J., HADDEN, G. G., JONES, C. O. and WALTON, W. H. (1971) *Inhaled Particles III* (edited by WALTON, W. H.) vol. II, pp. 757–781. Unwin Bros., Old Woking, Surrey.

DODGSON, J. and WHITTAKER, W. (1974) *Ann. occup. Hyg.* **16**, 373–387.

JACOBSEN, M. (1972) *Trans. Soc. occup. Med.* **22**, 88–94.

JACOBSEN, M. (1975) In *Recent Advances in the Assessment of the Health Effects of Environmental Pollution.* vol. I, pp. 211–229. C.E.C., Luxembourg.

JACOBSEN, M., RAE, S., WALTON, W. H. and ROGAN, J. M. (1971) *Inhaled Particles III* (edited by WALTON, W. H.) vol. II, pp. 903–917. Unwin Bros., Old Woking, Surrey.

LE BOUFFANT, L., MARTIN, J. C. and DANIEL, H. (1973) *Conference on Technical Measures of Dust Prevention and Suppression in Mines, Luxembourg, 11–13 October, 1972* (edited by Director General for Dissemination of Information) pp. 127–128. EUR 4957. C.E.C., Luxembourg.

LEITERITZ, H., BAUER, D. and BRUCKMANN, E. (1971) *Inhaled Particles III* (edited by WALTON, W. H.) vol. II, pp. 729–743. Unwin Bros., Old Woking, Surrey.

LIDDELL, F. D. K. and LINDARS, D. C. (1969) *Br. J. ind. Med.* **26**, 89–100.

MCLINTOCK, J. S., RAE, S. and JACOBSEN, M. (1971) *Inhaled Particles III* (edited by WALTON, W. H.) vol. II, pp. 933–952. Unwin Bros., Old Woking, Surrey.

RAE, S. (1967) *Inhaled Particles and Vapours II* (edited by DAVIES, C. N.) pp. 467–477. Pergamon Press, Oxford.

REISNER, M. T. R. (1971) *Inhaled Particles III* (edited by WALTON, W. H.) vol. II, pp. 921–931. Unwin Bros., Old Woking, Surrey.

ROBOCK, K. and KLOSTERKÖTTER, W. (1971) *Inhaled Particles III* (edited by WALTON, W. H.) vol. I, pp. 453–464. Unwin Bros., Old Woking, Surrey.

ROGAN, J. M., RAE, S. and WALTON, W. H. (1967) *Inhaled Particles and Vapours II* (edited by DAVIES, C. N.) pp. 493–508. Pergamon Press, Oxford.

SCHLIPKÖTER, H. W., HILSCHER, W., POTT, F. and BECK, E. G. (1971) *Inhaled Particles III* (edited by WALTON, W. H.) vol. I, pp. 379–390. Unwin Bros., Old Woking, Surrey.

APPENDIX

The models described in this paper were of the linear form

$$P = y = a_0 + \Sigma a_X E_X + a_{XY} E_{XY} + a_T T$$

where the a's are constants, E_X is the 10-year exposure to constituent X, E_{XY} is an interaction term involving constituents X and Y, and T represents age or years of previous work. Interaction terms examined included $E_Q \times E_K$ and $E_Q \times E_K/E_D$ (Table 2).

In earlier analyses by M. Jacobsen, M.D. Attfield and Miss A. M. Skrimshire other more complex relationships between P and y (including angular and logistic transformations) were examined, also many more combinations of the exposure variables than are quoted here. Their results have guided our selection of models. The curve fits were least squares regressions of binary responses (progression or not) on individuals exposure parameters, y.

The variables used, with their symbols and coefficients, were:

Variable	*Symbol*	*Coefficient*
Dust exposure (gh/m³)	E_D	a_D
Non-coal exposure (gh/m³)	E_N	a_N
Coal exposure (gh/m³)	E_C (= $E_D - E_N$)	a_C
Quartz exposure (gh/m³)	E_Q	a_Q
Kaolin + mica exposure (gh/m³)	E_K	a_K
Age at first survey (yr)	A	a_A
Constant		a_0

In the models containing coal rank, the coal exposure was in the form $a_C E_C(\%\ \text{carbon} - k)$, where k is a constant. To simplify the analysis, this was rewritten $a_C E_C\%$ carbon $+ b_C E_C$, $k = -b_C/a_C$. Per cent carbon relates to dry mineral-matter-free coal.

The models fitted and the resulting values of the coefficients are shown on the opposite page.

Binary regressions: Values of coefficients n = 3154

Model	Const., a_0	Age, a_A	Dust, a_D	Coal × % carbon, a_C	Coal, b_C	Non-coal, a_N	Quartz, a_Q	Kaolin and mica, a_K	$E_Q \times E_K$ a_{QK}	R^2
B0	−0.004188	—	0.001127	—	—	—	—			0.0347
B1	−0.06923	0.001684	0.001203	—	—	—	—			0.0378
B2	−0.07363	0.001889	0.001746	—	—	−0.001488	—			0.0431
B3	−0.06673	0.001771	0.001524	—	—	—	−0.01071			0.0410
B4	−0.07384	0.001890	0.001747	—	—	−0.001525	0.000424			0.0431
B7	−0.09884	0.001856	0.001625	—	—	—	0.005302	−0.000520	−0.000284	0.0466
R_1	−0.07191	0.001877	—	0.000211	−0.01763	0.001831	—			0.0501
R_3	−0.09498	0.001859	—	0.000197	−0.01643	0.002659	0.006543	−0.000104	−0.000264	0.0525

DISCUSSION

S. J. ROTHENBERG: You show an interesting correlation of coalworkers' pneumoconiosis (CWP) with exposure to dust as measured by mass concentration and duration of exposure. May I suggest that if other measures of concentration such as surface area/cm^3 or no./cm^3 were available correlations with CWP would also be found? Before it can be stated that simple mass concentration is the best measure, data of all types must be accumulated in several mines over a number of years, and the correlations with each measure of dust exposure compared.

MR WALTON: Earlier work reported at the third Symposium (JACOBSEN *et al.*, 1971) showed that the respirable mass concentration of dust correlates with the pneumoconiosis risk much better than does the particle number concentration. That is the main reason why the British coal industry changed from number to mass dust standards in 1970.

F. D. K. LIDDELL: It is stated that initial category was either 0/– or 0/0. What was the definition of "attack" or "progression"—both terms are used?

MR WALTON: A change of one or more steps from either 0/– or 0/0 was considered to constitute progression. In reality, there were very few 0/- cases.

F. D. K. LIDDELL: Your correlations were between progression and dust exposure. However, with variable periods of study, as here, it is important to base correlations on the rate of change and dust concentration. This will lead to lower coefficients of correlation of the sort seen in Fig. 1, as was shown in preliminary work on the same population, carried out for rather different purposes (LIDDELL, 1972, *N. Y. Acad. Sci.*). Moreover, if studies are to be based on individuals, it is essential that they be carried out within collieries, or at the very least by standardizing for collieries (by use of dummy variables in the regression analyses). I saw no evidence of such standardization; was it in fact carried out?

MR. WALTON. The period of observation differed slightly between collieries and if we had used dust concentrations in the analysis we would, of course, have standardized for these differences. However, we used cumulative exposures (*ct*), not concentrations, which take time into account, and we do not think that any further independent effect of the time period would be important within the range of our values. More significant, perhaps, would be fluctuations of concentration within the approximate 10-year period of observation (i.e. whether the greater part of the exposure was received early or late in the period) but we were not able to examine this.

I agree with your point about individual collieries and indeed this is emphasized in the paper. That is why we have presented data by collieries as well as the pooled data. The numbers at individual collieries are usually too small for reliable conclusions to be drawn.

F. D. K. LIDDELL: The values of R^2 in the Appendix are presumably the squared multiple correlation coefficients. Your "binomial regression" technique is exactly analogous to discriminant analysis, where the upper bound of R^2 is unity. Thus even the best of the reported fits, which are associated with $R^2 = 0.05$, means that only 5% of the variation between subjects has been accounted for by the exposure variables.

MR. WALTON: Our model assumes that the *probability* of pneumoconiosis progression is a continuous function of dust exposure and the validity of this is demonstrated by the high correlation between % progression and mean exposure for the groups in Table 2 and Fig. 2 ($R^2 = 0.93$ for Model B0). The lower values of R^2 for the binomial regressions based on the "yes" or "no" responses of individuals are to be expected and are consistent with the model. They reflect the fact that our data cannot explain why one individual may be "attacked" whereas another with equal dust exposure is not.

M. REISNER: This is the second time that good agreement has been found between the results of epidemiological investigations in British and German coal mines. Five years ago we agreed fairly well on the risk of contracting pneumoconiosis as a function of dust exposure; now the results on the effect of quartz are similar (see this Symposium, p. 703). We are glad to note this and expect that you are too.

MR. WALTON: Yes, indeed.

THE EFFECT OF QUARTZ AND OTHER NON-COAL DUSTS IN COALWORKERS' PNEUMOCONIOSIS.

PART II. LUNG AUTOPSY STUDY

J. M. G. DAVIS, J. OTTERY and ANNE LE ROUX

Institute of Occupational Medicine, Edinburgh, Scotland

Abstract—Preliminary pathological and mineralogical studies are reported on seventy-four sets of lungs from British coal miners who have been employed at the collieries included in the National Coal Board's Pneumoconiosis Field Research. The degree of lung damage was considered in relation to the lung dust content and to the known dust exposures of the men concerned. Lungs were classified as having soft macules, fibrotic nodules or PMF. Those with soft macules had the lowest dust content but there was no significant difference between the dust contents of the lungs with fibrotic lesions and those with PMF. The percentage of non-coal minerals in the lung dust appeared to increase with the pathological classification from soft macules to PMF, and comparisons with the exposure data indicated a preferential retention of non-coal minerals, and especially of quartz, in the cases with the more severe lesions. Histological examination of the lesions showed the packing of dust was less close and the cellular response more vigorous with the lungs with the highest quartz content.

INTRODUCTION

The pathogenesis of progressive massive fibrosis (PMF) in coal workers' lungs has been the subject of extensive studies for a number of years. The different theories of aetiology of PMF have been reviewed by ROGAN (1970).

The silica theory of the origin of PMF remains the most widely held hypothesis and has been examined in a previous study by NAGELSCHMIDT *et al.* (1963). These workers excised PMF lesions from pneumoconiotic lungs and analysed the dust contents separately from the rest of the lungs. They reported that although the dust load in PMF lesions was higher than in the rest of the lungs, the compositions of the dusts did not differ significantly in their quartz contents. Furthermore, no significant differences were observed in the percentage quartz composition of dusts from PMF and simple pneumoconiotic lungs. They concluded that the silica theory of the origin of the PMF was not supported by their study. However, PRATT (1968) has recalculated the data reported by NAGELSCHMIDT *et al.* (1963) and suggested that if the total weight of silica per lung is considered rather than the percentage of silica in the lung, then there is an association between high silica values and the presence of PMF.

Since 1953 the dust exposures of mine workers employed at selected British collieries have been measured by the National Coal Board as part of the Pneumoconiosis Field Research. Detailed information on the dust exposures of some 38 000 individuals is consequently available and forms the basis of the present study (JACOBSEN *et al.*, 1971). Lungs collected at autopsy from mine workers covered by the Pneumoconiosis Field Research have been examined and the lung pathology and dust contents determined. The present paper reports the preliminary findings of the study and relates the dust content and dust composition of the first seventy-four sets of lungs examined to the lung pathology and to the quantity and composition of the dust to which the coal-workers were exposed during their working lives.

MATERIALS AND METHODS

The lungs examined in the present study were received by courtesy of the Pneumoconiosis Medical Panels. These panels, which are situated in each of the main mining areas, examine all miners claiming compensation for pneumoconiosis. Compensation for the disease after death is only payable if post-mortem evidence of disease is found by the Panels. The Panels have been provided with index cards for all miners involved in the Pneumoconiosis Field Research and can, therefore, identify any case coming to autopsy which was included in this study. After examination by the medical Panels the lungs were made available for pathological examination and analysis of their mineral contents.

The cases selected in this way will, therefore, tend to be a biased sample with respect to age and extent of lung disease. This situation is unavoidable but, even so, the cases received encompass the range of normal and pneumoconiotic lungs one would expect in an unbiased sample.

The lungs were received after fixation with formalin. For pathological examination they were sliced to a thickness of 1 cm in the sagittal plane. All types of coal-dust lesion as well as areas of emphysema were carefully mapped and estimated, and blocks of tissue for histological examination were taken from every area of the lung. One complete slice of lung tissue was retained from each case for possible further studies, while samples of the remaining tissue were digested to liberate the retained dust.

This tissue was finely sliced and allowed to drain prior to weighing and mincing. The minced lungs were dried *in vacuo* at 105°C and ground in an end runner mill to give particles about 200 μm diameter. The dried ground lungs were weighed and stored until required. The procedure employed for the recovery of dust from representative samples of the dried lung was a modification of the method reported by RIVERS *et al.* (1963), in which the tissue is removed by hydrolysis with concentrated hydrochloric acid at 60°C. The dusts recovered from the tissue digestion procedure were ashed for 3 days to constant weight in a muffle furnace at 380°C and the coal content calculated from the weight loss. The quartz, kaolin and mica content of the residual ashes were determined by infrared spectrophotometry using the potassium bromide disc method (DODGSON and WHITTAKER, 1973).

The weight of each mineral in one lung was calculated by multiplying the total dried weight of the lung by the percentage of the mineral in the sample of lung taken for analysis.

From a complete set of lungs, one lung had been randomly selected and a stock slice retained. The other lung was used for mineral analysis. When calculating the dust content of both lungs, corrections were applied to the dust weight in the lung analysed to account for the different ventilation of the right and left lungs (SVANBERG, 1957). In cases where the right lung was analysed the weights of mineral present were multiplied by 1.85, where left lungs were analysed the correction factor was 2.17. The weight of blood in the formalin-fixed lungs was determined by the method of BERGMAN and LOXLEY (1971).

For the seventy-four cases reported in the present study it was possible to obtain chest X-rays taken within 2 years of death in forty-five instances. These were read by seven doctors from the National Coal Board's Radiological Services using the I.L.O. 1968 standard films for classification.

RESULTS

In order to correlate the pathology of coal workers' pneumoconiosis with the results of dust analysis it was decided to classify the lungs into three groups. The first group contained cases where all the coal-dust lesions consisted of soft macules with minimal fibrosis. The second group contained those cases where, in addition to soft macules, there were hard fibrotic nodules present with diameters below 1 cm. The third group consisted of cases where fibrotic nodules larger than 1 cm were present in the lung. These were classified as progressive massive fibrosis.

A comparison of the radiological classification with the pathological classification is shown in Table 1 for the forty-five cases in which chest radiographs taken within two years of death were available.

TABLE 1. A COMPARISON OF THE RADIOLOGICAL CLASSIFICATION OF CASES WITH THE CORRESPONDING PATHOLOGICAL ASSESSMENT

<table>
<tr><th></th><th colspan="11">Radiological category (N.C.B. elaboration of I.L.O. classification)</th></tr>
<tr><th>Pathological classification</th><th>0/0</th><th>0/1</th><th>1/0</th><th>1/1</th><th>1/2</th><th>2/1</th><th>2/2</th><th>2/3</th><th>3/2</th><th>3/3</th><th>PMF</th></tr>
<tr><td>Soft macules</td><td colspan="2">6</td><td colspan="3">–</td><td colspan="3">–</td><td colspan="2">–</td><td>1</td></tr>
<tr><td>Fibrotic lesions</td><td colspan="2">7</td><td colspan="3">5</td><td colspan="3">3</td><td colspan="2">1</td><td>1</td></tr>
<tr><td>PMF</td><td colspan="2">1</td><td colspan="3">1</td><td colspan="3">–</td><td colspan="2">–</td><td>19</td></tr>
</table>

Six out of seven cases with only soft dust macules in the lungs were classified as Category 0. Of the cases that contained fibrotic nodules, seven out of seventeen were still classed as Category 0, but the remainder were placed in higher categories that showed good correlation with the number and size of the nodules found in the lung. Twenty-one cases were classified radiologically as PMF. Of these cases nineteen contained fibrotic lesions larger than 1 cm in diameter, one case contained a large number of small fibrotic lesions and the remaining case proved to contain an atypical patch of pneumonia associated with large amounts of mine dust. Those figures indicated that direct examination of lung tissue was a more accurate method of estimating the presence of early pneumoconiosis lesions than categorization from X-ray photographs, and therefore for comparison with dust data this direct pathological classification was adopted. All cases containing recognizable dust lesions were considered to have pneumoconiosis.

A comparison of X-ray categories of simple pneumoconiosis with the dust content of the lungs indicated an association between the total dust content and X-ray category consistent with previous work (ROSSITER *et al.*, 1967), but no apparent relationship between X-ray category and any mineral type. However, only seventeen cases of simple pneumoconiosis with recent X-ray data were available. A more detailed comparison of X-ray categories, pathology and dust content will be made when more cases have been studied.

When the seventy-four cases classified into pathological classes were considered in relation to their dust content, the results were as follows.

The mean weights of minerals found in the lungs of mine workers are shown in Fig. 1. The results indicate significantly lower weights of total dust and non-coal minerals in

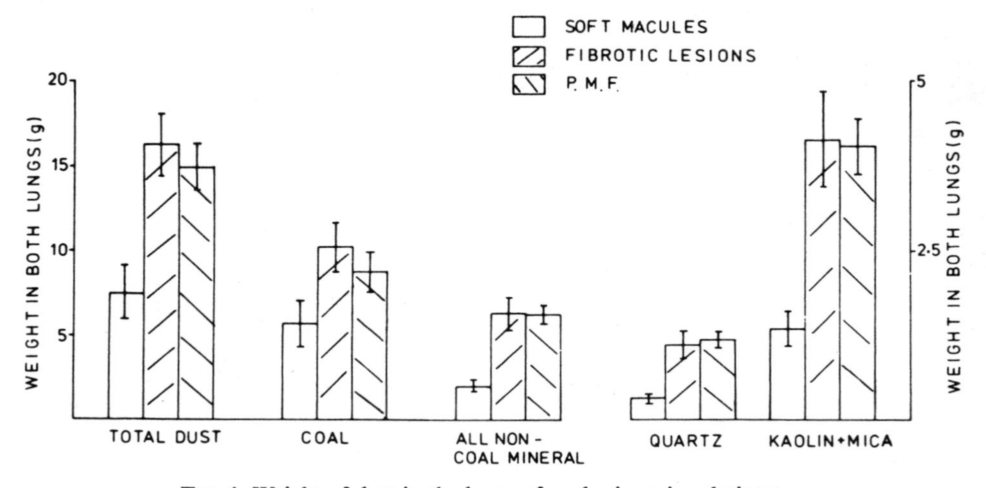

FIG. 1. Weight of dust in the lungs of coal miners in relation to the type of pneumoconiosis lesion.

the lungs containing soft macules than in those lungs with small fibrotic lesions or PMF. No statistical differences were detected between the weights of the various minerals in lungs with small fibrotic lesions and in lungs with PMF.

The percentage mineral compositions of the lung dusts for the three pathological classes are shown in Fig. 2. There was a tendency for the proportion of non-coal minerals in the dust to increase with increasing severity of pneumoconiosis. The composition of the dust from lungs with soft macules was significantly different from that of the dust from PMF cases, the percentage ash, quartz, kaolin and mica being higher in the dust from PMF cases ($P < 0.01$).

In ten cases it was possible to excise the PMF lesions from the lungs and to analyse the dust contents separately from the rest of the lung. The dust concentration in the PMF lesions was found to be 2–3 times higher, on average, than the concentration in the rest of the lung. There were, however, no differences in the dust composition between these two groups of samples.

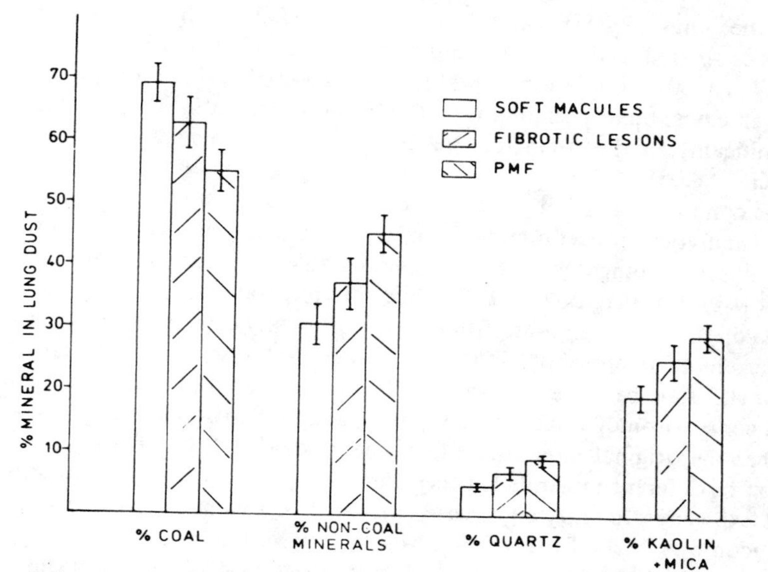

FIG. 2. Percentage composition of dust from the lungs of coal miners in relation to the type of pneumoconiosis lesion.

A comparison of the composition of the dust recovered from individual lungs with the composition of the mine dust to which the individual was exposed is shown in Fig. 3. The data are expressed as ratios of the percentage mineral in lung dust to the percentage mineral in mine dust. The expression of the data in this manner allows one to assess the "enrichment" of any particular mineral in lung dust. It is apparent that the

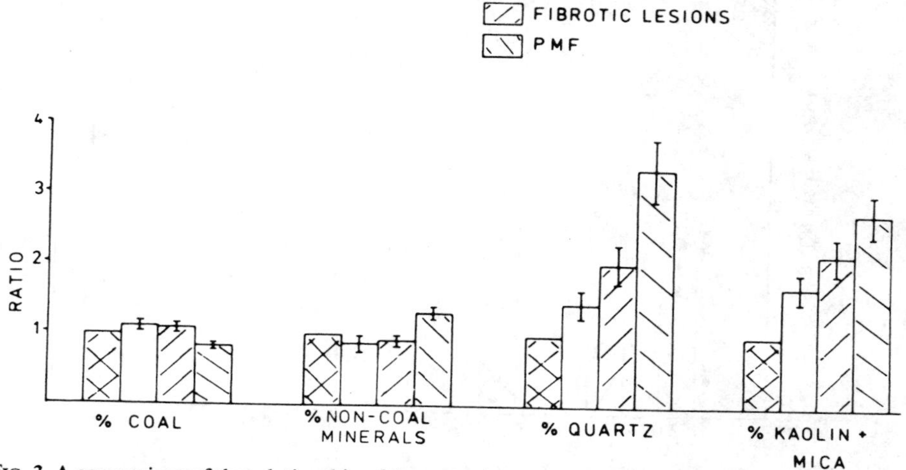

FIG. 3. A comparison of the relationship of the type of pneumoconiosis to the relative composition of lung dust and mine dust expressed as a ratio.

dust in the lungs of PMF cases has been "enriched" with respect to the non-coal minerals compared to the dust in lungs which have soft macules ($P < 0.01$) or fibrotic lesions ($P < 0.001$). There were notable increases in the ratios for quartz, kaolin and mica in all cases, but especially in the PMF lungs. The ratio for quartz in PMF lungs was significantly higher than for the lungs with soft macules ($P < 0.01$) or fibrotic lesions ($P < 0.05$).

In this comparison of lung-dust and mine-dust compositions it must be noted that different analytical procedures were used to determine the composition of the two types of dust. The lung dusts were analysed by an infrared spectrophotometric method (DODGSON and WHITTAKER, 1973) while the mineral compositions of mine dusts, collected on thermal precipitator slides, were originally determined by light microscopy and interference microscopy (DODGSON, 1963). At present the original thermal precipitator slides are being reanalysed by the infrared spectrophotometric method so that a direct comparison of values will soon be available. However, even if these studies do show that the original mine dust figures need revision, the differences in percentage retention of different minerals between the three groups of lungs must still remain.

Dust exposures for fifty-eight cases included in this study were derived from the Pneumoconiosis Field Research records. The investigation of dust exposures was restricted to those men who had spent more than 50% of their working lives in the PFR collieries. Since the majority of men under consideration had spent some years underground prior to the commencement of the PFR investigation it was necessary to assume that the dust levels at the collieries during these years were similar to those in the first 5 years of the study. In practice the proportion of the working lifetime dust exposure actually measured varied between 15 and 40%. A preliminary examination of

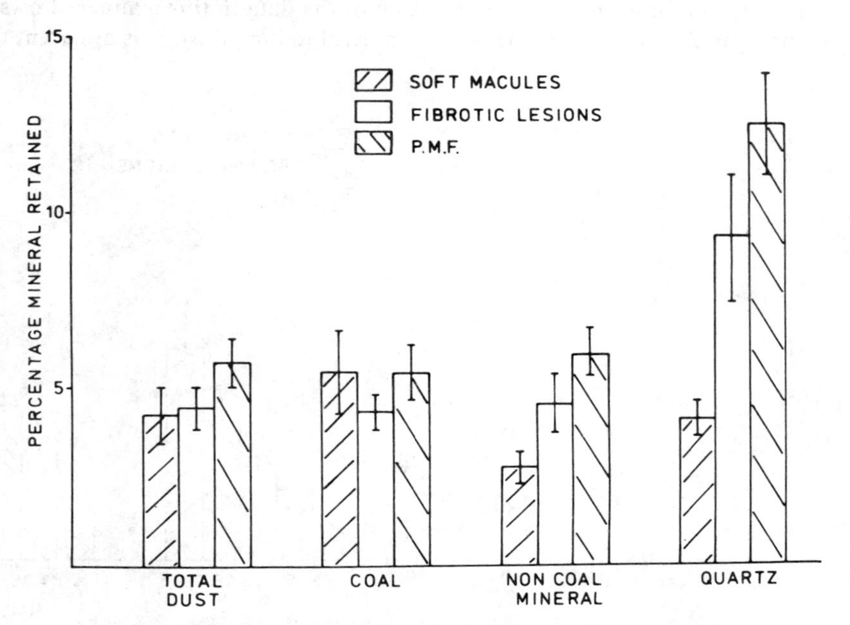

FIG. 4. The percentage retention of inhaled minerals compared to the severity of pneumoconiosis lesions.

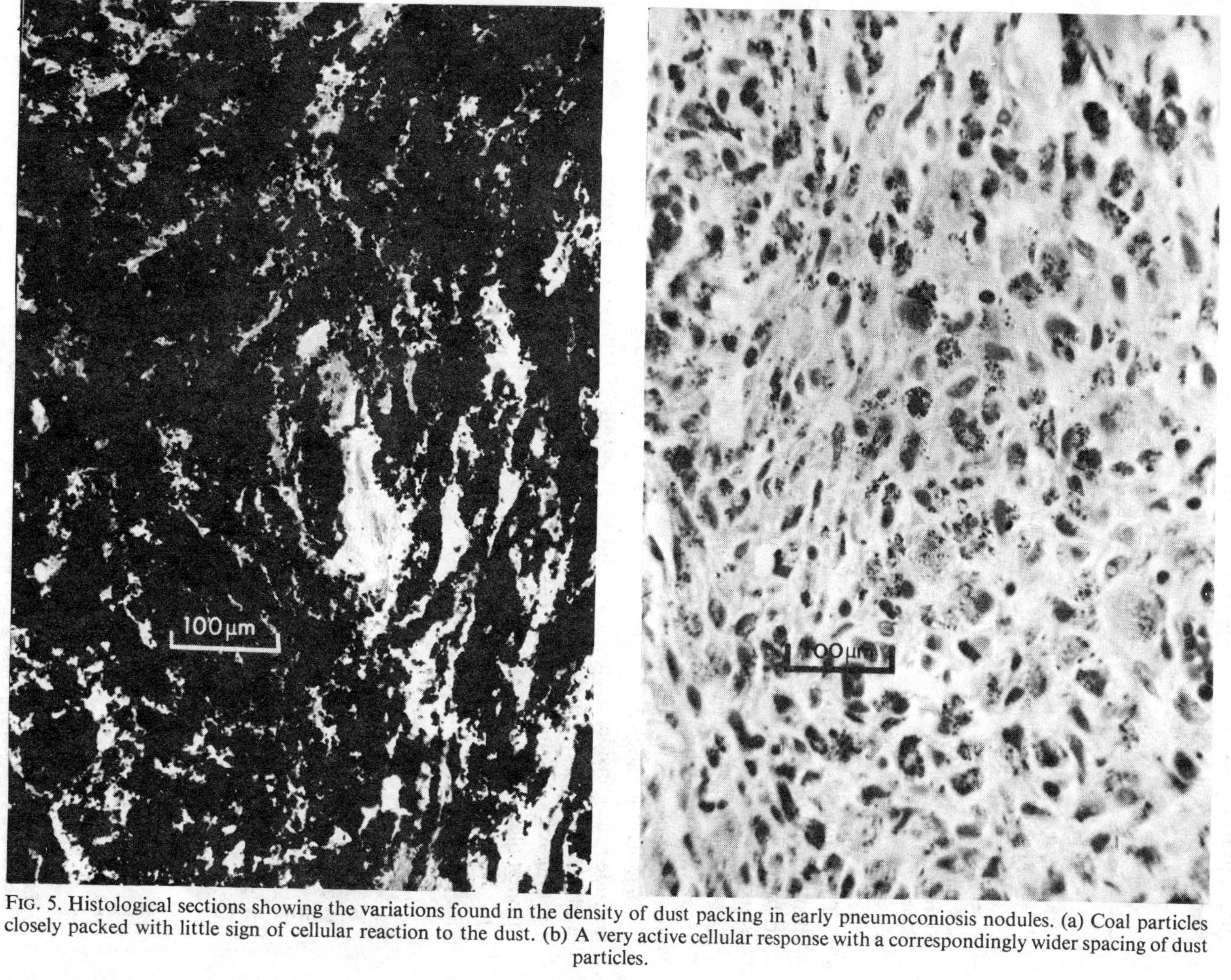

FIG. 5. Histological sections showing the variations found in the density of dust packing in early pneumoconiosis nodules. (a) Coal particles closely packed with little sign of cellular reaction to the dust. (b) A very active cellular response with a correspondingly wider spacing of dust particles.

these dust exposures showed a tendency for increased exposure to total dust, coal and quartz to be associated with increased severity of lung disease, these differences, however, proved not to be statistically significant (Table 2).

TABLE 2. MINERAL EXPOSURES OF CASES IN THE THREE PATHOLOGICAL GROUPS

Pathological classification	Mean age at death	Number of cases	Mean exposure (g) ± s.e			
			Total dust	Coal	Non-coal minerals	Quartz
Soft macules	66	12	196.7 ± 24.5	114.0 ± 16.6	82.7 ± 8.7	7.9 ± 1.4
Fibrotic lesions	69	19	243.1 ± 17.4	128.0 ± 12.0	119.1 ± 14.5	10.4 ± 1.6
PMF	69	27	283.7 ± 26.1	165.0 ± 16.3	118.5 ± 14.8	11.3 ± 1.5

The amount of dust retained in the lungs expressed as a percentage of the amount of dust inhaled during work is shown in Fig. 4. The percentage non-coal mineral retained in lungs where only soft macules were present was significantly lower than in lungs with PMF ($P < 0.01$). The percentage quartz retention of lungs with soft macules was also lower than those cases with fibrotic nodules ($P < 0.05$) or PMF ($P < 0.001$). While there was a tendency for cases with PMF to have retained more non-coal minerals and quartz than cases with fibrotic lesions, these differences were not statistically significant.

Detailed histological examination of slides from the lungs involved in this study has included the consideration of many different parameters involving the coal-dust lesion and other forms of tissue damage. Among the parameters it was noticed that the packing of coal-dust particles in the early dust deposits surrounding respiratory bronchioles varied considerably and corresponded to the degree of tissue reaction to the dust. Where the tissue reaction was minimal the coal-dust particles were very

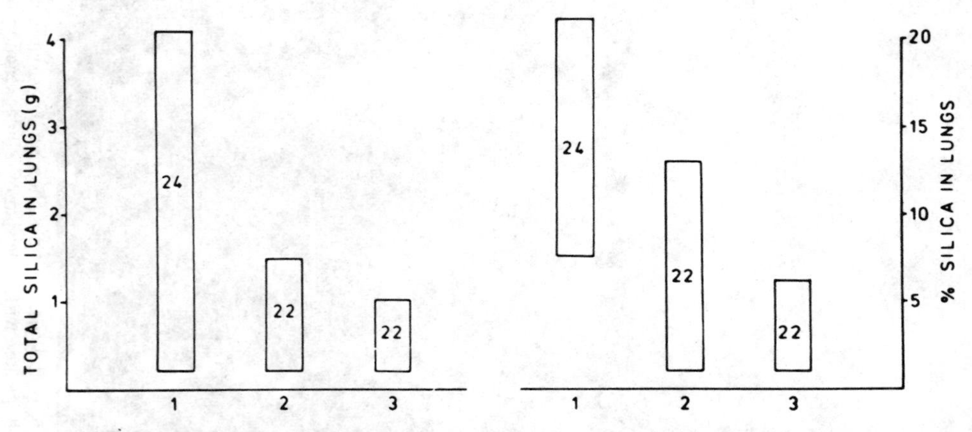

FIG. 6. Ranges of total and percentage silica content in dust from the lungs of coal miners classified according to the dust packing and cellular response in the early dust lesions. (1) Low dust packing, vigorous cellular responses. (2) Intermediate dust packing and cellular response. (3) High dust packing, minimal cellular response. Figures in blocks show number of cases in each group.

densely packed, while a vigorous cellular response was linked with much wider spacing of the dust particles. The extremes of this dust aggregation are shown in Fig. 5. In an attempt to quantify this effect, dust lesions were classified into three groups, those with the least dust per square millimetre of tissue, an intermediate group, and those with the most dust. These results have been plotted against the total weights of minerals contained in the extracted dust and also the percentage composition of the various components.

The results show a close correlation with dust components considered by weight and an even better correlation when considered by percentage composition. The lesions with widely spaced dust particles and a vigorous cellular response are those where the coal content of the dust is low and the mineral content high. Those with densely packed dust and poor cellular response are those with the highest content of coal and the lowest levels of all types of minerals. Of all minerals the content of quartz correlated most closely with the histological observations and there was no overlap between the high and low levels of tissue reaction when related to the percentage silica in the dust (Fig. 6).

DISCUSSION

The present study has confirmed many findings from previous pathological and mineralogical examinations of coal miners' lungs, but has also shown some marked differences. Most significant of these is the fact that the dust levels from the seventy-four cases under consideration were approximately half those reported by Bergman and Casswell, 1972. It is true that the analytical methods used were different in the two studies, but the procedures adopted by Bergman and Casswell have been tried in our own laboratory and were found to give identical results to our own for any sample of lung tissue. It would appear, therefore, that there were real differences in dust content between the cases in the two studies. Both were collected from a wide range of British coalfields so that the differing dust levels in the different mining areas was not the cause. However, Bergman and Casswell's cases were collected between 1952 and 1964 while the cases included in the present study were collected from 1971 to 1974. It may be that dust-abatement procedures have indeed begun to reduce the dust load that has accumulated in the lungs of most coal miners.

So far in the present study it has been possible to dissect out complete PMF lesions in ten out of thirty-four cases with this stage of the disease. In the remaining specimens the lesions were either too indistinct or the central areas had liquefied and cavitation had occurred. Dust analysis of the PMF specimens compared to the rest of the lung tissue for the ten cases confirmed the findings of Nagelschmidt *et al.* (1963) that the dust composition was identical throughout the lung, but the weight of dust per gram of dried tissue was much higher in the PMF lesion. Pratt (1968) pointed out that a strict comparison of dust accumulation in various lung areas is not possible by these methods since the amount of solid fibrous tissue is much higher in the PMF nodules than in the rest of the lung. However, this excess of fibrous tissue would in fact reduce the figures for dust accumulation in the areas of PMF rather than exaggerate them.

Examination of the data from the first seventy-four cases of the present study shows clear evidence that there is some association between the quartz content of the lungs and the presence of PMF. However, it is difficult to determine cause and effect in these circumstances. Dust-exposure data indicate that men with the highest dust exposures tend to develop the most severe pneumoconiosis but the differences in exposure levels, especially to quartz, are by no means marked. Similarly, the weights of dust retained in lungs differs little between the more severe cases of simple pneumoconiosis and those with PMF. It would appear, therefore, that for the cases under consideration, the mass of quartz inhaled was not an important factor in the development of PMF.

When, however, the percentage composition of lung dust is compared to that of the original mine dust and also to the levels of each mineral type that exposure data would indicate ought to be present, then a marked differential retention of some minerals becomes noticeable. Whereas the percentage retention of coal is roughly similar for all three pathological grades, the retention of quartz is much greater in PMF cases than in those with only simple pneumoconiosis.

A similar observation was reported by LEITERITZ *et al.* (1967), who concluded that this effect was due to the different particle sizes of the mineral types concerned. They suggested that the larger coal particles were cleared from the lung more effectively than the smaller non-coal-mineral particles, including quartz.

Further studies of the association between lung damage and dust retention will take into account the rank of coal (see Part I, p. 669) and size distribution of the dust to which the individual was exposed.

In the present study some of the cases of PMF had a very low quartz content so that it seems unlikely that quartz accumulation is the only cause of this condition. It may be that the accumulation of quartz even in small areas of the lung might stimulate either an auto-immune response or the development of some form of infection in certain individuals. In this way all three of the most frequently quoted hypotheses of PMF development could be involved in the development of this condition. It is hoped that an analysis of the complete series of lungs from the present study, coupled with figures from the past dust exposure of the men involved, might give a clearer indication of the importance of quartz in coalworkers' pneumoconiosis.

REFERENCES

BERGMAN, I. and LOXLEY, R. (1971) *Analyt. Chem.* **43,** 1204–1206.
BERGMAN, I. and CASSWELL, C. (1972) *Br. J. ind. Med.* **29,** 160–168.
DODGSON, J. (1963) *Nature, Lond.* **199,** 245–247.
DODGSON, J. and WHITTAKER, W. (1973) *Ann. occup. Hyg.* **16,** 373–387.
JACOBSEN, M., RAE, S., WALTON, W. H. and ROGAN, J. (1971) *Inhaled Particles III* (edited by WALTON, W. H.) vol. II, pp. 903–917. Unwin Bros., Old Woking, Surrey.
LEITERITZ, H., EINBRODT, H. J. and KLOSTERKÖTTER, W. (1967) *Inhaled Particles and Vapours II* (edited by DAVIES, C. N.) pp. 381–390. Pergamon Press, Oxford.
NAGELSCHMIDT, G., RIVERS, D., KING, E. J. and TREVELLA, W. (1963) *Br. J. ind. Med.* **20,** 181–191.
PRATT, P. C. (1968) *Archs envir. Hlth* **16,** 734–737.
RIVERS, D., MORRIS, T. G., WISE, M. E., COOKE, T. H. and ROBERTS, W. H. (1963) *Br. J. ind. Med.* **20,** 13–23.
ROGAN, J. M. (1970) *Encyclopaedia of Occupational Safety and Health*, pp. 307–309. International Labour Office, Geneva.
ROSSITER, C. E., RIVERS, D., BERGMAN, I., CASSWELL, C. and NAGELSCHMIDT, G. (1967) *Inhaled Particles and Vapours II* (edited by DAVIES, C. N.) pp. 419–437. Pergamon Press, Oxford.
SVANBERG, L. (1957) *Scand. J. clin. Lab. Invest.* **9,** suppl. 25.

DISCUSSION

M. T. R. Reisner: Do you think that the higher percentage of quartz in the dust found in the lungs of miners is more related to a biological enrichment process in the lung or to a change in dust conditions? Analyses of lung dusts from coal workers in Germany showed the same results. But these miners were exposed to dust mostly in the period between 1920 and 1950. At that time, because of lack of water (no water mains) especially in stone drifts and gateroads, we had a higher percentage of quartz in the respirable dust than we find today.

Dr Davis: In the small group of miners included in this preliminary report, some of the men had worked for some years before accurate dust monitoring began. It is possible, therefore, that some of these could have been exposed to a higher level of quartz dust than we have estimated. This point will be settled when we have a larger group available, and men with poor dust figures can be excluded. However, previous animal experimental studies (King, E. J. *et al.*, *Br. J. ind. Med.*, 1958, **15,** 172–177) do indicate a definite biological enrichment process for coal–quartz dust mixtures, and we believe that this is the most likely explanation for our present findings.

G. Knight: (i) Is the quantity of quartz found in PMF lungs comparable to that found in silicotic lungs? (ii) Does the progression to PMF increase after ceasing exposure to coalmine dust?

In Canadian hard rock mines we have found that the concept of quartz percentage can be misleading because it is variable from occupation to occupation for a number of reasons: (1) variations in rock composition; (2) quartz percentage can be dependent on dust size; (3) dilution of mineral dust by non-mineral dusts can be large—we find diesel exhaust particulates and oil mists from compressed-air-operated equipment contribute, on average, half to three-quarters of the weight of respirable dust collected on the filters. Thus it is desirable to talk in terms of quartz dust concentrations.

In British coal mines it appears that respirable quartz concentrations can reach 1 mg/m^3, a level likely to result in a high percentage of silicotics in South African gold mines or Canadian uranium mines. To explain the low incidence of fibrogenic reactions to quartz in British coal miners it seems necessary to postulate the presence of an inhibitor. Some inhibitors such as aluminium compounds seem likely to have only a limited life in the lungs and if this is general it would seem possible that as the quartz load builds up in the lung the supply of fresh inhibitor might at some stage be insufficient to prevent the fibrogenic action of quartz.

If inhibitors are widespread, i.e. present to varying extents in most mines, this could also explain the variable dependence of silicosis on time as well as dose.

Dr Davis: (i) It is true that the percentage of quartz in the lung dust from our PMF cases was well below that reported by Nagelschmidt from cases of pure silicosis. However, the total quartz in many of these cases was much higher than in silicotics. We know from cell culture studies that pure quartz dust mixed with coal is much less cytotoxic than the same weight of quartz on its own. However, the coal–quartz mixtures are still more cytotoxic than pure coal. It seems likely that quartz might still prove an important factor in the development of some cases of coal workers' pneumoconiosis even although its percentage in the inhaled dust is relatively small.

(ii) At present we have no data relating to the progression of PMF after the cessation of dust exposure. It is hoped, however, that information on this aspect of the problem will be included in the final report of this study.

A. G. Heppleston: (i) Fibrotic lesions appear to partake of the histological characters of PMF and hence these two categories might better be grouped for analytical purposes.

(ii) In taking lung samples for dust extraction a few areas of PMF were excised, but were fibrotic foci and macules also excised and analysed as individual lesions? Without such analyses it seems that no conclusion can be reached on the significance of a cellular reaction in some macules.

(iii) Your data are held to show "some association between the quartz content of the lungs and the presence of PMF". How can this claim be sustained when some of your cases of PMF had a very low quartz content and when other examples of PMF, reported elsewhere, have occurred in the absence or near absence of quartz in the lung dust? It is also difficult to accept comparisons of the dust content of lesions with the amount of dust inhaled during work when only 15–40% of the working lifetime dust exposure was actually sampled.

(iv) Only passing reference is made to the part an infective factor may play in the genesis of PMF. I find it hard to overlook the evidence which has been adduced on this aspect, more particularly in regard to tuberculosis, quiescent foci of which may simulate nodular silicotic lesions pathologically. The interplay of dust, infective and immunological factors has been discussed elsewhere (Heppleston, A. G., 1969, in *Pigments and Pathology* (edited by Wolman, M.), pp. 33–73).

(v) An important feature of lung disease in coal workers, to which I would like to draw attention, concerns the relation between dust and the occurrence of emphysema, the analysis of which is a complex exercise (Heppleston, A. G., *Ann. N.Y. Acad. Sci.*, 1972, **200,** 347–369).

DR DAVIS: (i) The histological similarity in the fibrotic nodules and PMF is accepted. We separated the two groups on the size of nodules to co-ordinate results with X-ray categories. Results combining the PMF cases with those containing only fibrotic nodules will be included in the final report of this project.

(ii) We considered that many of the smaller lesions were too indistinct for isolation by dissection. We are, however, developing a microanalysis method which we hope will permit dust analysis from histological sections.

(iii) It must be accepted that quartz cannot be the only factor in the development of PMF since a few such cases contain very little of this material. However, the fact that there was a high quartz level and evidence of differential quartz retention in many of our cases did indicate that quartz might be an important factor in these instances. It is accepted that dust records for some of the men are not satisfactory. However, it is hoped that taken as a whole the records for groups of men will be sufficiently detailed to show trends in dust-retention and disease relationships. When the final series of cases is examined it is hoped that sufficient of these will have reliable dust figures to validate our suggestions regarding differential quartz retention.

(iv) So far no one factor has been proved definitely to cause PMF. It seems most likely that a combination of factors is involved which may differ from case to case. Quartz, infection and auto-immunity may all be involved.

(v) Our studies do include estimations of emphysema in the lungs examined. These results will be reported separately.

RESULTS OF EPIDEMIOLOGICAL, MINERALOGICAL AND CYTOTOXICOLOGICAL STUDIES ON THE PATHOGENICITY OF COAL-MINE DUSTS*

M. T. R. REISNER
Steinkohlenbergbauverein, Essen

and

K. ROBOCK
Wirtschaftsverband Asbestzement, Neuss, Fed. Rep. Germany

Abstract—Risks of developing abnormalities on chest X-rays differ widely between collieries in the Ruhr, despite comparable dust exposures. Simple pneumoconiosis hazard indices have been determined for thirteen collieries, taking into consideration variations in miners' individual cumulative dust exposures, their ages at start of dust exposure, the residence time of dust in their lungs, and the mineral content of the dust.

Fine dust samples were taken in five collieries at places selected as representative of seams worked during the past 20 years. They were used for mineralogical and physical analyses and for cell and animal studies. Cytotoxicity of dusts with comparable composition increased with geological age and rank of coal seams. This finding is consistent with results from epidemiological studies.

INTRODUCTION

Prevalence rates of simple pneumoconiosis at individual collieries of the German Federal Republic differ markedly. They have varied between 2 and 40% during recent years (REISNER, 1968). Epidemiological studies have demonstrated that risks of developing simple pneumoconiosis differ between collieries, despite miners' comparable dust exposures and similar levels of other relevant variables (REISNER, 1968, 1971a, 1975b; LAUFHÜTTE *et al.*, 1971). The variations are not explained by differences in the mineral content of the dust. No increase in hazard with increasing quartz content has been detectable. Indeed, higher gravimetric concentrations of fine quartz dust ("fine" dust in this paper refers to dust collected by BAT I or BAT II sampler) were found in collieries with relatively low pneumoconiosis hazard (REISNER, 1971b). Variation in specific noxiousness of fine dusts was therefore postulated.

To investigate this question, fine dust samples were taken at five selected Ruhr collieries. The samples had to be large enough to permit cell and animal tests as well as physical and mineralogical analyses. The aim was to compare cytotoxicity, as deter-

*Report No. 22/75 of the Centre for Dust and Silicosis Suppression of Steinkohlenbergbauverein in Essen. Research project with the financial aid of the Commission of the European Communities and the Land Nordrhein-Westfalen.

mined from relatively short-term cell tests, with fibrotic effects in animals, and also with results from epidemiological studies, i.e. the effect in man. It has been suggested (ROBOCK and KLOSTERKÖTTER, 1973; ROBOCK, 1974) that certain semiconductor properties of minerals may be responsible for biological mechanisms related to pathogenicity of dusts. It was hoped therefore also to develop a physical method for measuring the specific pathogenicity of fine dusts. These studies are being conducted at various Institutes.* The present report refers only to results from cell tests and attempts to relate them to the dust source, the dust composition, and to epidemiological data..

EPIDEMIOLOGICAL STUDIES

REISNER (1975b) has reported on results from the recently completed third phase of epidemiological studies in the Ruhr coal field. Radiological and dust exposure data relating to more than 18 000 miners from thirteen collieries were examined; observation periods were up to 14 years. Individual cumulative dust exposures were calculated from monthly records of tyndallometric fine dust concentrations at the work place (k) and the number of shifts worked (S). These records have been kept since 1954. Individual exposures were expressed as the sum of products $\Sigma(kS)$. Numerous comparative dust measurements at individual collieries permitted conversion of the tyndallometric concentrations (k) into equivalent mass concentrations (c) of fine dust, expressed as mg/m^3. These conversions thus allowed calculation of cumulative dust exposures in gravimetric units, $\Sigma(cS)$.

Probabilities of developing simple pneumoconiosis were estimated from a multiple regression analysis of data from more than 4500 miners. Cumulative dust exposure for these men referred to periods up to 18 years and were based in the main on measured dust concentrations. They included also estimates of exposures prior to the start of dust measurements in 1954, but these latter estimates contributed only a small proportion to the cumulative exposures concerned. Explanatory variables considered were cumulative dust exposure, mineral content of the dust, age at first exposure to dust, and an estimate of the residence time of the dust burden in the lung. The computer program used (developed by G. Kotitschke of Aachen) provided also estimates of residual effects associated with differences between collieries. These "colliery factors" (Z) were scaled to have values between -1 and $+1$.

Figure 1 shows estimated probabilities of developing simple pneumoconiosis as a function of cumulative dust exposure, for various values of the colliery factor, Z. For illustrative purposes, the curves in Fig. 1 are based on equations in which other explanatory variables are held constant (ash content of the fine dust, $a = 20\%$, by weight; age at first exposure, $A_a = 23$ years; mean residence time of dust in the lungs, $T_v = 84$ months). The mass-exposure abscissa in Fig. 1 refers to fine dust as

* Abteilung Hygiene und Arbeitsmedizin der Medizinischen Fakultät der Rheinisch-Westfälischen Technischen Hochschule Aachen,
Medizinisches Institut für Lufthygiene und Silikoseforschung an der Universität Düsseldorf,
Institut für Hygiene und Arbeitsmedizin am Klinikum der Universität Essen-Gesamthochschule,
Max-Planck-Institut für Immunbiologie in Freiburg-Zähringen,
I. Physikalisches Institut der Justus-Liebig-Universität Giessen,
Abteilung für Pneumokonioseforschung der Bezirkshygienestation in Ostrau/ČSSR.

measured by the BAT I sampling instrument. "Respirable" dust concentrations measured with the MRE gravimetric sampler would be 4.5 times greater (HAMILTON *et al.*, 1967; REISNER, 1975a).

Figure 1 illustrates the wide range of the effect associated with the colliery factor *Z*. Although it is recognized that this may reflect, partially, variations in diagnostic criteria between doctors at the various collieries, it is nevertheless tempting to speculate that the differences shown are associated primarily with the specific noxiousness of the dusts concerned. The aim was to test this hypothesis using results from the biological tests.

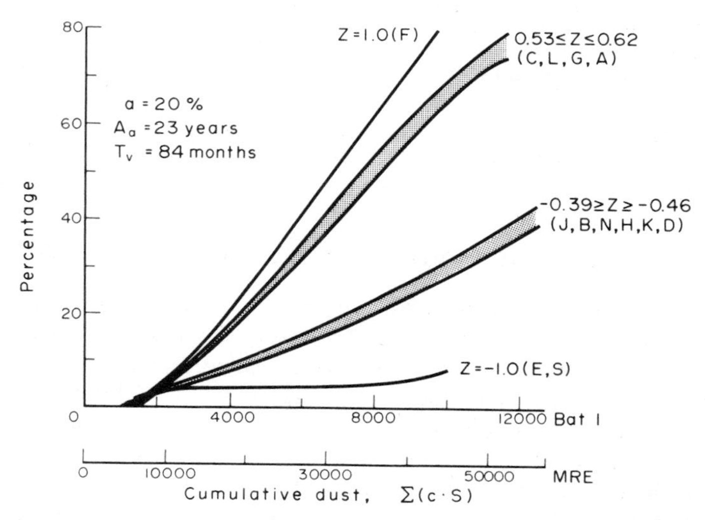

FIG. 1. The risk of simple pneumoconiosis as a function of cumulative fine dust exposure at thirteen collieries (result of a regression analysis).

Four of the thirteen collieries contributing to Fig. 1 and another colliery with a very low prevalence of simple pneumoconiosis had been included in the special dust sampling programme mentioned above. Prevalence of definite pneumoconiotic changes, as measured in 1966, varied between 25.7% and 2.5%. Pneumoconiosis incidence in the period 1956 to 1968 showed colliery-related trends similar to the prevalence results (Table 1). Collieries G, H and D had been included in earlier studies (REISNER, 1968). It will be seen from Table 1 that estimates of colliery factors from this first phase of the research differ from those derived from later (third phase) data. Nevertheless, the gradient in *Z* from collieries G to D is similar in direction. Colliery N was included only at a later stage in the epidemiological research. The estimated value of *Z* for this colliery should be regarded with caution firstly because the exposure times concerned did not exceed 11 years, and secondly, because the relatively low cumulative dust exposures for the men implied zero risk due to this factor.

In summary it appears that the highest risks of pneumoconiosis are associated with colliery G and the lowest with collieries N and V; collieries H and D take intermediary positions.

TABLE 1. PREVALENCE AND INCIDENCE OF PNEUMOCONIOSIS IN FIVE RUHR COLLIERIES

	Colliery				
	G	H	D	N	V
Percentage of underground workers with simple pneumoconiosis in 1966 (%)	25.7	18.2	22.9	3.9	2.5
Incidence of simple pneumoconiosis, 1956 to 1968, for miners in their 15th and	6.0	5.3	3.6	0.6	0.4
20th year of employment (%)	8.2	6.5	4.5	1.0	0.4
Colliery factor (first phase)	0.26	−0.19	−0.75	—	—
(third phase)	0.54	−0.45	−0.46	(−0.45)	—

SAMPLING AND ANALYSIS OF FINE DUST

Samples were taken only from coal faces where dust conditions were considered to be characteristic of those likely to have occurred in the mines concerned over the past 10 to 20 years. The seams had been worked repeatedly and consistently during this period. Two fine dust samplers, the BAT I with an air throughput of 12 m^3/h and the BAT II with an air throughput of 160 m^3/h, were mounted simultaneously in return roadways about 40 to 50 m behind the face with another BAT I in the coal face itself, about 10 m in front of the face end situated on the return air side. Sampling was carried out on 4 to 6 days during coal getting. The sampling period was 4 to 5 hours within one shift. Thus several hundred milligrams of BAT I respirable dust and several grams of BAT II fine dust could be collected per working point.

Table 2 shows the samples collected at working points by sampler, measuring point, seam and type of coal. An implosion of a desiccator, errors of analysis and the repetition of individual measurements were the reason that, in four cases, not all measurements per working point are included in Table 2.

The seam codes in Table 2 refer to geological age: the higher the number, the younger the seam. The first integer in the code indicates the geological strata in terms of Ruhr Carboniferous Measures, with 3 indicating the Witten strata, 4 the Bochum strata, 5 the Essen strata, and 6 the Horst strata. Extremely young or old strata seams at the selected collieries had been worked only rarely or not at all. The two middle integers in the seam code indicate the order of workability within the relevant strata code. The last integer refers to the type and rank of the coal; with 3 indicating low volatile steam coal, 4 bituminous medium volatile coal, 5 medium volatile gas coal, and 6 high volatile gas flame coal. The rank is dependent on the volatile matter in the coal (d.m.m.f.). The latter values were determined from coal samples taken and are recorded in Table 2.

Mineral analysis was by infrared spectrography (GADE and REISNER, 1970). Individual mineral components were related to the ash content which was determined by weigh-

TABLE 2. DUST SAMPLING PROCEDURE. CHARACTERISTICS OF THE SEAM, FINE DUST COMPOSITION AND CELL TEST RESULTS

Sample code	Sampler	Sampling site F = face R = return roadway	Seam code	Volatile matter (d.m.m.f.), % by weight	Mineral content of the fine dust, % by weight				TTC–RA, %
					Total	Quartz	Mica	Kaolin	
Mine G									
310921	BAT I	F	3094	20.5	10.9	1.6	6.0	3.0	73.0
310922	BAT I	R	3094	20.5	9.0	1.5	5.9	1.4	71.3
310E22	BAT II	R	3094	20.5	8.6	1.4	5.7	1.4	71.6
310931	BAT I	F	3014	21.2	13.9	1.4	9.1	3.2	67.9
310932	BAT I	R	3014	21.2	14.2	1.4	9.4	3.0	73.3
310E32	BAT II	R	3014	21.2	13.4	1.4	9.6	2.1	65.0
310E42	BAT II	R	4104	24.0	11.4	1.3	7.8	2.1	68.2
310951	BAT I	F	4204	28.1	13.1	1.9	8.1	2.8	78.9
310952	BAT I	R	4204	28.1	14.3	2.3	8.1	3.4	66.5
310E52	BAT II	R	4204	28.1	16.8	3.3	9.7	3.3	84.6
310961	BAT I	F	3014	21.2	12.8	1.2	8.5	2.7	72.6
310962	BAT I	R	3014	21.2	12.8	1.4	8.4	2.6	77.8
Mine H									
320921	BAT I	F	4074	21.6	7.8	1.1	5.6	1.1	68.6
320922	BAT I	R	4074	21.6	9.1	1.1	6.4	1.6	73.6
320E22	BAT II	R	4074	21.6	8.7	0.9	5.4	2.3	69.6
320931	BAT I	F	4074	18.1	20.7	2.3	13.3	4.6	71.2
320932	BAT I	R	4074	18.1	19.8	2.2	12.3	4.7	84.4
320E32	BAT II	R	4074	18.1	21.5	2.2	13.6	4.6	75.9
320941	BAT I	F	4404	21.3	15.2	1.8	11.1	2.2	77.3
320942	BAT I	R	4404	21.3	17.3	1.6	10.7	4.6	72.9
320E42	BAT II	R	4404	21.3	16.3	1.7	11.7	2.7	61.6
320953	BAT I	F	4314	19.6	9.2	1.4	5.0	2.6	81.0
320954	BAT I	R	4314	19.6	12.3	2.5	7.6	2.0	74.1
320E54	BAT II	R	4314	19.6	14.8	3.2	9.6	1.6	74.3
320963	BAT I	F	4203	15.3	7.4	0.6	4.4	2.5	71.6
320964	BAT I	R	4203	15.3	9.8	1.2	6.3	2.2	76.3
320E64	BAT II	R	4203	15.3	9.1	0.8	6.1	2.2	68.7
Mine N									
108922	BAT I	R	6076	35.9	62.1	9.0	37.0	14.0	52.5
108E22	BAT II	R	6076	35.9	59.2	9.3	34.3	14.8	58.4
108931	BAT I	F	5195	32.9	38.2	3.9	23.8	10.0	45.8
108932	BAT I	R	5195	32.9	33.8	2.9	21.6	8.5	59.6
108E32	BAT II	R	5195	32.9	34.8	3.2	21.3	9.3	59.9
108941	BAT I	F	5195	30.6	24.0	3.9	13.7	6.3	75.2
108942	BAT I	R	5195	30.6	19.5	3.7	10.9	4.5	81.4
108E42	BAT II	R	5195	30.6	18.4	3.4	10.9	3.8	64.4
108951	BAT I	F	6076	35.6	54.9	6.3	33.8	14.0	61.6
108952	BAT I	R	6076	35.6	54.5	6.7	35.3	11.9	57.0
108E52	BAT II	R	6076	35.6	50.3	6.5	29.8	13.2	67.5

TABLE 2 (*continued*)

Sample code	Sampler	Sampling site F = face R = return roadway	Seam code	Volatile matter (d.m.m.f.), % by weight	Mineral content of the fine dust, % by weight				TTC–RA, %
					Total	Quartz	Mica	Kaolin	
Mine D									
330921	BAT I	F	5176	36.0	34.2	5.0	19.1	9.3	74.7
330922	BAT I	R	5176	36.0	36.0	5.3	19.1	10.2	76.6
330E22	BAT II	R	5176	36.0	33.5	4.8	17.7	9.9	75.5
330931	BAT I	F	4384	25.5	14.5	1.6	9.0	3.7	76.2
330932	BAT I	R	4384	25.5	16.7	1.5	9.3	5.3	77.0
330E32	BAT II	R	4384	25.5	17.9	1.9	10.9	4.6	88.0
330941	BAT I	F	5064	27.2	25.3	2.0	13.8	9.6	72.5
330942	BAT I	R	5064	27.2	25.5	2.2	14.4	8.9	79.3
330E42	BAT II	R	5064	27.2	26.8	2.4	14.3	10.1	74.0
330951	BAT I	F	4574	21.4	9.7	1.3	5.6	2.7	91.7
330952	BAT I	R	4574	21.4	13.7	2.0	8.4	3.0	73.8
330E52	BAT II	R	4574	21.4	14.6	1.9	8.2	4.0	77.8
Mine V									
137901	BAT I	F	4504	26.8	24.5	3.2	16.4	3.8	68.7
137902	BAT I	R	4504	26.8	22.5	3.1	15.0	3.3	67.8
137E02	BAT II	R	4504	26.8	20.2	2.5	13.7	3.2	70.0
137911	BAT I	F	5085	30.8	19.2	1.8	10.6	6.2	62.5
137912	BAT I	R	5085	30.8	14.7	1.3	8.3	4.7	70.9
137E12	BAT II	R	5085	30.8	13.7	1.2	7.9	4.2	67.1
137915	BAT I	F	5085	30.8	16.9	1.5	9.3	5.6	62.9
137916	BAT I	R	5085	30.8	14.8	1.4	8.1	4.7	66.1
137E16	BAT II	R	5085	30.8	15.2	1.4	8.9	4.7	64.5
137921	BAT I	F	5095	31.8	17.5	1.7	11.3	4.1	68.0
137922	BAT I	R	5095	31.8	18.3	1.7	11.4	4.4	71.8
137E22	BAT II	R	5095	31.8	20.2	1.8	12.5	4.9	67.2
137931	BAT I	F	5235	34.4	21.6	2.7	9.8	6.5	78.8
137932	BAT I	R	5235	34.4	22.6	2.7	10.9	6.8	88.0
137E32	BAT II	R	5235	34.4	27.3	3.7	13.4	9.4	75.3
137941	BAT I	F	5255	32.5	37.4	5.6	16.3	14.5	64.9
137942	BAT I	R	5255	32.5	37.5	6.0	17.1	14.0	65.2
137E42	BAT II	R	5255	32.5	40.7	6.2	18.5	15.3	53.9
137951	BAT I	F	6116	34.9	47.9	5.9	21.2	18.2	61.8
137952	BAT I	R	6116	34.9	51.0	6.0	24.1	20.1	68.7
137E52	BAT II	R	6116	34.9	54.9	6.3	27.1	19.6	52.7
137961	BAT I	F	5175	32.0	28.6	4.0	15.1	8.6	64.8
137962	BAT I	R	5175	32.0	27.4	3.5	15.1	8.5	68.8
137E62	BAT II	R	5175	32.0	27.2	3.5	15.3	8.0	68.2
137971	BAT I	F	5075	29.9	27.9	3.4	15.6	8.7	52.0
137972	BAT I	R	5075	29.9	21.2	2.5	11.2	6.6	60.2
137E72	BAT II	R	5075	29.9	31.8	4.5	17.7	9.4	69.5
137E74	BAT II	R	5075	29.9	27.0	4.2	13.8	7.8	72.0

ing prior to and after incineration at 800°C. The small percentages of other minerals not shown in Table 2 were identified as feldspar, carbonates and FeO(OH).

The small variability in mineral content of the ashed samples should be noted. This is reflected in the high correlations between ash content and mineral composition, as well as the correlations between the mineral components themselves (Table 3).

TABLE 3. CORRELATION COEFFICIENTS BETWEEN ASH AND MINERAL COMPONENTS ($n = 78$)

Mineral content of the fine dust (% by weight)	Quartz	Mica	Kaolin	Other minerals
Ash	0.94	0.97	0.93	0.55
Quartz		0.90	0.85	0.52
Mica			0.82	0.47
Kaolin				0.52

Size analyses of the fine dusts by means of the Coulter Counter showed that in both samplers hardly any dust particles with an equivalent spherical diameter >7 μm were retained on the filter (Fig. 2). This corresponds to the cut-off characteristic of these

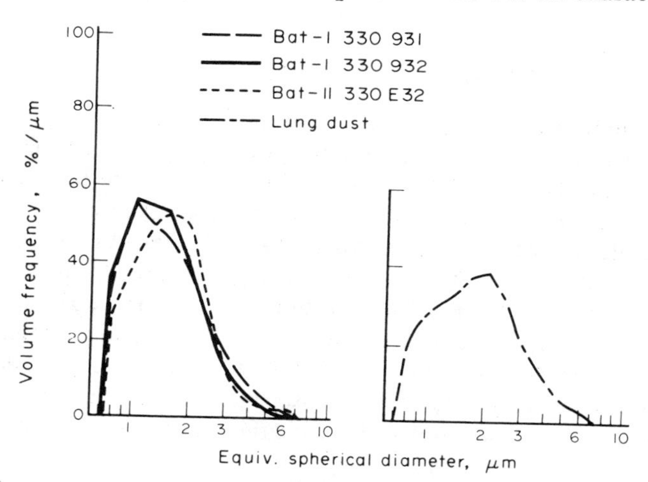

FIG. 2. Coulter counter volume size frequency distributions of BAT I and BAT II fine dusts from a working point and of lung dust isolated post-mortem from a coal miner with silicosis.

samplers for fine dust (BREUER, 1964; LEITERITZ *et al.*, 1967) which approximate to the retention conditions of the dust in the lung alveoli. The maximum volume size frequency distribution of the dusts is between 1 and 2 μm. Thus, the distributions are similar for all fine dust samples and provide a basis for determining the specific pathogenicity in the cell test. Figure 2 shows also the volume size distribution of lung dust isolated post-mortem from the lung of a coal miner with silicosis. It will be seen that there is good agreement between the size distribution of the collected fine dusts and those of the retained lung dust.

CELL TESTS

The TTC method (Klosterkötter and Robock, 1967; Robock, 1974) was used as a measure of dust cytotoxicity. This method determines the inhibition of reduction activity of peritoneal macrophages of guinea pigs using 2, 3, 5-triphenyltetrazolium chloride. In these initial trials, 0.6 mg of dust per 4.6 mm^3 of cells was used. This cell volume was obtained using a Coulter Counter particle size analysis in the range 10.5 to 26.5 μm equivalent spherical diameter. (The dust was not given to a definite number of cells, as has been reported in earlier work, since this approach makes no allowance for the variability of cell volume (Robock, 1974).) The dust samples were dispersed using ultrasound in a tyrode nutritive solution to which a surfactant (RBS 25) had been added as wetting agent at a non-noxious concentration (0.01 %). Each dust sample was tested in quadruplicate for at least 3 days, with dust-free cells as controls. Residual TTC-reduction activity was determined after immersion for 120 min at 37°C in a shaking water bath. Results are shown in Table 2 (TTC–RA) as percentages of control values. Each result shown is a mean of at least twelve separate measurements; the lower the residual TTC–RA, the more cytotoxic the dust concerned. It will be seen from Table 2 that TTC–RA values for different dust samples vary between 46 and 92 %.

RESULTS AND DISCUSSION

A statistical analysis (Table 4) showed no clear effects on cytotoxicity attributable to sampling site (coal face or return roadway) or sampling instrument (BAT I or BAT II). It is clear also that there is no significant difference between results from samples taken at collieries H and G, or between those taken at collieries V and N. Regrouping results in the manner shown in Table 4 indicates significant contrasts, some at the 0.1 % level, which suggest the following rank order. Dusts from colliery D have low toxicity (mean TTC–RA, 78.2 %); those from collieries H and G a moderate toxicity (73.1 %); and those from collieries N and V a fairly high toxicity (65.6 %).

At first sight this ordering is not consistent with the epidemiological data in Table 1. There, collieries N and V are shown to be associated with the lowest pneumoconiosis hazards, while fine dust from colliery G, with the highest prevalence and incidence, depressed TTC–RA only moderately.

The individual collieries produce coal from seams with varying rank and varying geological horizon. This suggests consideration of a further contrast, between dusts from the higher rank coals in the older Witten and Bochum strata, against the lower rank coals from the younger Essen and Horst strata. The statistical test showed a significant difference (Table 4). Fine dusts from seams in the Essen and Horst strata were more toxic (mean TTC–RA 66.8 %) than those from the Witten and Bochum strata (74.1 %). This result also appears at variance with earlier findings in the Ruhr (Reisner, 1971b) and elsewhere (e.g. Great Britain; see Hicks *et al.*, 1961) where pneumoconiosis prevalence has been greater in collieries working high rank coal.

Figure 3a alters the picture, however. In that Figure, TTC–RA results are plotted against the mineral content of the dust, separately for each stratigraphical horizon.

TABLE 4. STATISTICAL COMPARISON OF THE MEAN TTC–RA VALUES FROM FINE DUSTS OF DIFFERENT ORIGIN ($n = 78$)

Origin of samples	Number of samples	Mean TTC–RA, %	Standard deviation, %	Difference of the means, %	Confidence range of difference, %	Degree of freedom	Student's t	P
BAT I roadway	25	71.1	8.2					
BAT II roadway	25	69.1	8.4	2.0	2.3	48	0.85	>0.1
BAT I roadway	25	72.1	7.4					
BAT I coal face	25	69.9	9.4	2.2	2.4	48	0.92	>0.1
Colliery H	15	73.5	5.2					
Colliery G	12	72.7	5.7	0.8	2.1	25	0.38	>0.1
Colliery V	28	67.0	7.4					
Colliery N	11	62.2	9.8	4.8	2.9	37	1.67	>0.1
Colliery D	12	78.2	5.8					
Collieries H + G	27	73.1	5.4	5.1	1.9	37	2.67	<0.05
Colliery D	12	78.2	5.8					
Collieries N + V	39	65.6	8.3	12.6	2.6	49	4.90	<0.001
Collieries H + G	27	73.1	5.4					
Collieries N + V	39	65.6	8.3	7.5	1.8	64	4.14	<0.001
Witten and Bochum strata	36	74.1	6.3					
Essen and Horst strata	42	66.8	8.7	7.3	1.8	76	4.17	<0.001

The Bochum and Essen strata are divided into upper and lower horizons. Within particular seam horizons, an increase in cytotoxicity with increasing mineral content is clearly evident. Moreover, the individual horizons appear to be well differentiated as is indicated by the dashed lines in Fig. 3a. Although the mineral and quartz contents of the dusts were highly correlated in general (Table 3), the effects illustrated in Fig. 3a are not so obvious when the TTC–RA results are plotted against the quartz content of the dusts (Fig. 3b).

Equivalent cytotoxic effects in strata of increasing age are associated with reducing mineral content in the dust. Thus the Horst strata, with a mineral content of nearly 50% (by weight), caused a 35% depression of the biological activity (TTC–RA = 65%). Similar depressions were caused by upper Essen strata dusts with 33% mineral;

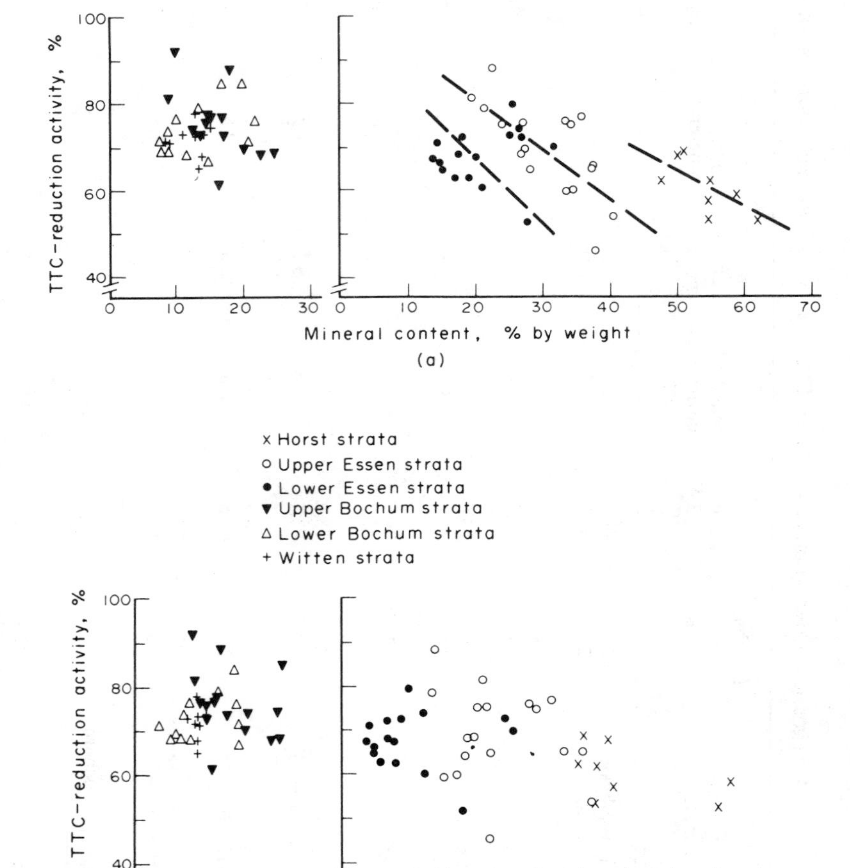

FIG. 3. TTC reduction activity of macrophages after an incubation period of 120 min of fine dust from seams of different horizons (related to the cell control). (a) As a function of the mineral content. (b) As a function of the quartz content.

by lower Essen and Bochum strata dusts (mineral ≃ 20%) and by Witten strata dusts (mineral ≃ 15%). This is illustrated in Fig. 4. Note that differences between the (older) lower Essen, Bochum and Witten strata are small, while the differences between the younger strata are very marked.

It will be noted also that given the same mineral content, dusts from older strata cause more cell damage than dusts from younger strata. This statement must be qualified, however, since it is based on some extrapolation from the range of observed data. Thus, for example, no samples from the Horst strata had mineral levels below

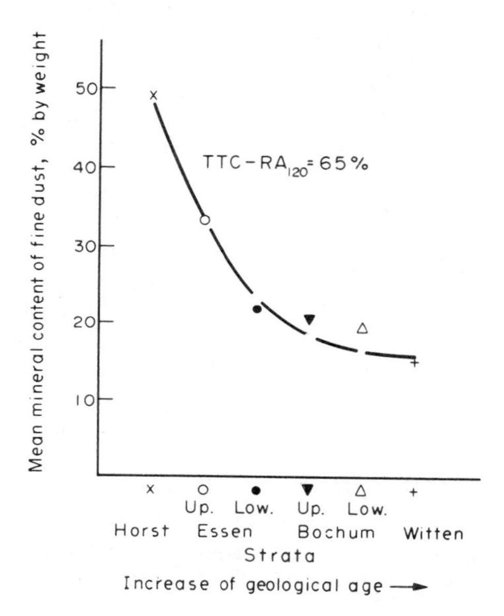

FIG. 4. Mineral contents of fine dusts from seams of different horizons causing the same cytotoxicity (depression of the TTC–RA_{120} by 35%).

47%, while no samples from the Witten and Bochum strata seams exceeded 25% mineral.

Figure 5 shows the cytotoxicity of the dusts in relation to their mineral content, separately for different values of coal rank; the latter variable is expressed as the percentage volatiles in the coal. Differences depending on coal rank are apparent. Samples from seams with more than 34% volatiles are clearly different from the others. A similar difference is observable when considering data from higher rank seams with low volatile coals. Results from the Essen strata seams with relatively high volatiles follow the same trend as observed with Horst strata sample. This illustrates the overlapping effects of the variables considered.

The results to date suggest higher specific noxiousness of fine dust from higher rank seams of older strata. This is consistent with results from cell tests on dust from the Saar district (LAUFHÜTTE *et al.*, 1971). If it is argued that the noxious effect on cells is due primarily to the minerals, including quartz, in the dust, then this would imply that equivalent damage from older strata dusts requires lower concentrations of the noxious agent. Alternatively, it could be argued that a particular concentration of the noxious agent in older strata dust causes more cell damage than the same concentration in dusts from younger strata. Thus, either higher specific noxiousness is attributed to minerals in the older strata, or one could postulate an inhibiting effect of certain minerals in the younger strata. In addition, a possible strengthening or potentiating effect associated with the coal itself (as reflected in its rank) cannot be excluded.

It appears now that the results are more consistent with the epidemiological findings. Thus, fine dusts from collieries N and V (originating mainly from the Essen and Horst strata) have lower specific noxiousness by virtue of their mineral content, while dusts from collieries G and H have the highest specific noxiousness. Finally, the analysis has

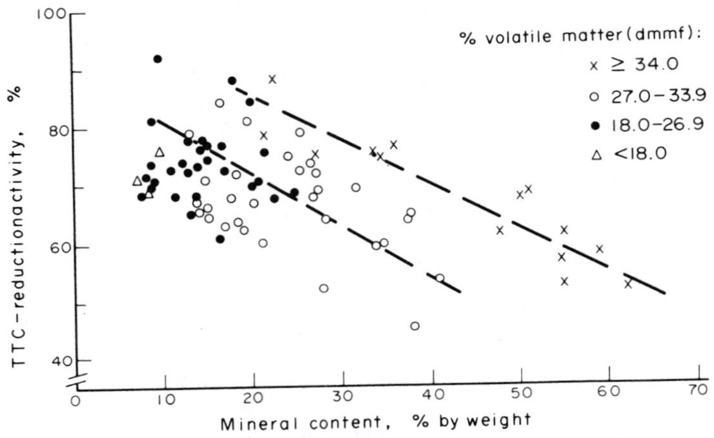

FIG. 5. TTC reduction activity of macrophages after an incubation period of 120 min of fine dust from seams of different rank (related to the cell control), as a function of the mineral content.

permitted determination of colliery factors reflecting colliery-associated variations in hazard at comparable fine dust exposure and for similar mineral content.

It appears that cell damage caused by fine dusts from West German coal mines increases both with the mineral and quartz content of the dust, and with the geological age and rank of the coals (positive correlations). However, these factors are themselves correlated negatively (Fig. 6). The mineral and quartz content of dust is, on average, lower in the older and higher rank seams than in the younger and lower rank seams (REISNER, 1971b). This explains the partly contradictory findings from the epidemiological, animal and cytotoxicological studies. Thus the epidemiologically determined pneumoconiosis hazard is related primarily to the age of the strata and the associated noxiousness, resulting in a negative correlation between the pneumoconiosis hazard and the mineral and quartz contents of the dusts. Measurement of the cytotoxic properties of the mine dusts has permitted unambiguous clarification of this problem for the first time. Nevertheless, experimental studies may often show an increase of toxicity with increasing quartz or mineral content, that is, whenever these components originate from the same coal deposits and have the same specific properties.

These results indicate that the specific noxious properties of coal-mine dusts cannot be characterized simply by their quartz or mineral content, although these variables

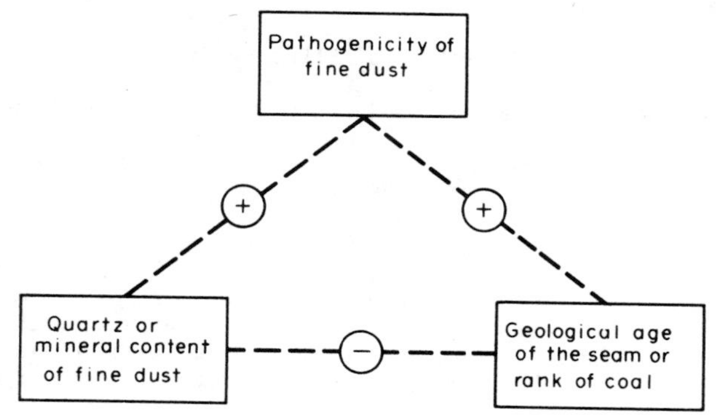

FIG. 6. Correlations.

correlate positively with noxiousness when considering dusts from the same source. An as yet unknown factor, associated with the age or rank of the seams, affects the issue to a considerable extent. It remains to determine this "specific noxicity factor" quantitatively, particularly by utilizing semiconductor properties in electron transfer reactions.

REFERENCES

BREUER, H. (1964) *Staub* **24,** 324–329.

GADE, M. and REISNER, M. T. R. (1970) *Pneumoconiosis. Proceedings of the International Conference, Johannesburg, 1969* (edited by SHAPIRO, H.A.) pp. 636–639. Oxford University Press, Cape Town.

HAMILTON, R. J., MORGAN, G. D. and WALTON, W. H. (1967) *Inhaled Particles and Vapours II* (edited by DAVIES, C. N.) pp. 533–546. Pergamon Press, Oxford.

HICKS, D., FAY, J. W. J., ASHFORD, J. R. and RAE, S. (1961) *The Relation between Pneumoconiosis and Environmental Conditions.* National Coal Board, London.

KLOSTERKÖTTER, W. and ROBOCK, K. (1967) *Ergebn. Unters. Staub- Silikosebekämpf Steinkohlenbergbau* **6,** 51–54.

LAUFHÜTTE, D. W., ROBOCK, K. and KLOSTERKÖTTER, W. (1971) *Ergebn. Unters. Staub-Silikosebekämpf. Steinkohlenbergbau* **8,** 131–138.

LEITERITZ, H., EINBRODT, H. J. and KLOSTERKÖTTER, W. (1967) *Inhaled Particles and Vapours II* (edited by DAVIES, C. N.) pp. 381–390. Pergamon Press, Oxford.

REISNER, M. (1968) *Beitr. Silikoseforsch.* (95), 1–112.

REISNER, M. T. R. (1971a) *Inhaled Particles III,* (edited by WALTON, W. H.) vol. II, pp. 921–929. Unwin Bros., Old Woking, Surrey.

REISNER, M. T. R. (1971b) *Ergebn. Unters. Staub- Silikosebekämpf. Steinkohlenbergbau* **8,** 215–219.

REISNER, M. T. R. (1975a) *Ergebn. Unters. Staub- Silikosebekämpf. Steinkohlenbergbau* **10,** 89–100.

REISNER, M. T. R. (1975b) *Ergebn. Unters. Staub- Silikosebekämpf. Steinkohlenbergbau.* **10,** 209–231.

ROBOCK, K. (1974) *Beitr. Silikoseforsch.* **26,** 111–262.

ROBOCK, K. and KLOSTERKÖTTER, W. (1973) *Staub* **33,** 60–63.

DISCUSSION

J. FERIN: Could you briefly describe your TTC-test? How is the cytotoxicity measured related to other dust effects?

DR ROBOCK: By TTC-test we mean the reduction activity of macrophages *in vitro* against 2,3,5-triphenyltetrazolium chloride. The TTC- reduction activity of the cell control, of macrophages without dust, is set up 100% on every test day. The depression of the TTC-reduction activity of the macrophages after addition of dust percentually related to the value of the cell control then is to be considered as a measure for the cytotoxicity of the respective dusts. The cytotoxicity so investigated is correlating with the depression of the oxygen consumption of the macrophages and with the extent of released enzymes resp. pigment uptake of macrophages by the action of all dusts tested till now. Furthermore, for the SiO_2 dusts a good correlation between TTC-test and biochemical parameters (hydroxyproline and phospholipids) in regard to a fibrogenic effect in animal experiments could be proved.

J. FERIN: I had the impression that the line drawn through the points of the lower seams would fit equally a line of the opposite direction?

DR ROBOCK: I agree with you that it would have been better not to draw the dotted line for the dust samples from the oldest horizons for these dust samples do not show a dependence of the cytotoxicity from the mineral content which is very low, anyway. But for the dust samples out of the younger horizons the drawn dependence is clearly visible. Figure 3a illustrates this clearlyin accordance with the results of epidemiological investigations.

DR REISNER: Because of the small variation of the mineral content of the fine dusts from seams of the lower Essen and, especially, of the Bochum and Witten strata, and the scatter of the TTC–RA values, the hypothesized relation from the results of the younger strata was hardly apparent. We shall continue to examine the existing variation in TTC–RA values and will concentrate our studies on dusts from those older strata with large variation in mineral content.

T. L. OGDEN: How was the "lung residence time" of the dust measured?

DR REISNER: The mean residence time t of the dust retained in the lungs is a calculated term and means the average of the exposure time in months weighted by the monthly dust exposure (cS):

$$t = \frac{\sum_{i=1}^{n} [c_i S_i (n - i)]}{\sum_{i=1}^{n} (c_i S_i)}$$

(c = respirable dust concentration, S = number of shifts, n = number of months within a period).

The mean residence time of the dust in the lungs of a miner who has been exposed to dust for a certain period, e.g. 10 years, would be half of the exposure time, i.e. 60 months, if the dust exposure over all the 120 months had been the same. The mean residence time would be longer, if the dust exposure had been higher in the first years, and shorter, if the dust exposure had been higher in the late years of this period.

J. BRUCH: It is noteworthy that the cytotoxic effect of the fine dust cannot be inhibited by PVNO. The causative link to fibrogenicity seems to be the influence of the cytotoxicity on the amount of dust which penetrates into the septal and lymphatic spaces, i.e. the retention of the dusts. On the other hand, after penetration the dusts are likely to become fibrogenic by virtue of their quartz content. This hypothesis has been developed in the parallel animal experiments I reported on p. 373 of this Symposium.

DR REISNER: We have found some relation between our experience with men in epidemiological studies and the results of cell tests, i.e. the cytotoxicity of dusts. We hope to establish the relationship between cytotoxicity and fibrogenicity (both indices of pathogenicity of dust) by further animal experiments. In future, therefore, we shall use these three methods to study the biological mechanisms of pneumoconiosis.

CHARACTERISTICS OF LUNG DUSTS AND THEIR RELATION TO DUST EXPOSURE AND PATHOLOGICAL FINDINGS IN THE LUNGS

M. DOBREVA, T. BURILKOV, K. KOLEV and P. LALOVA

Centre of Hygiene, Sofia, Bulgaria

Abstract—Lung dusts were investigated, post-mortem, in twenty-five miners from mixed metal mines, tunnels, and quarries who had been exposed to high concentrations of mixed dust containing about 20–25% free crystalline silica. The character of the relations found between the amount of quartz per 100 g dry tissue and the clinical, X-ray and pathological findings is similar to that established in coal miners. The difference lies in the fact that with equal amounts of quartz per 100 g dry tissue, there is less silicosis in coal miners than in our cases; the average residence time of retained dust is longer in coal miners, but its quartz per cent is lower.

INTRODUCTION

Nowadays there is no doubt of the dominating role of crystalline free silica in the origin of lung fibrosis in workers exposed to mixed dust. In most countries the standards adopted for these dusts are based primarily on quartz concentration. The role of the amounts and nature of the other dust components in the occurrence and progress of fibrosis is still disputable.

Investigations of lung dusts, coupled with post-mortem and X-ray findings, have contributed greatly to the elucidation of this problem. Many of the investigations have covered miners exposed to coal dust in the Ruhr and Saar regions (HÖER *et al.*, 1967; LEITERITZ *et al.*, 1967; WORTH *et al.*, 1967; EINBRODT and KLOSTERKÖTTER, 1965). Systematic investigations on workers employed in the ceramic industry were carried out by OTTO (1960).

The results obtained show a clear-cut relationship between the quartz content in milligrams per 100 g of dry lung tissue and the degree of fibrosis. In the cases without lesions or initial changes, small quantities are found—of the order of 150 mg/100 g—and only light silicosis is observed in cases with a content up to 500 mg/100 g. EINBRODT and KLOSTERKÖTTER (1965) tabulated the relation between quartz content in lungs, the average residence time of retained dusts and degree of silicosis. Some extreme cases with large quartz amounts but no silicosis have also been reported (WORTH *et al.*, 1967).

The number of investigations of individuals exposed to ore or other industrial dusts of high quartz percentage is relatively small. STRECKER and EINBRODT (1958) point out that in cases of exposure to different mixed dusts or in different branches of industry the relationship between retained dust and pathological changes is considerably less distinct than for coal miners. LANDWEHR and BRUCKMANN (1969) examined a mixed group including ore and coal miners and did not find a clear relationship between quartz content and the degree of pathological change. Nevertheless, the authors drew the conclusion, based on all cases examined, that there was usually between 440 and 480 mg quartz per 100 g tissue in moderate silicosis confirmed post-mortem. EINBRODT and GRUSSENDORF (1973) reported three cases of workers exposed to diatomaceous earth dust whose lung dust contained an average of over 15% quartz and cristoballite, and whose degree of nodulation was higher than in coal miners with the same amount of crystalline free silica. The authors suggested that these results might be explained by a potentiating effect of amorphous silica on quartz.

MATERIAL

Our investigation was on the lungs of twenty-five deceased workers exposed at work to dust with high quartz content. Details of dust exposure are presented in Table 1. The subjects are divided into three groups according to the post-mortem diagnosis:—(a) without silicosis, (b) with reticular and nodular silicosis forms, and (c) with large opacities.

The exposure of all underground miners included a period of from 2 to 6 years in the very dusty conditions produced by dry drilling of blasting holes followed by a period of markedly improved working conditions. Eight of the subjects worked exclusively, and one (no. 2) predominantly in uranium mines during the period 1947–1964. With the exception of no. 33, who was a mine surveyor and timber worker, all were diggers. Six persons worked in tunnel construction and quarries, five were miners solely in lead/zinc mines, three mainly in barytes mines, and the rest had a mixed exposure. The twenty-five subjects were followed up for between 7 and 18 years at the silicosis ward at the Institute. Detailed medical histories were available for all twenty-five, including X-ray records, tests of lung function and circulation, occupational history including a description of the working environment, case histories, and details of each hospitalization.

The lungs of twenty-four individuals were investigated at the Clinic of Occupational Diseases after their death, and the other after a fatal accident at work. All necropsies were performed by the same pathologist (Dr K. Kolev).

METHODS

After dissection, each lung was weighed separately. Density and size of silicotic nodules, the presence and size of massive lesions, pleural adhesions, emphysema, and enlargement of bronchopulmonary and mediastinal lymph nodes were also determined. The lungs were sent for digestion after material had been taken for the histological examination of each lobe and massive lesion. The histological sections were stained for collagen with haematoxylin eosin and saturn red using the extremely selective method of HOLUŠA (1963).

Dust was extracted from the lungs by the formamide method of THOMAS and STEGEMANN (1954). Dust quantity was determined as constant weight at 150°C, and

TABLE 1. DURATION AND NATURE OF DUST EXPOSURES

Case no.	Dust exposure duration (years)	Place of work	Life span from the beginning of dust exposure till death (years)
		No silicosis	
27	6	Dams	18
4	10	Lead/zinc mines	21
33	21	Uranium mines	25
23	6	Tunnels	44
		With reticular and nodular forms	
21	5	Lead/zinc mines	21
6	17	Barytes mines	27
17	41	Quarries and grinding of quartz sand	53
3	14	Barytes and zinc mines	20
16	8	Quarries and tunnels	39
		Large opacities	
9	10	Lead/zinc mines	18
14	10	Uranium mines	19
11	15	Barytes and copper mines	26
25	8	Uranium mines	20
15	8.5	Lead/zinc and coal	18
18	7	Quarries and tunnels	21
1	13	Lead/zinc mines	20
2	12	Uranium, lead/zinc and coal mines	22
19	16	Uranium mines	25
26	6.5	Barytes and copper mines	18
13	3.5	Tunnels and coal mines	26
7	14.5	Uranium mines	24
8	11	Uranium mines	23
12	8.5	Uranium mines	20
5	12.5	Copper mines	20
10	13	Uranium mines	19

the mineral residue was obtained by heating the dust at 360°C. The quantity of total silica was determined by the method of PEREGUD and GERNET (1973), and of crystalline silica by the microchemical method of DOBREVA and IVANOVA (1969).

Considerable difficulties were met in the accurate determination of the average residence time of retained dust in lungs. Average dustiness varied substantially with time depending on whether there was dry drilling or not, and it also varied with working place. Some of the individuals had dust exposure interrupted by periods of non-dusty employment. In these cases the Einbrodt formula for determining average residence time of retained dust in the lungs proved to be insufficiently accurate.

We calculated an exposure index and average lung residence time (t_w) of retained quartz dust in terms of the total retained quantity of quartz (Q) in grams per 100 g of dry lung tissue, the time between end of exposure and death (T), and exposure history. To quantify this, the subject's working life was divided into periods for which dust concentration had been roughly constant; for the ith period, the average respirable quartz concentration in the air was K_i, and the period's duration was t_i. The total number of periods was n. For most of the subjects, there were four such periods: (1) a period of dry drilling, (2) a transition period of introduction of wet drilling, (3) a period of wet drilling and introduction of other dust-suppression methods, and (4) a period of fully implemented dust suppression.

If q_i is the quartz quantity retained in the lungs per year in the ith period,

$$Q = \sum_{i=1}^{i=n} t_i q_i$$

q_i is a constant fraction P of K_i, and can be determined for each subject from

$$Q = P \sum_{i=1}^{i=n} t_i K_i$$

so that each q_i can be determined from the measured K_i.

We define the residence time of retained dust t_w from the summed (lung burden × time) for each of the i periods (total duration τ) and the man's retirement.

$$t_w Q = TQ + t_1\left(\frac{q_1 t_1}{2}\right) + (\tau - t_1)\, q_1 t_1$$

$$+ t_2\left(\frac{q_2 t_2}{2}\right) + (\tau - [t_1 + t_2])\, q_2 t_2 + t_n\left(\frac{q_n t_n}{2}\right).$$

This assumes uniform exposure to dust during each period.

The product $t_w Q$ is our exposure index, which should correlate with degree of silicosis.

The clinical data, comprising diagnosis while alive, the character of X-ray changes (ILO–U/C, 1971), the decrease in ventilatory indices (vital capacity, Tiffenau index, maximal minute ventilation), and the degree of disability, were compared with the post-mortem diagnosis and lung-dust measurements.

RESULTS

The basic data from the lung-dust analysis are presented in Table 2. The cases are divided into three groups: without silicosis, nodular and reticular silicosis, and massive silicosis, and within the groups they are arranged in ascending order according to our exposure index.

The quantity of dust isolated from the lungs varied from 0.8 to 8 g per 100 g dry lung tissue, and the mineral residue from 0.3 to 7 g/100 g. The total silica was about 35 to 40% of the mineral residue, while its absolute quantity ranged from 0.16 to 2.7 g/100 g. The average free crystalline silica content was between 20 and 25% and the quantity was from 0.02 to 1.81 g/100 g. The average residence time of retained dust was about 17.4 years at an average dust-exposure duration of 11 years.

TABLE 2. QUANTITY AND MINERAL COMPOSITION OF DUST ISOLATED FROM THE LUNGS

Case no.	Dust quantity at 105°C g/100 g dry tissue	Mineral residue at 360° C g/100 g dry tissue	Total SiO_2 g/100 g dry tissue	Free cryst. SiO_2 % of mineral residue at 360°C	Free cryst. SiO_2 g/100 g dry tissue	Lung residence time of retained dust (years)	Index of silicosis risk
27	0.84	0.34	—	6.1	0.021	17.4	0.4
4	1.86	0.64	0.157	15.9	0.102	14.5	1.5
33	1.68	1.09	—	17.0	0.185	12.0	2.2
23	2.90	1.50	0.296	9.5	0.142	38.0	5.4
21	2.11	1.51	0.479	20.4	0.308	18.4	5.7
6	3.40	2.42	0.995	14.6	0.354	17.5	6.2
17	3.05	2.45	0.939	27.2	0.620	16.0	9.9
3	6.11	4.38	1.257	14.2	0.624	16.8	10.5
16	3.63	2.85	1.104	26.0	0.741	33.8	25.0
9	2.07	1.41	0.419	19.7	0.275	16.2	4.4
14	2.62	1.94	0.716	22.8	0.443	16.4	7.3
11	3.36	2.51	0.787	23.4	0.590	18.5	10.9
25	3.75	2.94	1.083	20.9	0.615	18.7	11.5
15	3.84	3.01	1.238	29.9	0.899	13.2	11.9
18	4.25	3.24	1.187	23.2	0.752	18.0	13.5
1	3.32	2.20	1.573	34.3	0.933	17.1	16.0
2	6.20	5.17	2.323	21.1	1.097	15.8	17.3
19	5.11	3.70	1.411	23.3	0.864	20.9	18.0
26	6.77	6.73	2.585	19.7	1.128	16.0	18.0
13	3.32	2.69	0.914	28.4	0.771	24.1	18.5
7	7.84	6.67	2.330	15.2	1.005	18.7	18.8
8	7.40	6.21	2.353	16.1	1.002	20.9	20.9
12	5.97	5.20	1.857	24.8	1.290	17.8	23.0
5	7.19	6.01	2.400	24.8	1.487	17.2	25.5
10	8.09	7.15	2.710	25.5	1.811	17.0	30.8

Quartz quantity per 100 g did not show a statistically significant correlation with total duration of exposure or with duration of work with dry drilling of blasting-holes. The relations between quartz quantity, average residence time of retained dust determined according to the formula given above, and the X-ray morphological diagnosis of the cases are presented in Fig. 1. In the individuals without silicosis the average residence time of retained dust did not differ from that in the other groups and quartz quantity did not exceed 200 mg/100 g. The second group–individuals with reticular or nodular silicosis—had quartz values from 250 to 760 mg. The subject with an average residence time of retained dust over 30 years was a worker at an open sandstone quarry. The third group, with advanced silicosis, showed the most marked clustering around the average residence time, while quartz quantity varied from 400 to 1800 mg/100 g.

The good agreement between clinical (with X-ray) diagnosis and post-mortem

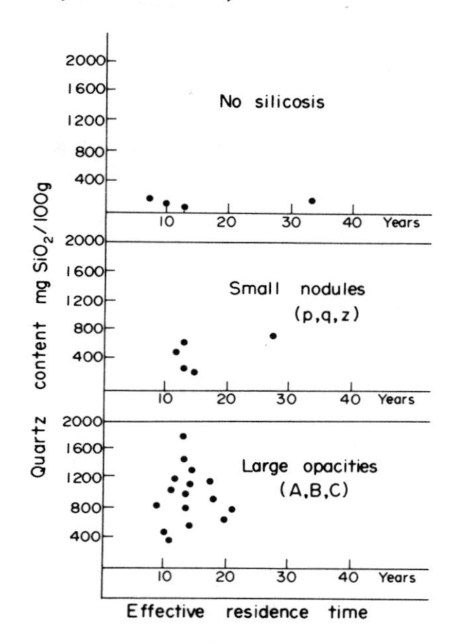

FIG. 1. Relation between quartz content, average residence time of retained dust in lungs, and X-ray morphological diagnosis of the subjects.

diagnosis and their relation to quartz quantity per 100 g tissue is shown in Fig. 2. The post-mortem diagnosis in one case failed to agree with the clinical diagnosis of reticular silicosis—the pathologist admitted only the presence of moderate non-specific fibrosis. There was complete agreement of diagnosis of massive forms. We subdivided these severe cases into two sub-groups: by X-ray, according to whether the large opacities were on a nodular (p, q, r) or a reticular (s, t, u) background; and post-mortem, according to whether the massive spread over more or less than a quarter of

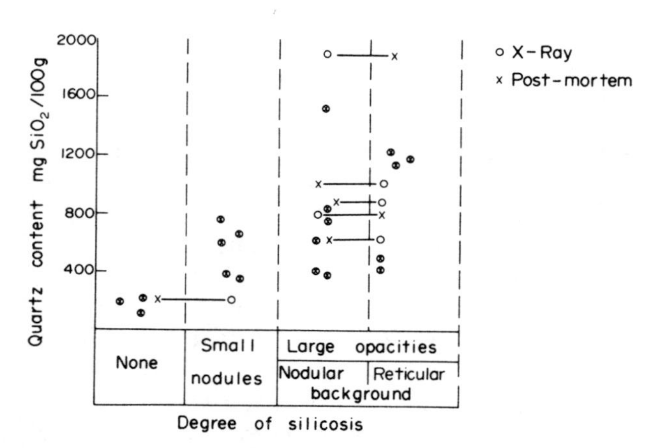

FIG. 2. The agreement between X-ray and post-mortem diagnoses and their relation to quartz content per 100 g tissue.

the pulmonary field. This classification revealed that a nodular background with massive lesions occupying less than a quarter of the field was found in miners with a higher percentage of quartz in the deposited dust (cases 1, 10, 5, 9, 13, 14, 15, 19). Reticular background prevailed in dusts with lower quartz percentage, and more massive lesions also formed.

The schematic distribution of the cases according to their X-ray classification (ILO U/C, 1971), based on the last X-ray before death (5 days to 3 months before, except for no. 33), is presented in Table 3.

TABLE 3. SCHEMATIZED X-RAY FINDINGS ACCORDING TO ILO–U/C CLASSIFICATION

X-ray findings	Case number
Irregular opacities (s, t, u)	17, 23, 27, 33
Mixed, nodular and irregular opacities (p, q, r + s, t, u)	3, 4, 6, 16, 21
Large opacities (A, B, C)	
id + (p, q, r)	5, 9, 13, 14, 15, 19
id + (s, t, u)	2, 8, 11, 12, 18, 25, 26
wd + (p, q, r)	1, 10
wd + (s, t, u)	7

There was no statistically significant correlation between quartz quantity and ventilatory disturbance in the last year of the patients' life.

DISCUSSION

Generally our results confirm the relation of degree of silicosis and lung content of quartz established by many other authors.

A very good agreement is established between clinical and post-mortem diagnosis, and there is a positive correlation between silicosis and lung quartz content. That correlation is best shown in the classification of the cases by our dust exposure index, since this takes into account both quartz amount and residence time of dust retained in the lungs. The detailed analysis of clinical and post-mortem data of the cases in the two silicosis classes, listed in order of exposure index, reveals that the less severe cases appear at the top and the more severe cases at the end of each group. Thus, the first three cases of the group of massive forms have early opacities in one lung only. The only exception is case no. 5, where the high index and the large amount of quartz in pulmonary tissue fail to agree with the clinical and X-ray picture and the length of exposure. This was a case of the Caplan form of pneumoconiosis, where an immunobiological model of reaction seems to be present, unlike the other cases.

In this study we could not get a complete picture of the role played by the proportion of quartz in the dust. Nevertheless, some differences can be seen between our results and those obtained in coal miners. Miners in this study, exposed predominantly to ore and rock dust of high quartz percentage, have in general developed severe silicosis with less quartz in the lungs (in one case less than 275 and on average 500 to 1000 mg/100 g) and at a considerably shorter average residence time of retained dust (17 years). For comparison, coal miners with about 4 to 5% quartz in the lung dust develop severe silicosis after an average residence time of retained dust of over 20 years, and with a quartz content of over 1000 mg/100 g. The question arises as to why approximately equal quartz amounts lead to more rapid progress of massive silicosis in ore miners in Bulgaria than in coal miners in the Ruhr. An explanation of this discrepancy might involve the different percentage quartz content in the dust, the different biological activity of quartz from coal and ore beds, and the effect of other components present in the dust. One other factor should not be neglected, namely the rate of deposition of dust in the lungs. In the majority of our cases it occurred in massive doses for a very short period. If the proportion of quartz in the dust is important, a change of 10 in the quartz percentage might be necessary before any effect is seen, and this might well explain why no manifestations have been observed in our relatively homogenous group. The data of EINBRODT and GRUSSENDORF (1973) about cases exposed to diatomaceous earth dust support this explanation.

Because of the limited data available for the group "without silicosis" we are not prepared to adopt unreservedly the acceptable critical value for lung quartz content of 150–200 mg/100 g dry tissue established by EINBRODT and KLOSTERKÖTTER (1965). This may not be valid for our dusts with their high quartz percentages, although our results are in good agreement with this value.

Some authors (KNAGGE *et al.*, 1971; AMORT and EINBRODT, 1970) give evidence about the cytotoxicity of lead and zinc and their possible role in silicosis development. These observations, mainly on coal miners, suggest that our workers should be studied with this in mind since a number of them had worked in lead/zinc mines and with some other metals. The lead/zinc miners show, for an equal stage of silicosis lesions, a lower quartz content than the uranium miners, although the difference is not statistically significant. Statistical evaluation of considerably more cases is necessary before arriving at a definite conclusion.

Acknowledgement—I am indebted to Dr T. L. Ogden for revising the English of this paper and presenting it at the Symposium.

REFERENCES

AMORT, H. and EINBRODT, H. J. (1970) *Int. Arch. Arbeitsmed.* **26**, 25–29.
DOBREVA, M. and IVANOVA, St. (1969) *Higiena i zdraveopazvane* **4**, 375–379.
EINBRODT, H. J. and GRUSSENDORF, J. (1973) *Staub* **33**, 273–276.
EINBRODT, H. J. and KLOSTERKÖTTER, W. (1965) *Ergebn. Unters. Staub- Silikosebekämpf. Steinkohlenbergbau* **5**, 97–99.
HÖER, P. W., EINBRODT, H. J. and LEITERITZ, H. (1967) *Fortschr. Staublungenforsch.* **2**, 607–611.
HOLUŠA, R. (1963) *Stain Technol.* **38**, 204–205.
KNAGGE-RUHE, B., STECHER, W. and EINBRODT, H. J. (1971) *Beitr. Silikoseforsch.* **23**, 157–171.
LANDWEHR, M. and BRUCKMANN, E. (1969) *Staub* **29**, 5.
LEITERITZ, H., EINBRODT, H. J. and KLOSTERKÖTTER, W. (1967) *Inhaled Particles and Vapours* (edited by DAVIES, C. N.) pp. 381–390. Pergamon Press, Oxford.
OTTO, H. (1960) *Berufskr. keram. Glasindustr.* **7**, 304–306.
PEREGUD, E. and GERNET, E. (1973) *Air Chemical Analysis in Industry*. Himia, Leningrad.
STRECKER, F. J. and EINBRODT, H. J. (1958) *Die Staublungenerkrankungen* (edited by JÖTTEN, K. W. and KLOSTERKÖTTER, W.) vol. 3, pp. 298–307. Steinkopff, Darmstadt.
THOMAS, K. and STEGEMANN, H. (1954) *Beitr. Silikoseforsch.* (28), 1–30.
WORTH, G., MUYSERS, H. and EINBRODT, H. J. (1967) *Fortschr. Staublungenforsch.* **2**, 443–449.

DISCUSSION

J. C. GILSON: Could the author tell us:

1. The ages of the subjects.
2. Was tuberculosis present in men with massive lesions?
3. What was the *total weight* of dust in each lung? It is difficult to interpret figures for *dust per gram dry weight*, because the lung dry weight is raised by the pathological processes.

Mme DOBREVA: The answers to queries 1 and 3 are given in the following table:

Case no.	27	4	33	23	21	6	17	3	16	9	14	11	25
Age	70	68	44	70	65	59	77	50	65	64	63	57	45
Total weight of dust (g)	1.60	5.6	3.4	5.7	5.2	9.1	7.6	14.7	8.4	4.3	6.9	8.7	14.9

Case no.	18	1	2	19	26	13	7	8	12	5	10
Age	60	47	44	49	46	60	62	47	43	45	52
Total weight of dust (g)	8.5	8.2	12.4	15.4	22.8	8.6	21.9	18.3	18.9	30.2	31.3

Query 2: Neither clinical nor X-ray or pathological data for active tuberculosis were found in any of the cases.

CHRONIC OBSTRUCTIVE LUNG DISEASE IN GOLD MINERS

F. J. WILES and M. H. FAURE

Medical Bureau for Occupational Diseases, Johannesburg, R.S.A

Abstract—A survey has been made of 2209 gold miners in the Republic of South Africa. The result showed that there is a significant dose–response relationship between dust inhaled and both chronic bronchitis and airways obstruction. This is found in smokers, ex-smokers and non-smokers. The effect of smoking is more potent than that of dust but there does not appear to be a dose–response relationship in regard to smoking. The effect of smoking differs from the effect of dust in that ex-smokers show less bronchitis and less airways obstruction than smokers, but ex-miners do not show a similar advantage over working miners.

THIS is a report on a survey of 2209 gold miners in the Republic of South Africa. The object of the study was to determine whether there is a dose–response relationship between chronic obstructive lung disease and occupational exposure to dust. Dust counts vary with occupation between 70 and 250 particles per cm^3 and the dust in the gold mines contains about 75% free silica.

Every miner is compelled by law to undergo an annual medical examination as long as he is working in a dusty occupation. Most men who have left the mines continue to come for medical examinations because of the hope of being awarded compensation. The Medical Bureau for Occupational Diseases, therefore, has regular contact with all working miners and irregular contact with the majority of ex-miners. Every man who attended the Bureau during the 4-year period 1968 to 1971 was included in the study provided that he met the criteria laid down:

1. Bureau number within the block of Bureau numbers B.9000 to C.8999.
2. Age between 45 and 54.
3. Minimum of 10 years' service underground.
4. Resident in South Africa for not less than 20 years.

METHODS

A shortened and adapted version of the British Medical Research Council Bronchitis questionnaire was used. A detailed smoking history was obtained. As smoking habits have been recorded annually since 1959, it was possible to compare answers to the smoking questionnaire with the evidence on the man's Bureau file. It was found that 80% of men gave reliable smoking histories, but in 20% their accuracy was improved by referring back to answers given in previous years.

For every man a spirogram was recorded on a Godart spirometer. All spirograms were checked by a pulmonary physiologist and 8 % of the total were excluded because they were considered to be sub-maximal efforts. The numbers in the tables which analyse the forced expiratory volume in one second (FEV_1) and the maximum mid-expiratory flow (MMF) are therefore smaller than the numbers in the tables dealing with chronic bronchitis.

A chest radiograph was read by a single reader without knowledge of the occupational history.

Each man was asked to cough and expectorate as much as possible into a jar for a period of 5 min. The volume produced was measured and 1 ml or more of mucus or mucopus (but not saliva) was recorded as "sputum produced". Early morning or 24-h sputum could not be obtained, and the actual specimens were produced at any time between 2 h and 6 h after rising.

An analysis of the mining service of each man was made from records kept by the Chamber of Mines. These records show the exact number of shifts worked in each occupation. About 200 occupations are listed and the dust count for each of these was measured by technicians who followed men in the various occupations throughout a number of shifts. On the basis of these dust counts BEADLE (1971) classified all occupations into eleven groups. He used these data to study the relationship of radiological silicosis to dust exposure and reported his results in *Inhaled Particles III*. The fact that Beadle was able to show a significant relationship between silicosis and his grouping of occupations lends validity to his observations. The same occupational groups have been used for estimating dust exposure in this paper.

For every man in the survey the number of shifts worked in each occupation was multiplied by the mean dust count (expressed as respirable surface area) for that occupation. The sum of the products gives total dust exposure which for convenience has been converted to particle-years.

RESULTS

Because they may be motivated by hopes of compensation, it is often suspected that miners tend to exaggerate their symptoms. A strict criterion for a diagnosis of chronic bronchitis was therefore adopted, six positive answers being required: cough in the early morning, cough at other times during the day and cough for 3 months in the year as well as positive answers to the equivalent questions about sputum. Even if symptoms are exaggerated, there is no reason to suppose that the tendency is greater among men with high dust exposure than among men with low dust exposure. We have, therefore, assumed that the answers to the questionnaire given by men in the various sub-groups are comparable.

In the tables, total dust exposure is shown as particle-years divided by 1000.

Table 1 shows the prevalence of chronic bronchitis in relation to total dust exposure as well as the percentage of men who produced sputum (as defined above). It is surprising that the number of men who produced sputum is larger than the number who had chronic bronchitis as revealed by the questionnaire. This suggests that our suspicion that miners exaggerate their symptoms is unjustified.

TABLE 1. BRONCHITIS RELATED TO TOTAL DUST EXPOSURE

Total dust (10^3 RSA–years)	Number in group	% with bronchitis	% with sputum
10	169	20.7	32.0
17	457	27.4	35.4
24	464	37.1	42.2
31	443	40.6	43.6
38	353	41.9	41.9
45	185	39.5	44.9
52	138	38.4	42.7
Total	2209		
Significance		$P<0.001$	$P<0.01$

Table 2 shows the prevalence of chronic bronchitis in relation to total dust exposure for non-smokers, ex-smokers and smokers separately. It is clear from Tables 1 and 2 that there is a dose–response relationship between dust and chronic bronchitis irrespective of the smoking habits. In the group of twenty-four non-smokers in the lowest dust category none had chronic bronchitis. The figure was about 20% in non-smokers with high dust exposure and about 35% in smokers with the lowest dust exposure. It appears that the effect of smoking is greater than that of dust.

TABLE 2. BRONCHITIS RELATED TO TOTAL DUST EXPOSURE

(Separate smoking groups)

	Non-smokers		Ex-smokers		Smokers	
Total dust (10^3 RSA–years)	No. in group	% with bronchitis	No. in group	% with bronchitis	No. in group	% with bronchitis
10	24	0	57	7.0	88	35.2
17	58	3.4	106	11.3	293	37.8
24	53	17.0	98	23.4	313	44.7
31	50	20.0	96	26.0	297	48.8
38	36	19.4	76	26.3	241	50.2
45	25	16.0	50	20.0	110	53.6
52	14	14.3	31	12.9	93	50.5
Total	260		514		1435	
Significance		$P<0.05$		$P<0.05$		$P<0.001$

The increase in the percentage of men with chronic bronchitis in all three smoking groups reaches a peak at a total dust exposure of 38 000 particle-years and then levels off or tends to fall. Possible reasons for this will be discussed below.

Table 3 shows both the FEV_1 and the MMF in relation to total dust exposure. The figures given are absolute values. Neither the mean height nor the mean age were significantly different in any of the sub-groups. Both the FEV_1 and the MMF decline progressively with increasing dust exposure. The more rapid decline of the MMF shows, as would be expected, that it is a more sensitive indicator of early airways obstruction than the FEV_1.

TABLE 3. LUNG FUNCTION RELATED TO TOTAL DUST EXPOSURE

Total dust (10^3 RSA–years)	Number in group	Mean MMF (l./s)	Mean FEV_1 (l.)
10	164	3.23	3.40
17	432	2.91	3.24
24	429	2.78	3.15
31	394	2.63	3.04
38	313	2.49	2.97
45	160	2.66	3.03
52	128	2.60	3.04
Total	2020		
Significance		$P<0.01$	$P<0.001$

Table 4 shows the mean MMF in relation to total dust exposure for non-smokers, ex-smokers and smokers separately. The effect of dust is apparent in all smoking

TABLE 4. MAXIMUM MID-EXPIRATORY FLOW RELATED TO TOTAL DUST EXPOSURE (Separate smoking groups)

	Non-smokers		Ex-smokers		Smokers	
Total dust (10^3 RSA–years)	No. in group	Mean MMF (l./s)	No. in group	Mean MMF (l./s)	No. in group	Mean MMF (l./s)
10	24	4.20	56	3.22	84	2.96
17	57	3.70	101	3.26	274	2.61
24	46	3.66	89	2.91	294	2.61
31	46	3.23	82	2.67	266	2.52
38	28	3.08	72	2.75	213	2.32
45	22	3.60	45	2.92	93	2.30
52	14	3.59	27	2.89	87	2.36
Total	237		472		1311	
Significance		$P<0.05$		$P<0.05$		$P<0.001$

groups. In non-smokers in the lowest dust category the mean MMF is 4.20 l./s. This falls to 3.08 l./s in non-smokers with high dust exposure and to 2.96 l./s in smokers with the lowest dust exposure. In contrast to the situation with chronic bronchitis, dust exposure seems to be very nearly as potent as smoking as a cause of airways obstruction.

The increase in airways obstruction follows the same pattern as the rising prevalence of chronic bronchitis. Both reach a peak at or about a total dust exposure of 38 000 particle-years and then level off. This point represents about 25 years' service with a konimeter dust count of the order of 200 particles per cm^3. The fact that both the bronchitis prevalence and the MMF level off at the same point, and that this occurs in all smoking groups suggests that this is a real phenomenon. The reason for it is obscure. In view of the composition of the sample it is unlikely that the levelling off is caused by ill men leaving the industry and healthy men remaining. As 30% of those included had already left the mines, the sample is not heavily biased by movement out of the industry.

A more probable explanation is that 25 years of moderate dust exposure is a sufficient insult to the bronchial tree to cause chronic obstructive bronchitis in all men who are susceptible. Men who have not been affected by then may be presumed to be immune to any further increase in the dust load.

It should be noted that the size of the groups beyond the point where levelling off occurs is small compared with the groups before that point. The general trend over the whole range of dust exposure is therefore statistically significant at the levels indicated in the tables.

Average Dust Level

Dust exposure has also been analysed in terms of the mean level of dust to which each man was exposed ignoring years of service. Table 5 shows the increase of chronic bronchitis with increasing dust levels expressed as respirable surface area. Table 6 shows an inverse relationship between mean MMF and mean dust levels.

TABLE 5. BRONCHITIS RELATED TO MEAN DUST LEVEL EXPRESSED AS RESPIRABLE SURFACE AREA

Mean dust level	No. in group	% with bronchitis
700	371	17.5
900	374	32.6
1100	312	37.8
1300	256	44.9
1500	524	42.7
1700	155	34.2
1900	127	45.7
2100	90	34.4
Total	2209	
Significance		$P < 0.001$

TABLE 6. MAXIMUM MID-EXPIRATORY FLOW RELATED TO MEAN DUST LEVEL EXPRESSED AS RESPIRABLE SURFACE AREA

Mean dust level	No. in group	Mean MMF
700	364	3.07
900	347	2.93
1100	297	2.74
1300	219	2.59
1500	462	2.50
1700	139	2.64
1900	113	2.71
2100	79	2.66
Total	2020	
Significance		$P<0.001$

As in the previous tables there is a levelling off both in the prevalence of chronic bronchitis and in the mean MMF. A comparison of mean dust levels with total dust exposure expressed as particle-years indicates a correlation between the two measurements. From our data it is not possible to determine which of the two is the more important causative factor.

Level of Smoking

A comparison between light smokers and heavy smokers is given in Table 7. Ex-smokers were excluded from this analysis. The level of smoking was calculated by the

TABLE 7. COMPARISON OF LIGHT AND HEAVY SMOKERS

	Light smokers	Heavy smokers
Number	663	772
Percentage with bronchitis	45.1%	46.0%
Mean MMF (l./s)	2.31	2.32

formula: Total smoking = Present number of cigarettes (or grams of tobacco for pipe smokers) daily × years × 365. The upper limit for light smokers was the equivalent of 15 cigarettes daily for 25 years. The pattern of total dust exposure for the light and heavy smoking groups is approximately the same. Both for the prevalence of chronic bronchitis and for the mean MMF there is almost no difference between light and heavy smokers. In contrast to dust, therefore, a dose–response relationship for tobacco smoking seems to be lacking.

The precise method of assessing smoking habits does not affect this conclusion. Two other methods were tried:

(1) If a man used to smoke more heavily than at present, a mean figure for daily smoking was estimated. The formula then became: Total smoking = Mean daily smoking × years × 365.
(2) The amount smoked daily at present ignoring the total duration. These methods gave very nearly the same figures as those in Table 7.

Comparison of Working Miners with Ex-miners

Of the total sample, 653 men had been away from mine work for 1 year or longer at the time of examination. The prevalence of chronic bronchitis and the mean MMF for working miners and ex-miners are shown in Tables 8 and 9. The proportions of smokers, ex-smokers and non-smokers are the same for working miners and ex-miners. At most of the dust levels ex-miners have a somewhat higher prevalence of chronic

TABLE 8. CHRONIC BRONCHITIS IN WORKING MINERS AND EX-MINERS

	Working miners		Ex-miners	
Total dust (10^3 RSA–years)	No. in group	Bronchitis %	No. in group	Bronchitis %
10	35	14.3	134	22.4
17	281	26.7	176	28.4
24	322	34.2	142	43.7
31	332	41.0	111	39.6
38	294	41.5	59	44.1
45	292	38.0	31	47.6
Total	1556	35.8	653	34.7

TABLE 9. MAXIMUM MID-EXPIRATORY FLOW IN WORKING MINERS AND EX-MINERS

	Working miners		Ex-miners	
Total dust (10^3 RSA–years)	No. in group	Mean MMF (l./s)	No. in group	Mean MMF (l./s)
10	35	3.18	129	3.24
17	271	2.97	161	2.79
24	307	2.91	122	2.46
31	303	2.65	91	2.56
38	266	2.47	47	2.58
45	268	2.65	20	2.30
Total	1450	2.74	570	2.75

bronchitis and lower mean MMF. The ex-miners are certainly in no better condition than the working miners. It may be argued that chest trouble caused the ex-miners to leave the mines and on this account they are a selected group. We do not think that this is what occurs. Undoubtedly many of those who leave the mines between the ages of 40 and 55 do so for financial and social reasons or because non-respiratory diseases have made them unfit to work underground. Although we have no figures on this point, it is our impression that there is not a disproportionate number of complaints about chronic chest disease among ex-miners as compared with working miners.

We therefore conclude that removal from dust exposure does not delay or reverse the progress of chronic bronchitis. This is different from what has been shown in regard to smoking where the average condition of ex-smokers was found to be significantly better than that of smokers.

Several writers have suggested that pneumoconiosis is less common in men who have chronic bronchitis. GOUGH (1960) postulated that not only does excess mucus in the airways lessen the amount of dust reaching the alveoli, but even dust in the interstitial tissues may be removed by macrophages which are stimulated by inflammation in the bronchi. This would reduce the likelihood of pneumoconiosis. Table 10 shows the

TABLE 10. INCIDENCE OF SILICOSIS IN BRONCHITICS AND NON-BRONCHITICS

	No. in group	No. with silicosis	% with silicosis
Bronchitics	786	59	7.5
Non-bronchitics	1423	90	6.3

number of men with radiological silicosis among bronchitics and non-bronchitics. The proportion with silicosis is slightly higher in the men with chronic bronchitis, but the difference is not statistically significant at the 0.05 level. Our evidence does not support the hypothesis that there is a lower incidence of silicosis among men who have chronic bronchitis.

REFERENCES

BEADLE, D. G. (1971) *Inhaled Particles III* (edited by WALTON, W. H.) vol. II, pp. 953–966. Unwin Bros., Old Woking, Surrey.

GOUGH, J. (1960) *Ind. Med. Surg.* **29**, 283–285.

DISCUSSION

R. S. J. du Toit: I would like to point out that the figure of 75% for the free silica content of the dust refers to samples which have been heated to 550°C (to remove combustibles) and acid-treated to remove soluble salts. Also, the conversion from surface area to number of particles to express the dust concentration, involves division by a factor of about 7, which is the surface area (in μm^2) of a sphere of diameter 1.5 μm. This diameter in turn is the size of the surface area mean particle of airborne gold-mine dust in the diameter range 0.5 to 5 μm.

R. A. Francis: Could you please justify a little more fully the statement that the more rapid decline of MMF shows, as would be expected, that it is a more sensitive indicator of early airways obstruction than the FEV_1. In particular, is it known how the decline of MMF compares with that of the FEV_1 for a normal control group of the same race, sex, etc., as your study population?

Dr Wiles: Not being a pulmonary physiologist I hesitate to answer your question. It would perhaps be more accurate to say that the FEV_1 and the MMF are not measuring the same thing, but in practice we almost always find a reduction of the MMF before the FEV_1 is affected. I have no figures for the decline of the FEV_1 or MMF in a control group.

J. Jahr: How did you calculate the dose? Exposure over the years is rarely constant and a high exposure at the start of the exposure period should be given more weight than a high exposure nearer the end of a man's service. I have proposed a simple formula (Jahr, J. (1974) *Archs envir. Hlth* **29**, 338–340) which takes this into consideration. I wonder whether you made any allowance for this factor?

Dr Wiles: We have records of whether the higher dust exposure was in the early, middle or late part of a man's service, but these data have not yet been analysed.

C. E. Rossiter: I am concerned about the use of absolute values of FEV_1 and MMF. Even though the subjects were all 45–54 years old, there could still be large differences in average ages which could account for the differences in lung function shown in Table 3. How similar were the average ages in the total dust exposure groups?

Dr Wiles: The mean height and age in every cell were calculated. The mean height did not vary by more than 1 inch and the age by more than 1 year from cell to cell.

W. K. C. Morgan: The almost identical values for the mean MMF for the light and heavy smokers is surprising and I wonder whether the ethnic composition of the two groups was similar. In this regard, Dr Rossiter, Dr Weill and my own group have shown that black subjects have flow rates and lung volumes that are 12% lower than have whites of the same age and height. In response to the point that Dr Francis brought up, the difference persists throughout life.

Dr Wiles: We limit our studies to one race only to avoid the complications of race as a variable. This group were all white miners. Black miners have been described in a paper elsewhere.

W. T. Ulmer: There seems to be very good agreement between your results and those published by Worth *et al.* and by our group. In all dust-exposed workers—it does not matter what kind of dust—the FEV_1 and the arterial oxygen pressure are decreased and the functional residual capacity is increased. But we do not believe that these are signs of chronic obstructive airway disease, because airway resistance measurements show normal values in all these groups. The FEV_1 decrease depends on the collapsibility of the small airways under the high lung pressures (never used in normal breathing) required by the FEV_1 measurement procedure.

Dr Wiles: Unfortunately when this study began some years ago we did not have a plethysmograph. We are doing another survey now in which airways resistance is being measured.

G. Berry: I should like to raise a point concerning the grouping of the men into the different dust categories. Since the whole group was chosen to be homogeneous for age, presumably the higher cumulative dust groups contain disproportionately more men in jobs with higher dust concentrations. Is it possible, therefore, that this has introduced a selective mechanism, the more fit men carrying out the more arduous and more dusty jobs?

Whether this is so or not I would suggest that the explanation put forward for a peak in respiratory symptoms and function at 38 000 particle-years cannot be accepted on the basis of the data given. Whether it is reasonable to presume that men unaffected after 25 years of moderate dust exposure are immune to further increases in their dust load can only be determined by carrying out a longitudinal study on a group of such men.

Dr Wiles: Having already said that the reason for the levelling off phenomenon is obscure, I agree that my explanation is hypothetical. Nevertheless, I think it is a real phenomenon not caused by a selective mechanism and I welcome any suggestion about it.

FACTORS INFLUENCING EXPIRATORY FLOW RATES IN COAL MINERS

J. L. HANKINSON, R. B. REGER, R. P. FAIRMAN, N. L. LAPP and W. K. C. MORGAN

Appalachian Laboratory for Occupational Respiratory Diseases, National Institute for Occupational Safety and Health,

and the

Department of Medicine, West Virginia University Medical Center, Morgantown, W.V., U.S.A.

Abstract—The most commonly used tests of ventilatory capacity, viz. the forced expiratory volume in one second (FEV_1) and the forced vital capacity (FVC) are derived from a volume versus time record of a forced expiratory volume manoeuvre. Numerous studies have been unable to show a relationship between radiographic category of simple coal-workers' pneumoconiosis (CWP) and the FEV_1 and FVC. The explanation for this is related to the fact that coal dust responsible for pneumoconiosis is deposited in the alveoli and distal airways below 2 mm in diameter, and that marked increases in the air-flow resistance of these airways may be present without significantly affecting the FEV_1, FVC, or the total airways resistance.

The flow volume curve has been suggested as a means to detect disease in the small airways since it permits measurement of expiratory flow at both high and low lung volumes. To derive additional information about the effects of coal dust on the small airways, the maximal expiratory flow volume curves of 6014 working coal miners have been analysed. The influence of (1) age, (2) height, (3) weight, (4) underground exposure, and (5) cigarette smoking, on maximal expiratory flows at 75, 50, 25, and 10% of forced vital capacity as well as peak flow was analysed. Age and cigarette smoking had a highly significant effect on flows at all lung volumes. Also prolonged underground exposure had a significant effect on the flow rates at high lung volume and was especially noticeable among the non-smokers. Although previous work has shown that miners have lower flows than do comparable age-matched controls, in the present study neither category of CWP nor major workplace had any detectable effect on flow rates in excess of what may be attributable to age, height, weight, and years spent working underground. The decrement in flow rates at higher lung volumes due to prolonged underground exposure, when considered in conjunction with the absence of an effect on flows with increasing radiographic category, suggests that a dust-induced bronchitis is responsible.

INTRODUCTION

Although there is a definite relationship between the category of simple coal-workers' pneumoconiosis (CWP) and the coal content of the lung (ROSSITER, 1972), the transition from category 0 to category 1, and from category 1 to 2, and so on, is unassociated with a decrement in the standard tests of ventilatory capacity until progressive massive fibrosis supervenes (ROGAN *et al.*, 1961; COCHRANE and HIGGINS, 1961; MORGAN *et al.*, 1974). The location of the coal macule, around the first- and second-order respiratory bronchioles, explains why simple CWP does not affect ventilatory capacity (HEPPLESTON, 1953). The airways resistance of the lungs can be partitioned into central and peripheral components (MACKLEM and MEAD, 1967). The central component includes the resistance from the trachea to the eleventh generation of bronchi, while the peripheral component is composed of the resistance from the twelfth generation of bronchi (those airways with diameters of 2 mm or less) down to the gas-exchanging portions of the lung. In normal subjects the central resistance constitutes 85–90% of the total, leaving only 10–15% for the peripheral airways. It is therefore possible for a subject to have diffuse involvement of his small airways producing a doubling or tripling of the peripheral resistance, and yet for the total airways resistance still to be within normal limits (MEAD, 1970). Similarly, the most commonly used standard spirometric tests—namely, the forced vital capacity (FVC) and the forced expiratory volume in one second (FEV_1)—depend mainly on flow in the large airways during dynamic compression and, for this reason, the FEV_1 and FVC are usually little affected by changes in the peripheral airways resistance. Previous studies have shown that miners with normal spirometry may show frequency dependence of dynamic compliance suggesting involvement of the small airways (SEATON *et al.*, 1972).

The maximal expiratory flow volume curve has been advocated as a means of investigating the state of the peripheral airways (LAPP and HYATT, 1970). It has been suggested that the latter part of the curve reflects the geometry of the small airways and the mechanical properties of the surrounding lung, and is relatively unaffected by muscular effort. Accordingly, we have used the flow volume curve in our epidemiological studies of coal miners in order to test its usefulness as an index of disordered function in the peripheral airways. This paper describes the effects of radiographic category, bronchitis, underground exposure, age, smoking, and other factors on peak flow and also on expiratory flows at 75, 50, 25, and 10% of forced vital capacity.

METHODS

In 1973 and 1974 the U.S. Public Health Service conducted a study of the miners employed at thirty-six coal mines widely distributed throughout the United States. Thirty of these mines were part of an original study conducted in 1969. The mines were chosen to represent different mining methods and coal seams. Other criteria for inclusion were that the mines should have at least 100 employees and have an expected working life of approximately 10 years. Details of the survey have been previously described (MORGAN *et al.*, 1973).

All participating miners underwent a limited medical examination consisting of standard posteroanterior and lateral chest films and an administration of an adapted form of the Medical Research Council of Great Britain questionnaire on chronic respiratory symptoms, along with an occupational and smoking history (MEDICAL RESEARCH COUNCIL, 1965). In addition, at least five forced expiratory volume manoeuvres were performed using a high fidelity, waterless electronic spirometer (Ohio Medical Products, Madison, Wisconsin, Model No. 800).*

* Mention of brand name products does not constitute endorsement by the U.S. Public Health Service.

The flow and volume signals from the spirometer were recorded on FM analog tape (HANKINSON and ROSE, 1974) and later processed on a PDP-12 laboratory computer (Digital Equipment Corporation, Maynard, Massachusetts). The flow rates at 75, 50, 25, and 10% of the vital capacity were calculated from the flow volume curve which showed the best effort. The best effort manoeuvre was defined as the curve with the largest forced vital capacity (FVC) and a peak flow within 15% of the largest observed peak flow. If the curve with the largest FVC did not also have a peak flow within 15% of the largest observed peak flow, then the curve with the second largest FVC was tested, and so forth until a satisfactory curve was found. In approximately 75% of the miners, the flow volume curve with the largest FVC also had a peak flow within 15% of the largest peak flow.

For the purpose of this study, chronic bronchitis was defined as persistent phlegm production regardless of complaints of coughing. Smoking was considered qualitatively rather than in terms of pack-years or average daily consumption.

Although individual measurements of dust exposure were not available for the participants in this study, it can be assumed that the magnitude of their exposure to dust was related to their job and working place in the coal mines. Previous measurements by the Bureau of Mines (DOYLE, 1970) showed that face workers are exposed to the greatest, and surface workers to the least concentrations of respirable coal dust. In general, based on declining order of dust exposure, the working force can be divided into three groups; i.e. face, other underground, and surface workers.

All radiographs were classified using the I.L.O. U/C Classification System (U.I.C.C. COMMITTEE, 1972), and the results from one of five separate readers were used. Each interpreter had previously passed the U.S.P.H.S. proficiency examination (MORGAN *et al.*, 1973). Ex-smokers were excluded in order to emphasize the clear distinction between smokers and non-smokers, leaving 6014 miners in the study.

RESULTS

The mean flow rates, viz. peak flow, FEF_{75}, FEF_{50}, and FEF_{25}, according to underground exposure, age and smoking status are shown in Figs. 1–8. Table 1 also shows the mean flow rates at 50% of the vital capacity.

With minor exceptions, decreases in flow rates with age were evident for nearly all of the exposure by smoking status groups. Sharp decrements were particularly evident for the cigarette smokers, while declines for non-smoking miners were appreciably less. This was especially true for flow rates at high lung volumes, viz. peak flow and FEF_{75}. Slight decrements in flow rates existed within age categories with increasing dust exposure for the miners who were cigarette smokers; however, they were more striking for the non-smoking miners, particularly at higher lung volumes. For the flow rates at lower lung volumes, the decrements due to exposure were minimal for both smokers and non-smokers. The differences in flow rates between the smokers and non-smokers for each age/exposure group were nearly as great as the decrements due to age; the smokers showed markedly lower flows.

Although years spent working underground is only an indirect measure of dust exposure, it is the only index available to us, and we therefore decided to assess its

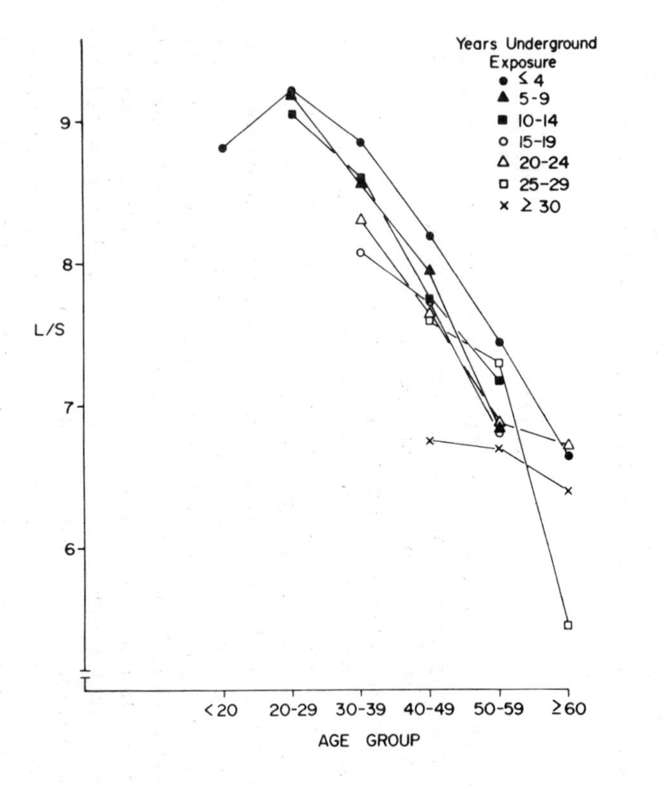

FIG. 1. Mean peak flow × age group × exposure group (smokers).

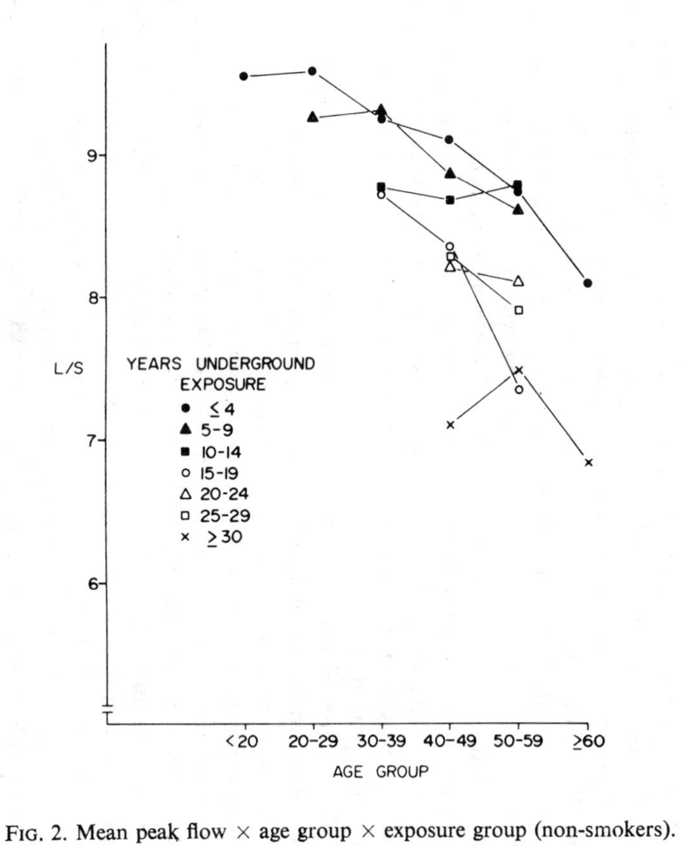

FIG. 2. Mean peak flow × age group × exposure group (non-smokers).

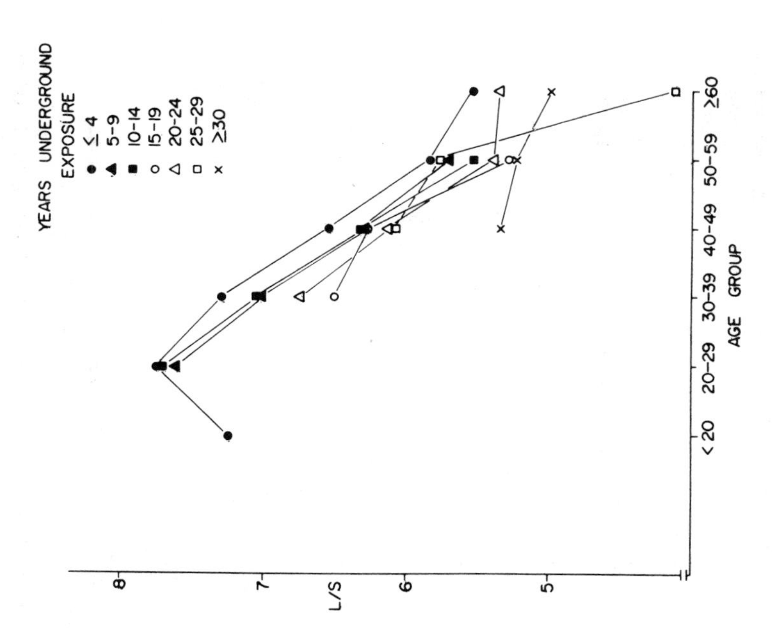

FIG. 3. Mean FEF_{75} × age group × exposure group (smokers).

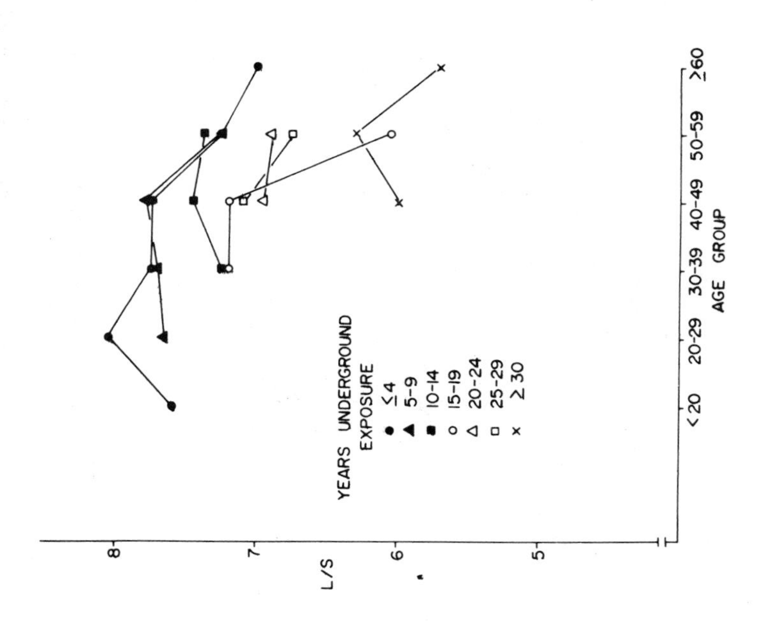

FIG. 4. Mean FEF_{75} × age group × exposure group (non-smokers).

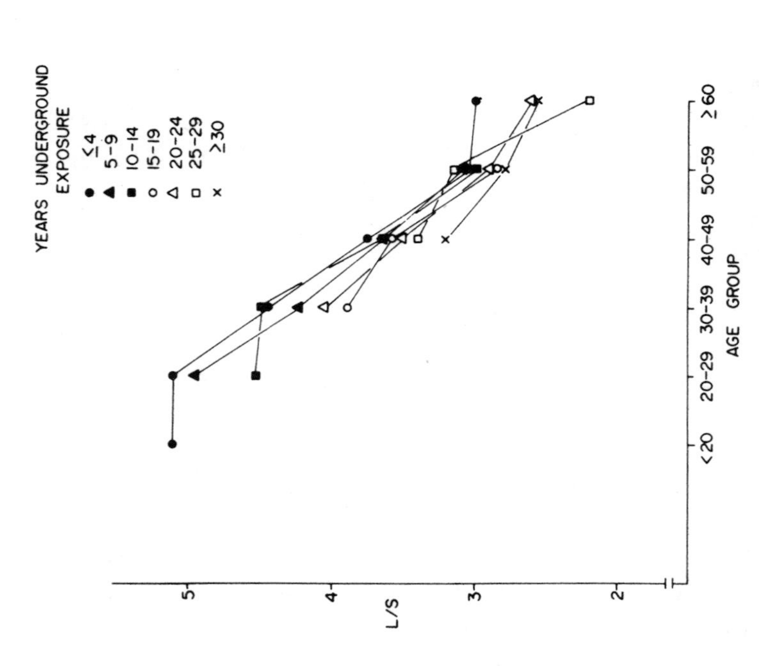

FIG. 5. Mean FEF_{50} × age group × exposure group (smokers).

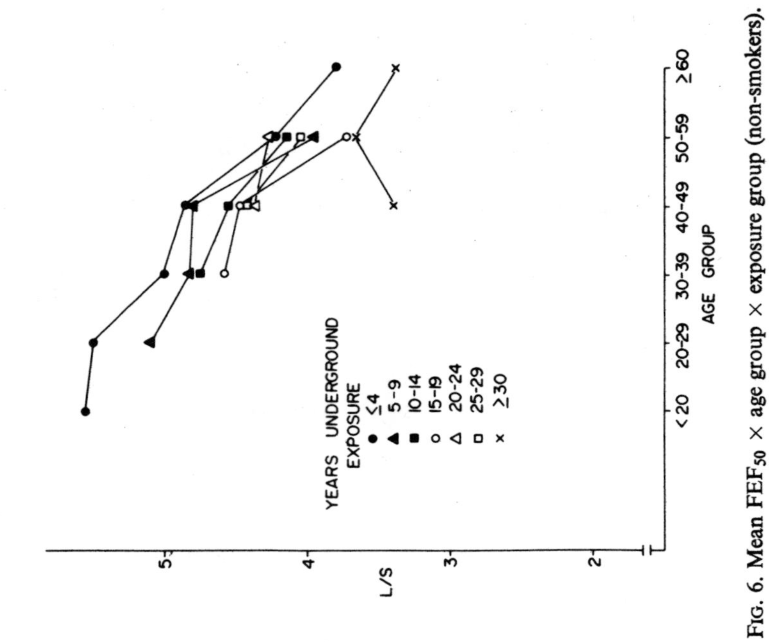

FIG. 6. Mean FEF_{50} × age group × exposure group (non-smokers).

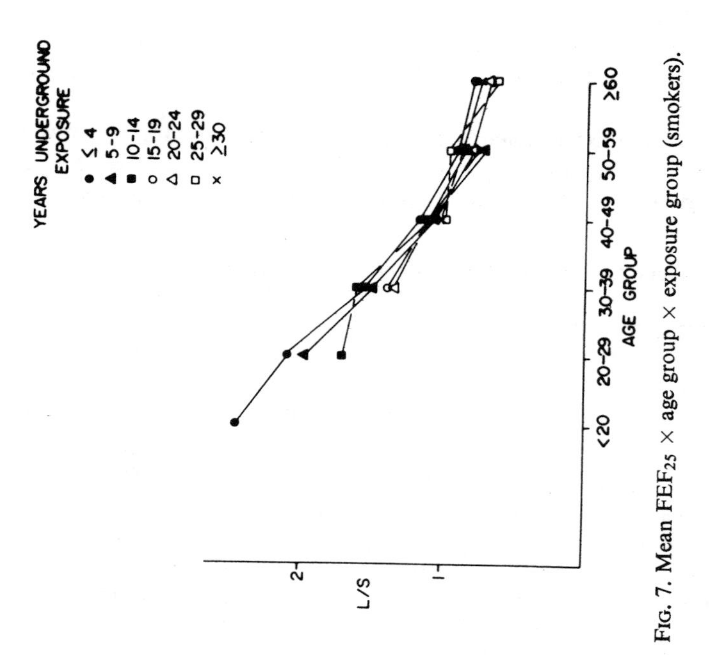

FIG. 7. Mean FEF_{25} × age group × exposure group (smokers).

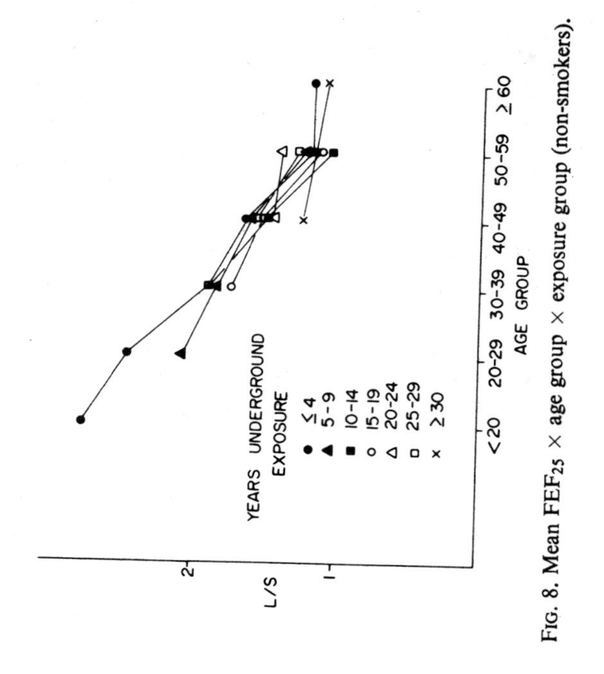

FIG. 8. Mean FEF_{25} × age group × exposure group (non-smokers).

TABLE 1. MEAN FEF_{50} FOR 6014 MINERS BY UNDERGROUND EXPOSURE, AGE, AND SMOKING STATUS[a]

Underground exposure (Years)	Age											
	20		20–29		30–39		40–49		50–59		$\geqslant$60	
	S	NS	S	NS	S	NS	S	NS	S	NS	S	NS
$\geqslant$ 4	5.12 (60)	5.56 (34)	5.11 (978)	5.51 (439)	4.45 (428)	5.00 (138)	3.75 (175)	4.86 (68)	3.04 (120)	4.23 (62)	2.99 (11)	3.81 (21)
5– 9	—	—	4.96 (207)	5.09 (82)	4.23 (280)	4.83 (92)	3.64 (94)	4.84 (28)	3.07 (29)	3.96 (16)	—	—
10–14	—	—	4.53 (16)	—	4.48 (115)	4.74 (31)	3.65 (90)	4.56 (35)	3.03 (43)	4.15 (16)	—	—
15–19	—	—	—	—	3.88 (83)	4.58 (25)	3.57 (133)	4.47 (39)	2.84 (55)	3.73 (17)	—	—
20–24	—	—	—	—	4.06 (26)	—	3.54 (204)	4.39 (75)	2.89 (104)	4.24 (41)	2.61 (13)	—
25–29	—	—	—	—	—	—	3.42 (214)	4.46 (68)	3.16 (240)	4.06 (74)	2.19 (23)	—
$\geqslant$ 30	—	—	—	—	—	—	3.22 (43)	3.41 (19)	2.83 (416)	3.69 (193)	2.57 (118)	3.38 (83)

[a]FEF_{50} in l./s. ( ) = no. of men per cell. S = smokers. NS = non-smokers.

importance relative to other variables presumed or known to affect flow rates. Tables 2 and 3 show the results of the stepwise multiple regression analyses for smokers and non-smokers. Details of the statistical methods may be found in the technical notes of this paper.

As expected, the coefficients for age were negative and for height were positive for all flow rates for both smokers and non-smokers. Weight had a very small but positive effect on flow rates at high and medium lung volumes but showed a reversal for FEF_{25}

TABLE 2. MULTIPLE REGRESSION ANALYSES REGRESSION COEFFICIENTS FOR FLOW RATES FROM 4318 MINERS (SMOKERS)

Variable	Peak flow	FEF_{75}[a]	FEF_{50}	FEF_{25}	FEF_{10}
Age (years)	−0.0569	−0.0611	−0.0670	−0.0443	−0.0166
Height (cm)	0.0439	0.0270	0.0146	0.0109	0.0085
Weight (kg)	0.0071	0.0097	0.0075	−0.0033	−0.0060
Underground exposure (years)	−0.0183	−0.0138	−0.0030[b]	0.0034	0.0034
Constant (l./s)	2.4317	3.7678	3.5472	1.4816	0.0345

[a] e.g. $FEF_{75} = 3.7678 - (\text{age} \times 0.0611) + (\text{height} \times 0.027) + (\text{weight} \times 0.0097) - (\text{exposure} \times 0.0138)$.

[b] Non-significant at the 0.05 level.

TABLE 3. MULTIPLE REGRESSION ANALYSES REGRESSION COEFFICIENTS FOR FLOW RATES FROM 1696 MINERS (NON-SMOKERS)

Variable	Peak flow	FEF_{75}	FEF_{50}[a]	FEF_{25}	FEF_{10}
Age (years)	−0.0278	−0.0197	−0.0366	−0.0358	−0.0139
Height (cm)	0.0339	0.0193	0.0144	0.0125	0.0085
Weight (kg)	0.0132	0.0132	0.0062	−0.0053	−0.0075
Underground exposure (years)	−0.0349	−0.0319	−0.0155	−0.0001[b]	−0.0012[b]
Constant (l./s)	3.2875	4.0725	3.3087	1.4550	0.2052

[a] e.g. $FEF_{50} = 3.3087 - (\text{age} \times 0.0366) + (\text{height} \times 0.0144) + (\text{weight} \times 0.0062) - (\text{exposure} \times 0.0155)$

[b] Non-significant at the 0.05 level

and FEF_{10}. The effect due to underground exposure, although not consistent, showed a general decline for flow rates at high lung volumes. While the effect was minimal (relative to age) for the smokers, it was highly significant for the non-smokers.

Both smokers and non-smokers without CWP demonstrated flow rates which were higher than for the groups with radiographic evidence of the condition (Table 4, Figs. 9–12). The difference may be attributed mainly to the fact that the miners with CWP were older and had been exposed longer. As a general rule there was no evidence that

TABLE 4. MEAN FEF_{50} BY CATEGORY OF COAL-WORKERS' PNEUMOCONIOSIS FOR 5853 MINERS[a]

	0	1	2 and 3	PMF
No. of miners (smokers)	(3832)	(260)	(66)	(37)
Observed	4.07	3.27	3.10	2.58
Expected[b]	4.07	3.20	2.97	2.79
No. of miners (non-smokers)	(1511)	(98)	(28)	(21)
Observed	4.74	4.18	4.21	2.37
Expected[c]	4.75	3.97	3.89	3.63

[a] 161 films of study group of 6014 miners judged unreadable.

[b] Obtained from regression in Table 2.

[c] Obtained from regression in Table 3.

miners with simple CWP suffered a decrement in their flow rates in excess of what may be attributed to their age, height, and years spent working underground. Nevertheless there were exceptions to this rule. First, the non-smoking miners with categories 2 and 3 had flow rates which were significantly higher than expected. This was probably the consequence of self-selection, whereby the healthy continue to work after the less fit have left mining. The second exception involves those subjects with progressive massive fibrosis (PMF), and again was most noticeable among the non-smokers. Their flow rates were significantly lower than what one might predict on the basis of their age,

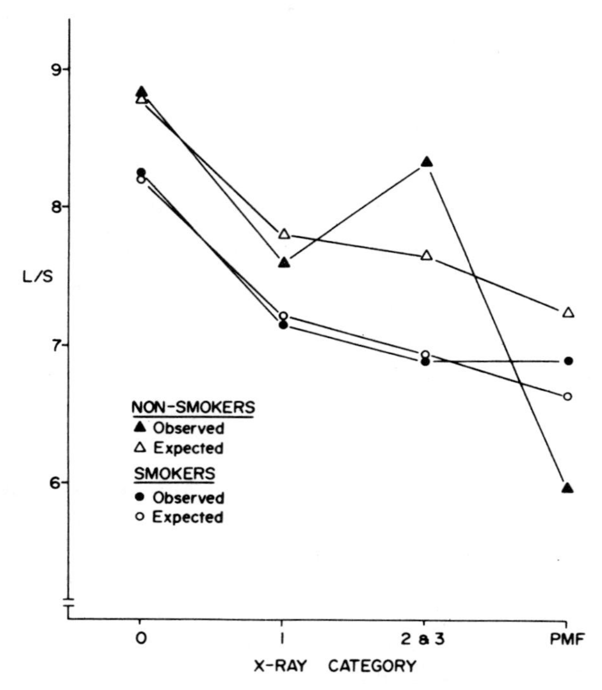

FIG. 9. Observed and expected peak flow by smoking status and by X-ray category of CWP (effect of years underground removed).

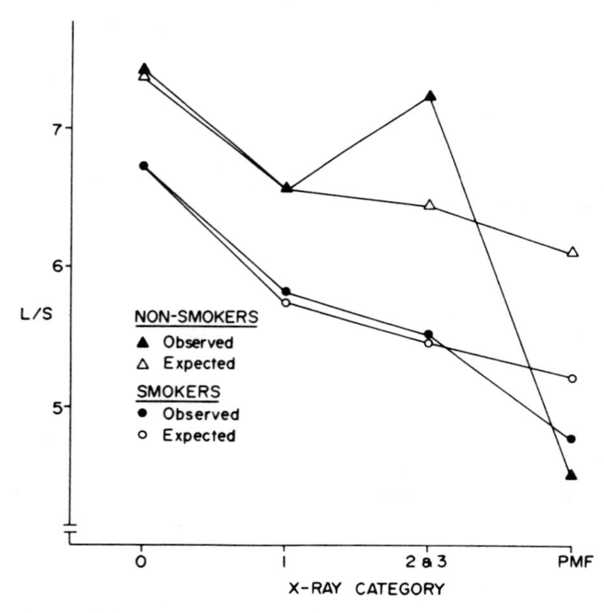

FIG. 10. Observed and expected FEF_{75} by smoking status and by X-ray category of CWP (effect of years underground removed).

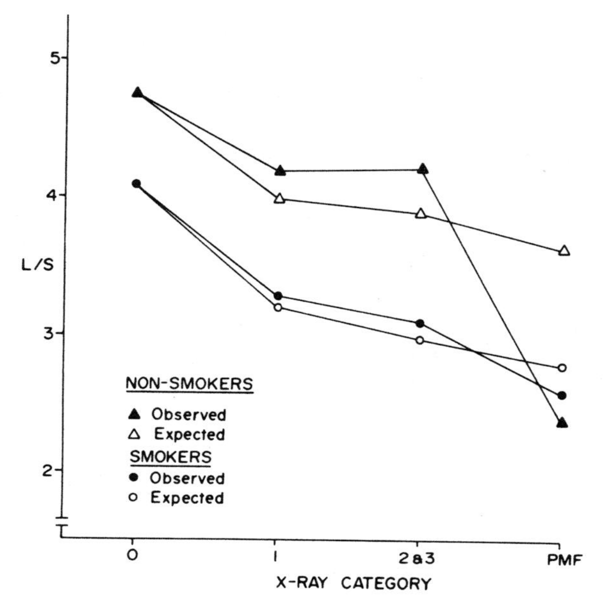

FIG. 11. Observed and expected FEF_{50} by smoking status and by X-ray category of CWP (effect of years underground removed).

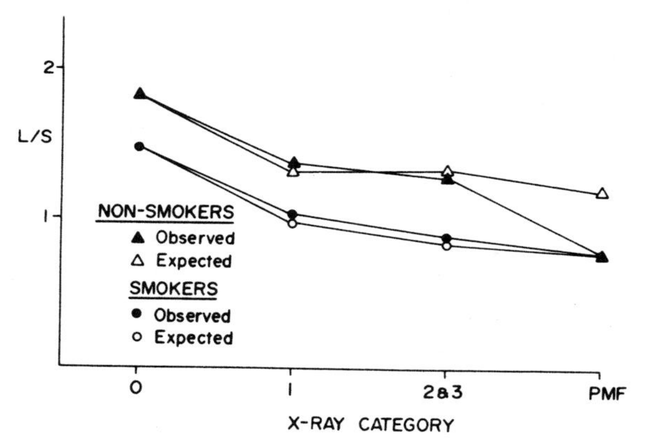

FIG. 12. Observed and expected FEF_{25} by smoking status and by X-ray category of CWP (effect of years underground removed).

height, and exposure. This was to be expected in that subjects with PMF have been shown to have a significant reduction in ventilatory capacity (ROGAN *et al.*, 1961; MORGAN *et al.*, 1974).

The relationship of bronchitis to the flow rates is shown in Table 5. As anticipated, bronchitics have lower flow rates than do non-bronchitics. The striking results of this portion of the analyses relate to the deviations of the observed from predicted flow rates (Fig. 13). In general, the deviations for the bronchitics were negative, while the

TABLE 5. MEAN FEF_{50} BY BRONCHITIS FOR 6014 MINERS

	Bronchitic	Non-bronchitic
No. of miners (smokers)	(1869)	(2499)
Observed	3.59	4.29
Expected[a]	3.70	4.20
No. of miners (non-smokers)	(459)	(1237)
Observed	4.22	4.83
Expected[b]	4.29	4.81

[a] Obtained from regression in Table 2.
[b] Obtained from regression in Table 3.

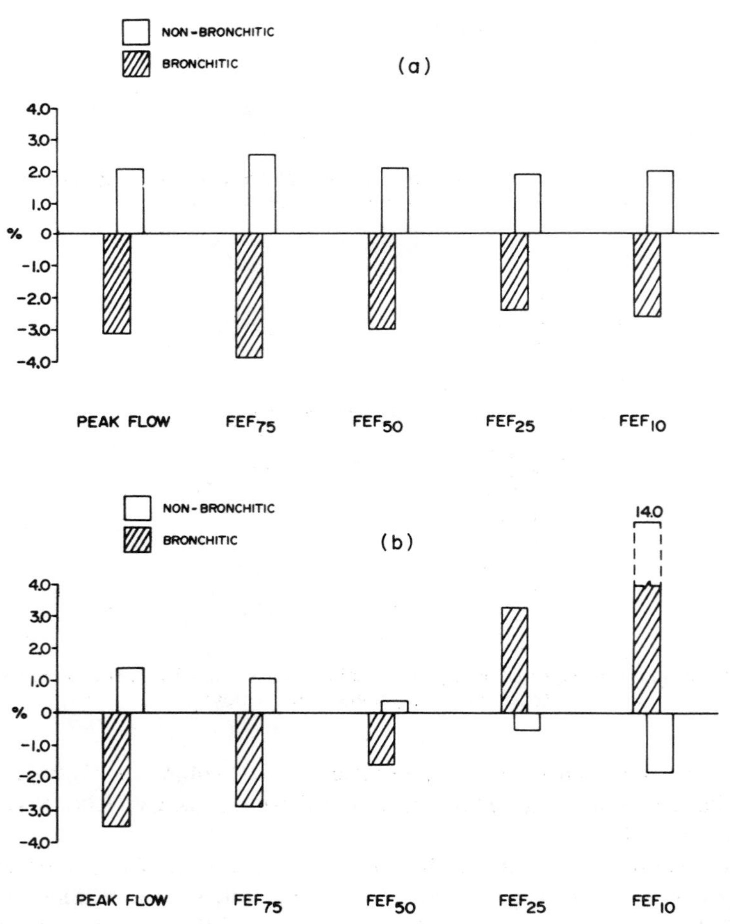

FIG. 13. Flow rate deviations (observed-expected) as a per cent of expected for bronchitics and non-bronchitics. (a) Smokers, (b) Non-smokers.

opposite was true for the non-bronchitics. This was especially evident in the smokers where the pattern existed for flows at all lung volumes. For the non-smokers, the pattern existed for the flow rates at high and medium lung volumes and reversed itself at FEF_{25} and FEF_{10}.

In underground miners, workplace, i.e. face or other underground, seemed to have little to no effect on flow rates over and above what may be accounted for by age, height, and years spent working underground. The results for FEF_{50} are illustrated in Table 6. Analysis of the FEV_1 showed results similar to those reported by others (ROGAN *et al.*, 1973) and which were comparable to those we observed for flows at higher lung volumes.

TABLE 6. MEAN FEF_{50} BY MAJOR WORK PLACE FOR 6014 MINERS

	Face	Other underground	Surface
No. of miner (smokers)	(1950)	(1916)	(452)
Observed	4.01	4.03	3.73
Expected[a]	4.02	4.02	3.74
No. of miners (non-smokers)	(732)	(712)	(252)
Observed	4.60	4.72	4.73
Expected[b]	4.67	4.67	4.68

[a] Obtained from regression in Table 2.
[b] Obtained from regression in Table 3.

DISCUSSION

Most industrial lung diseases, and in particular the pneumoconioses, affect what MEAD (1970) has aptly termed the quiet zone of the lungs, thereby making early detection difficult. However, previous studies from our laboratory have shown that non-smoking working coal miners with categories 2 and 3 simple CWP, but without evidence of large airways obstruction, often show frequency dependence of dynamic compliance (SEATON *et al.*, 1972) and an increased residual volume (MORGAN *et al.*, 1971). The clinical significance of these findings remains uncertain at the present time. The physiological abnormalities mentioned above are present only in the higher categories of simple CWP, and it can reasonably be inferred that their presence depends on an appreciable dust burden. The results of the present study also showed that certain flow rates seemed to be affected by exposure, but the reduction of flow rates was independent of the radiographic category when the effect of years underground was removed.

The decrement in flows associated with age was as obvious in this study as it has been in others (CHERNIACK and RABER, 1972). Cigarette smoking likewise exerted a detrimental effect on flow rates. In addition, in the non-smokers a significant decrement independent of age occurred with increasing years worked underground, which was not found in miners smoking cigarettes, probably because the effects of smoking were so much greater that they tended to override and mask the effects of dust. The decrement in flow rates that occurred with increasing years underground in the non-smokers mainly affected flows at higher lung volumes, thereby suggesting large airways involvement. Further support for this inference comes from the fact that the flows showed no additional decrement with increasing category of simple CWP, a condition which is characterized pathologically by lesions located in the distal airways.

The finding of greater than expected flow rates at lower lung volumes in the non-smoking bronchitics is difficult to explain. This seems to imply that dust-induced bronchitis helps to preserve function in the distal airways, but this is difficult to imagine. A better explanation for this anomaly relates to our method of expressing flow rates at a percentage of FVC. If flow rates had been expressed at absolute lung volumes, they probably would not have been as high in the non-smoking bronchitics since the latter may well have had an increased residual volume. However, it is clear that bronchitis caused by a combination of cigarette smoking and dust inhalation induces a much greater decrement in flow rates at lower lung volumes than does bronchitis which is caused by dust inhalation alone.

Since no comparable long-term dust measurements are available in the U.S., we have had to rely on indirect measures of dust exposure (MORGAN *et al.*, 1973). An overall indication of life-long dust exposure can be obtained by measuring the number of years that a miner has spent working underground or at the coal face. Indeed, several studies have shown that a definite relationship exists between radiographic category and increasing underground exposure (LAINHART, 1969; MORGAN *et al.*, 1973). Elsewhere we have shown that bronchitis, as defined by the presence of cough and sputum, occurs most often in the most dust-exposed miners; namely, face workers, and that the prevalence of bronchitis declines the further away from the face and the nearer to the surface that the miner works. Associated with this industrial bronchitis is a minimal decrement in FEV_1, which was significant only when the non-smoking face workers were compared with the non-smoking surface workers (KIBELSTIS *et al.*, 1973). Bearing in mind that ventilatory capacity as determined by the FEV_1 depends almost entirely on the resistance to flow in the large airways during dynamic compression (MEAD, 1970); whatever the process that is responsible for the decrease in FEV_1, it can be assumed that it must predominately affect the larger airways. The most reasonable inference to draw is that industrial bronchitis is the culprit. Since it is mainly the larger non-respirable particles that are deposited in the larger airways, it is logical to assume that the non-respirable dust fraction is mainly responsible for industrial bronchitis. Such a hypothesis explains why no relationship exists between FEV_1 and radiographic category when the effect of years underground had been removed. Larger particles, unlike those of respirable size, are completely removed by the muco-ciliary escalator and thus produce no radiographic changes. It is difficult not to conclude that bronchitis and simple CWP often occur independently and need not be necessarily related. The slight reduction of ventilatory capacity that is sometimes observed in miners as compared to control populations, and which is independent of radiographic category, is best explained by the concept of industrial bronchitis. The decrements in flow at high lung volumes that we observed in the study, and which showed a relationship to years worked underground, provided additional strong support for this concept.

In conclusion, we have shown that flow rates at higher lung volumes are related to years spent working underground. We believe the small reductions in flows that we observed are produced by industrial bronchitis and are often unaccompanied by radiographic evidence of CWP. Nevertheless, the clinical significance of such minor reductions in flow rates must remain *sub judice* until follow-up studies have been completed. Finally, flow rates at lower lung volumes, as far as this study is concerned, have proved disappointing in the detection of functional impairment of the small airways of the lung.

TECHNICAL NOTES

The purpose of the regression analyses in this paper was to quantify the effects of flow rates from person to person by observing the person's age, height, weight, smoking habits, and underground exposure time on expiratory flow rates. With five linear main effects, there were 10 two-way (e.g. age × height), 10 three-way (e.g. age × height × weight), 5 four-way, and 1 five-way interactions. Thus, when one considered the linear main effects and all possible interactions among these main effects, there were thirty-one "independent" variables. Because it would be difficult, if not impossible, to look at all possible equations, certain ones were selected. There are many methods for doing this (DRAPER and SMITH, 1966); however, we chose the stepwise procedure.

Basically, the procedure is as follows. The variable with the highest simple correlation with the flow rate is "stepped" into the equation if a sufficient amount of variation in the flow is explained. If no variable is stepped in, the selection is terminated. If a variable is stepped in, each variable (at this point there is only one) in the equation is checked to make sure it is still explaining sufficient variation. If not, it is removed from the equation. The process is repeated using partial rather than simple correlations until no more variables can be added to improve sufficiently the equation containing the "independent" variables. What is desired is an equation with only a few variables, but which has an R^2 almost as large as that for the equation containing all the "independent" variables.

A stepwise regression was performed using all thirty-one variables for each flow rate, and then the regression was repeated utilizing only the linear main effects. For a given number of variables in the model, the two regressions yielded similar values of R^2. However, in the regression involving all thirty-one variables, interactions involving smoking (a dichotomous variable that was 0 for non-smokers and 1 for smokers) were usually stepped in early and were highly significant; i.e. the regression lines for smokers and non-smokers were not parallel. Since it was easy to consider smokers and non-smokers separately, it was decided to do so.

For smokers and non-smokers, the equations involved four main effects and eleven interactions. Again, all fifteen variables were used in one regression analysis, and the four main effects were used in another. In addition, for the linear main effects which were included in the model after the second analysis, a third analysis was performed forcing those linear main effects into the equation and then employing a stepwise selection procedure on the interactions.

The results showed that the analyses involving only linear main effects yielded an R^2 which was essentially as large as those for the regressions involving the interactions. The most significant interactions were accounted for by separating the analyses into smoker and non-smoker groups.

The regression coefficients in the tables can be interpreted as follows: a coefficient, b_x, corresponding to an "independent" variable X is the amount the flow rate changes when X changes by one unit, given the other "independent" variables remain unchanged. For example, assume a particular flow-rate coefficient for age in the smoking group as −0.0441. Then, for two smokers with the same number of years in underground mining, the same height and the same weight, where one miner is 36 years old and the other is 35, the older miner's predicted flow rate would be 0.0441 litres per second less than that for the younger miner.

It is realized that a certain amount of confounding may exist between the measures of age and exposure as used in this paper. At the present time, there are no statistical manipulations that can totally separate these effects, and only when actual dust measures are used in conjunction with biological phenomena can the effects of age and dust exposure be completely untangled.

Detailed data on flow rates at all lung volumes are available upon request.

REFERENCES

CHERNIACK, R. M. and RABER, M. B. (1972) *Am. Rev. resp. Dis.* **106,** 38–46.
COCHRANE, A. L. and HIGGINS, I. T. T. (1961) *Br. J. prev. soc. Med.* **15,** 1–11.
DOYLE, H. N. (1970) *Dust Concentration in the Mines. Proceedings of the Symposium on Respirable Coal Mine Dust, Washington, DC, 1969* (edited by GOODING, R. M.) pp. 27–33. U.S. Bureau of Mines Information Circular 8458. Dept. of Interior, Washington, D.C.
DRAPER, N. R. and SMITH, H. (1966) *Applied Regression Analysis.* Wiley, New York.
HANKINSON, J. L. and ROSE, W. (1974) *Proc. San Diego Biomed. Symp.* **13,** 237–239.
HEPPLESTON, A. G. (1953) *J. Path. Bact.* **66,** 235–246.
KIBELSTIS, J. A., MORGAN, E. J., REGER, R. B., LAPP, N. L., SEATON, A. and MORGAN, W. K. C. (1973) *Am. Rev. resp. Dis.* **108,** 886–893.
LAINHART, W. S. (1969) *J. occup. Med.* **11,** 399–408.
LAPP, N. L. and HYATT, R. E. (1970) *Bull. Physiopath. resp.* **6,** 595–604.
MACKLEM, P. T. and MEAD, J. (1967) *J. appl. Physiol.* **22,** 395–401.
MEAD, J. (1970) *New Engl. J. Med.* **282,** 1318–1319.
MEDICAL RESEARCH COUNCIL (1965) *Lancet* **2,** 775–779.
MORGAN, W. K. C., BURGESS, D. B., LAPP, N. L. and SEATON, A. (1971) *Thorax* **26,** 585–590.
MORGAN, W. K. C., BURGESS, D. B., JACOBSON, G., O'BRIEN, R. J., PENDERGRASS, E. P., REGER, R. B. and SHOUB, E. P. (1973) *Archs envir. Hlth* **27,** 221–226.
MORGAN, W. K. C., HANDELSMAN, L., KIBELSTIS, J., LAPP, N. L. and REGER, R. B. (1974) *Archs envir. Hlth* **28,** 182–189.
ROGAN, J. M., ASHFORD, J. R., CHAPMAN, P. J., DUFFIELD, D. P., FAY, J. W. J. and RAE, S. (1961) *Br. med. J.* **1,** 1337–1342.
ROGAN, J. M., ATTFIELD, M. D., JACOBSEN, M., RAE, S., WALKER, D. D. and WALTON, W. H. (1973) *Br. J. ind. Med.* **30,** 217–226.
ROSSITER, C. E. (1972) *Ann. N.Y. Acad. Sci.* **200,** 465–477.
SEATON, A., LAPP, N. L. and MORGAN, W. K. C. (1972) *J. clin. Invest.* **51,** 1203–1211.
U.I.C.C. COMMITTEE (1972) *Med. Radiogr. Photogr.* **48,** 65–110.

DISCUSSION

D. LIDDELL: You have described stepwise regression analyses in which years of exposure had some influence. Was X-ray change also included in these analyses? If so, at what steps did these two variables enter the regression? In other words, have you any evidence from the regression analyses of the relative importance of these two variables?

Dr HANKINSON: We did perform multiple stepwise regression analysis with the X-ray reading as a variable. However, the X-ray coefficient was not significant, and we did not include it in our regression equations shown in these data.

M. McDERMOTT: It is disappointing that you have not also shown the results for the MEV and MLC so that the effect on these could be compared with that on the flow–volume curve. You state that the reduction in flow at higher lung volumes suggests changes in the larger airways, with which I agree. You then suggest that this is due to a dust-induced bronchitis. But would not this mainly affect either the middle or the end of the volume curve rather than the beginning? You also suggest that the flow at the terminal portion of the vital capacity curve is independent of muscular effort; I would have thought that this would be more likely in the middle range.

Dr HANKINSON: We feel that the least effort-dependent portion of the curve tends to be between 50 and 25% of forced vital capacity. The effect of an individual's effort will show up most at peak flow. Secondly, we did analyse the FEV_1, although we did not include these results in our paper. These results were very similar to those of Rogan *et al.*, referred to in our paper. We can provide the information, if you wish. Finally, the effect of dust-induced bronchitis would be primarily on the large airways and should affect the flows primarily at higher lung volumes. I would refer you to the article by Mead (1970) referenced in our paper.

D. C. F. MUIR: The term "respirable dust" appears to be used increasingly as if it were identical with alveolar dust. This leads to the supposition that there is a separate fraction causing bronchitis which could be measured. In fact, "respirable dust" refers to the aerodynamic size distribution of that fraction of the dust which could have access to the alveoli if inhaled deeply enough. Many such particles deposit in the airways during transit or, because of the anatomical dead space, never reach the alveoli in the first place. These two effects suggest that the mass distribution of dust particles causing bronchitis may not be very different from that causing pneumoconiosis and that the MRE gravimetric sampler provides a good measure of both.

It is pleasing to note that you confirm the findings of the National Coal Board, published by ROGAN *et al.*, in 1973 (*Br. J. ind. Med.* **30,** 217–226). The essence of that report was that dust exposure underground led to an impairment of ventilatory capacity but that there was little additional effect as a result of the appearance of radiographic simple pneumoconiosis. However, the radiograph does appear to be evidence of excessive dust exposure. Would you therefore accept that it should also be taken as evidence that some functional impairment has taken place—not as a result of the opacities themselves but simply as a result of the dust exposure which they indicate.

Dr MORGAN: I would agree with you that if a man has category 2 or 3 simple pneumoconiosis that he has had an appreciable dust burden. However, if we are going to accept that impaired function in simple pneumoconiosis is occupational in origin, then we should accept that similar impairment in a man with category 0 or 1 simple pneumoconiosis is also of occupational origin.

D. C. F. MUIR: The two cases are not comparable. If a man has an abnormal X-ray, then we know that he has been exposed to excessive dust. It is reasonable to presume that the dust has caused a functional impairment. If his radiograph is normal, there is no method of knowing, in the absence of a detailed occupational history with corresponding environmental measurements, whether he has been exposed to excessive dust or whether other factors, such as cigarette smoke, are the cause of any functional impairment.

D. LIDDELL: How can you be certain that a single X-ray reading of category 2 (or even 3) implies a dust burden? A further reading by another reader of a film taken on another occasion may not show such change. (Dr Dick points out that the reverse is also true!) There is plenty of evidence of such phenomena in the literature.

D. C. F. MUIR: It is not usual for coal workers whose radiographs show category 2 or 3 pneumoconiosis to have a normal film at a later date.

W. T. ULMER: Dr Muir has spoken as a clinician and emphasized the importance of the individual case. However, it is only the mean values of ventilatory capacity of groups of dust-exposed workers which show reductions below normal levels. There is a considerable scatter and many individual results are within the normal range. This makes the assessment of the individual case very difficult.

M. BUNDY: I think that the occupational history can indicate whether disability is due to previous environmental exposure. I do not accept that men with normal radiographs are different, in this respect, from those with evidence of pneumoconiosis.

R. A. FRANCIS: Do I understand that you took five or more curves, but subsequently measured values on only *one* of them?

Dr HANKINSON: We always obtained at least five trials, and more than five when the subject was having coaching problems, but never more than ten trials. Yes, we picked the best curve by our definition. If the curve with the largest FVC had a peak flow within 15% of the largest observed peak flow, we would use it. If not, we would use the curve with the second largest FVC. It is somewhat an arbitrary method and perhaps as more papers come out, a standardized method can be agreed upon. This is a difficult problem, and I would welcome any suggestions.

J. P. LYONS: It is important to remember that we are discussing ventilatory results in mainly working miners. We have recently looked at serial ventilatory capacity tests in miners and ex-miners in Cardiff and it is apparent that impairment continues to progress into the 60s and 70s in many of these cases, with eventual significant disablement.

Also I believe that when smokers and non-smokers are being compared, the normal values for non-smokers should be employed. I believe that there is a difference of almost one litre in the expected values, between smokers and non-smokers, and therefore such comparisons may be quite misleading.

Dr HANKINSON: I would agree with you. Unfortunately, normal values for flow data are not available; at least we have found that our normal values do not agree with those values from other laboratories. Some work needs to be done to establish normal flow rates for both smokers and non-smokers.

P. D. OLDHAM: While I sympathize with the reasons which led the authors to exclude ex-smokers from their presentation, I feel that the decision was regrettable. Men as a whole select themselves into smokers and non-smokers; smokers further select themselves into continuing smokers and ex-smokers. If we wish to have a representative sample, free from this form of self-selection, all three groups must be included.

Dr HANKINSON: We had only a limited amount of material which we could present because of the size of the paper, so ex-smokers were omitted. We did look at them and, in general, their flow rates fell somewhere between non-smokers and smokers. We can make the data available, if you are interested.

M. JACOBSEN: There are three major conclusions from this paper which are so remarkably consistent with results published by Rogan *et al*, in 1973 on the experience in British coal mines that I believe they deserve special emphasis.

Firstly, increasing impairment of lung function characteristic of damage to the larger airways has been related convincingly to an index of exposure to airborne dust.

Secondly, it has been shown that provided such exposures are taken into consideration then there is no *additional* decrement in lung function associated with increasing radiological category of simple pneumoconiosis. I agree with the interpretation of Mr Hankinson and his colleagues that this implies that impairment of lung function induced by exposure to airborne dust may occur independently of dust-related radiological simple pneumoconiosis. Indeed, we have both shown that dust-related reductions in lung function occur among men with category 0. I agree also with Mr Hankinson that these findings explain the previously reported relatively poor correlation between loss of lung function and radiological category. This low correlation must therefore *not* be interpreted as indicating that exposure to airborne coalmine dust has no important effect on lung function.

Thirdly, the results show that where there is evidence of respiratory symptoms characteristic of chronic bronchitis an *additional* reduction in lung function may be observed which is *not* attributable to dust exposure, age or anthropometric variables. We found the same results, and we suggested 2 years ago that this phenomenon is consistent with an hypothesis that if early bronchitic symptoms (persistent phlegm, persistent cough) are present, then the disease may progress and ventilatory capacity may deteriorate independently of factors initiating the disease process.

The authors of this paper have concluded that flow rates at low lung volumes appear not to be particularly useful for the detection of disease in the small airways of the lung. For this conclusion to be valid it is necessary to assume that small airways disease among coal miners occurs in a way which is related to either one or more of the variables considered. It is possible that "years underground" is not a sufficiently sensitive index of dust exposure to reflect what may be a real relationship between such exposure and reduced flow rates at low lung volumes. In any case, the lack of correlation between the measures used may explain the anomalous results at low lung volumes with respect to body weight among smokers (Table 2) and non-smokers (Table 3). The curious reversal of the algebraic sign for the bodyweight coefficient for FEF_{25} and FEF_{10} indicates that it would be premature to conclude from Fig. 14 that "dust-induced bronchitis helps to preserve function in the distal airways." Not only is this "difficult to imagine"; it seems an unjustified inference in a situation where the response variables concerned are exhibiting unexplained, suspiciously artefactual, correlations with fundamental physiological attributes such as body weight.

Perhaps one may be forgiven also for interpreting the results as evidence supporting the view of some epidemiologists that a simple Gaensler spirometer may be at least as useful for studying occupationally related respiratory impairment as some of the more sophisticated equipment now available.

Dr Hankinson: Although the flow-volume curve did not prove to be more useful than the FEV_1 in studying coal miners with dust-induced bronchitis, it may still prove useful in studying other occupationally exposed groups who may have small airways disease.

SESSION 10

Friday, 26th September

EPIDEMIOLOGICAL STUDIES (2)

SMOKING AND COALWORKERS' SIMPLE PNEUMOCONIOSIS

M. JACOBSEN, J. BURNS and M. D. ATTFIELD

Institute of Occupational Medicine, Edinburgh, Scotland

Abstract—The attack rate of simple pneumoconiosis in 2723 British coal miners is considered in relation to the men's dust exposures and smoking habits. A complementary analysis is presented, using less precise radiological data, of prevalence and attack rates in an independent group of miners. One of the analyses suggests that, at high dust exposures, smoking may be associated with an increased risk of developing pneumoconiosis: but the most sensitive statistical test used reveals that the apparent effect might well be due to chance factors (P not less than 0.09). The possibility is investigated that the net observed effect is the resultant of conflicting tendencies in sub-groups characterized by their responses to questions on phlegm production. There is no evidence to support this hypothesis. It is concluded that the main variable determining the development of simple pneumoconiosis is exposure to airborne dust, and that this effect is not modified appreciably by whether or not coal miners smoke.

1. INTRODUCTION

A quantitative relationship between the development of simple pneumoconiosis and measured exposures to respirable airborne coal-mine dust was reported 5 years ago (JACOBSEN *et al.*, 1971). In the discussion of these results BUNDY (1971) asked whether smoking history influenced the slope of the probability curve. The question stimulates formulation of four hypotheses concerning possible interactions between inhaled coal-mine dust and tobacco smoke, as follows.

(a) *Smoking plays no role in the aetiology of coalworkers' simple pneumoconiosis (CWP).*

(b) *Men who are exposed to airborne dust and who smoke are more likely to develop CWP than those who do not smoke.* If this were the case then the observation might be explained by a potentiating action of two insults: coal-mine dust and tobacco smoke. Alternatively, such an effect might be attributable to reduced activity of the cilia among smokers. Consequential delayed clearance of inhaled dust particles might result in an increased alveolar burden.

(c) *Men who are exposed to airborne coal-mine dust and who smoke are less likely to develop CWP.* This might be the case if hypersecretion of sputum associated with smoking increases the deposition of inhaled coal dust particles in the bronchi and thus prevents them from reaching the alveoli.

(d) *Two or more of the mechanisms hypothesized under* (b) *and* (c) *occur but the net observed effect, on average, is small or effectively zero.*

RAE *et al.* (1971) have presented data which permit a preliminary examination of the problem. In their table II these authors demonstrated a higher prevalence of persistent cough and phlegm (determined by questionnaire responses) among men with at least the earliest radiological signs of pneumoconiosis. These results can be rearranged as in Table 1 below. The numbers shown in Table 1 are percentages of men with pneumoconiosis as defined.

TABLE 1. PERCENTAGE OF MEN WITH AT LEAST THE EARLIEST SIGNS OF PNEUMOCONIOSIS (CATEGORY 0/1 OR HIGHER) IN THOSE WITH AND WITHOUT SYMPTOMS (PERSISTENT COUGH AND PHLEGM), BY AGE AND SMOKING HABIT; REARRANGEMENT OF DATA FROM TABLE II BY RAE *et al.* (1971)*

	Age group							
Symptoms	25–34		35–44		45–54		55–59	
No/Yes	NS	S	NS	S	NS	S	NS	S
NO	9.4 (138)	8.8 (386)	21.4 (210)	24.2 (633)	39.8 (191)	40.8 (404)	44.4 (36)	41.1 (73)
YES	25.0 (24)	12.0 (167)	38.1 (42)	31.6 (450)	60.0 (45)	45.7 (451)	61.1 (18)	51.4 (111)

NS = non-smokers; S = smokers.

(The figures in brackets are the numbers of men to whom the superior percentages relate, e.g. 9.4% of 138 non-smoking men with no symptoms aged between 25 and 34 years had pneumoconiosis).

* A typographical transposition error occurs in Table II of RAE *et al.* (1971). The percentage of men with "bronchitis" among 788 smokers with no pneumoconiosis in the 35–44 year age-group is 39.1, not 31.9 as printed. Results in Table 1 above are based on the correct figures.

Prevalence of pneumoconiosis among all 2675 smokers (30.2%) was very similar to the figure for the 704 non-smokers (29.8%). The higher prevalence of CWP among men who reported symptoms (smokers and non-smokers, in all age groups) is, of course, the mirror image of the result reported previously by RAE *et al.* (1971): more symptoms among men with CWP. However, the rearrangement of the figures shows that among the 1308 men who reported symptoms, CWP prevalence was lower for smokers in each age group. This observation might perhaps be regarded as consistent with the mechanism hypothesized under (c) above, in that men with cough and persistent phlegm associated with smoking may be protected from developing radiological signs of CWP to some degree, when compared with non-smokers who report these symptoms. (In the latter group the symptoms must be attributable to a cause or causes other than smoking, including occupational dust exposure.)

There are at least three reasons why the indications from Table 1 cannot be regarded as conclusive. Firstly, in that table, no account has been taken of the most important variable likely to affect variations in pneumoconiosis prevalence: differences in cumulative dust exposures. Secondly, there is ambiguity concerning the relevance of the classifications into the smoker and non-smoker groups. These classifications were based on reports of smoking habits at the time that the radiological surveys were made; no account was taken of variations in the number of cigarettes being smoked, and ex-smokers were included in the "smokers" group. Lastly, there is a similar difficulty concerning classification of men according to symptoms. For their analyses, RAE *et al.* (1971) excluded one sub-group who replied inconsistently to questions on symptoms at two consecutive surveys, but they included another such group. Further analyses are reported now with these difficulties in mind. The data are from the National Coal Board's Pneumoconiosis Field Research.

2. ATTACK RATE OF CWP OVER 10 YEARS

Results reported in this section are based on further analyses of data relating to 4122 coalminers described by JACOBSEN *et al.* (1971) and RAE *et al.* (1971). These authors provide details on how the sample was selected and on how the data were collected. The immediately relevant information is given below.

2.1 *Men Studied*

The men selected for study were from twenty British collieries in each of which three medical surveys had been made at approximately 5-year intervals. All men had worked at the coal face at the start and end of 5-year periods between the first and second surveys, and had worked either at the coal face or elsewhere underground at the third surveys (after a further 5-year period). For the present study of smoking in relation to simple pneumoconiosis, results were excluded from men for whom there was any evidence of the presence of complicated pneumoconiosis.

2.2 *Radiological Classifications*

Chest X-rays had been taken for each man at all three surveys. Film-pairs covering 10-year periods between the first and third surveys were classified for pneumoconiosis using the elaboration of the I.L.O. (1959) classification described by LIDDELL and LINDARS (1969). Each film-pair was examined by eight doctors experienced in the radiology of pneumoconiosis. Film readers worked independently and examined both films from a pair side-by-side on the viewing box with temporal order known. The eight classifications of each film for simple pneumoconiosis (small rounded opacities only) were averaged as described by JACOBSEN *et al.* (1971).

2.3 *Smoking Habits and Phlegm Production*

At the second and third medical surveys a questionnaire on respiratory symptoms and smoking habits was completed for all men in the sample. The questionnaire is similar to that recommended by the Medical Research Council. Details of its validity and reproducibility have been documented by RAE *et al.* (1971).

For the present analyses results were used only from men who replied consistently at both the second and third surveys to the questions: "*Do you smoke?*" and "*Have you ever smoked as much as one cigarette per day for one year?*" "Smokers" were defined as those who answered positively to the first question on both occasions. "Non-smokers" were defined as those who responded negatively to both questions on both occasions.

The questionnaire includes questions on cough and phlegm. A preliminary analysis of the data showed that 6% of the coal miners questioned may report either persistent cough ("on most days for as much as 3 months in the year") and deny persistent phlegm, or they may report persistent phlegm and deny persistent coughing. It must be remembered that the replies to the questionnaire refer to the respondents' conceptions of cough and phlegm rather than to clinically defined entities. The present investigation is concerned *inter alia* with evaluation of evidence, from replies to a questionnaire, concerning effects possibly associated with sputum production as such. For this reason replies to questions on coughing were ignored and concentration was focused on replies to questions dealing specifically with phlegm. There were four such questions, and they follow earlier questions concerning coughing: Q.3. "*Do you bring up phlegm when you get up or first thing in the morning?*" Q.3a. "*Do you bring up phlegm like this on most days for as much as* 3 *months in the year?*" Q.4. "*Do you bring up phlegm during the rest of the day?—I don't mean just at the end of your shift.*" Q.4a. "*Do you bring up phlegm like this on most days for as much as* 3 *months in the year?*" (Questions 3a and 4a were asked only if there was a positive reply to the relevant preceding question.)

"Persistent phlegm" at any one survey was defined as a positive response to question 4a. (Some men replied positively to question 4a and negatively to question 3a.)

2.4. *Dust Exposure*

During the 10-year period between the first and third medical surveys airborne dust measurements had been made close to randomly selected men in occupational groups. The measurements were made using the standard Thermal Precipitator. Mean concentrations for occupational groups over 10 years were expressed as particles per cubic centimetre and were converted subsequently to mass concentration units (mg/m^3) as described by JACOBSEN *et al.* (1971) and DODGSON *et al.* (1971). For all men in the collieries concerned records had been kept of the number of shifts worked in the occupational groups defined by the dust sampling programme. The number of shifts worked were converted into hours, depending on the shift length in the period and area concerned. Individuals' cumulative exposures to dust over 10 years were computed by summing the products of estimated mass concentrations in occupational groups and the number of hours worked in them. The exposure units were expressed as gram-hours per cubic metre (gh/m^3) of sampled air; they are equivalent to time weighted cumulative mass concentrations of dust particles in the "respirable size range" defined by Medical Research Council criteria (HAMILTON and WALTON, 1961).

2.5. *Results*

Among the 4122 men for whom data were available 954 had averaged radiological classifications higher than category 0/0 on the earlier film; a further 432 replied inconsistently at the second and third surveys to the questions on smoking; a further 13 had at least one X-ray where one or more film reader diagnosed rheumatoid lung or complicated pneumoconiosis or both. Results from these 1399 men were not included in the analyses that follow.

Table 2 shows attack rates of CWP over 10 years among 2335 smokers and 388 non-

TABLE 2. ATTACK RATE OF CWP OVER 10 YEARS (%) BY DUST EXPOSURE AND SMOKING HABITS (Number of men in group in brackets)

	10-year dust exposure (gh/m³)								
	−20	−40	−60	−80	−100	−150	−200	200+	All
Smokers	0.9 (110)	1.7 (630)	6.0 (504)	7.9 (393)	14.2 (281)	11.4 (298)	15.1 (93)	26.9 (26)	7.2 (2335)
Non-smokers	0.0 (13)	1.9 (108)	6.2 (81)	4.4 (68)	4.0 (50)	5.1 (39)	31.3 (16)	23.1 (13)	5.7 (388)

smokers whose earlier X-rays were classified as category 0/0 or 0/–. Average classification of X-rays from five of these men indicated that they progressed from category 0/– to category 0/0 on the 12-point scale of abnormality during the 10 years. These five sets of results were included among the "attacks" in the analyses that follow. All other "attacks" were movements from category 0/0 to category 0/1 or higher.

At dust exposures up to 60 gh/m³ (equivalent approximately to a mean exposure to 3.4 mg/m³ over 10 years) there was little difference between smokers and non-smokers. At higher dust exposures (60 to 150 gh/m³), however, attack rates were higher for smokers. Further analyses were made to investigate the statistical significance of the observed differences and to compare attack rates in smaller sub-groups who differed in their reports concerning phlegm production. This approach permits consideration of hypothesis (d): that a possible increased risk of developing CWP as a result of inhaling tobacco smoke may be counterbalanced partially by reductions in the amount of inhaled dust reaching the alveoli, as a result of the expectoration frequently associated with smoking.

Table 3 shows the numbers of men who developed CWP among smokers and non-smokers in relation to their reports of phlegm production at each of two medical

TABLE 3. ATTACKS OF CWP BY SMOKING HABITS AND REPORTS OF PERSISTENT PHLEGM AT TWO CONSECUTIVE SURVEYS

Sub-group	1	2	3	4	5	6	7	8
Persistent phlegm: 2nd surveys	Yes		Yes		No		No	
Persistent phlegm: 3rd surveys	Yes		No		Yes		No	
Smokers	No	Yes	No	Yes	No	Yes	No	Yes
Number of men in sub-group	12	189	14	147	33	314	329	1685
Attacks of CWP: Observed	1	13	0	9	4	25	17	121
Attacks of CWP: Expected	2.7	14.8	1.4	10.7	2.3	25.6	22.9	109.6
Standardized mean residuals	−1.29	−0.51	−1.18	−0.57	1.46	−0.18	−1.52	0.61

surveys. The influence of variations in dust exposure on the observed results is reflected in the numbers of attacks "expected" in each sub-group. These numbers have been calculated from an equation (1) described in an appendix. The statistical model embraces the influence of age at the initial survey (reflecting to some degree earlier dust exposure), exposure to mixed respirable coal-mine dust during the 10-year inter-survey period, and the exposure over the same period to certain mineral components in the dust. The variables considered have each been shown to influence the probability of developing CWP. The form in which they appear in the equation represents the most satisfactory explanation of the observed data when compared with many variants of the same basic model. The expected numbers in each sub-group were calculated by summing the individual estimates of probabilities within each sub-group.

Among the 2335 smokers considered, 168 developed CWP during 10 years as compared with the 161 expected on the basis of the equation which takes into account the ages and dust exposures of the men concerned. In contrast, 22 of the 388 non-smokers developed CWP, while equation (1) predicts 29. The net difference between smokers and non-smokers unexplained by the equation [$7 - (-7) = 14$] would be expected to have arisen by chance with a probability of about 13% ($\chi_1^2 = 2.33$). An alternative and perhaps more sensitive test of the apparently increased risk for smokers can be made by re-fitting the data to an equation which includes a binary variable differentiating between smokers and non-smokers (equation (2) in the appendix). The statistical significance of the smoking effect is then increased further to about 9% ($\chi_1^2 = 2.84$). If all variables in equation (2) are taken as the mean values observed for these 2723 miners then, for a non-smoker, the probability of an attack of CWP is estimated as 4.1%. The corresponding probability for a smoker is estimated as 6.0%.

The observed effect apparently associated with smoking may be the resultant of two or more conflicting tendencies as suggested by hypothesis (d). If so, this might explain the equivocal statistical significance of the observed smoking effect in the group as a whole. Such conflicting tendencies might be reflected in discrepancies between observed and expected attacks in one or more sub-groups. These discrepancies are expressed conveniently as standardized mean residuals shown in Table 3 and defined in the appendix. If the discrepancies are due simply to random variation then these statistics are equivalent approximately to standardized Normal variates: 95% of such values would lie in the range (-1.96, $+1.96$). The results show no convincing evidence of real differences between the attacks observed and those expected in any of the sub-groups. Probabilities of chance occurrence range from about 13% for sub-group 7 to 86% for sub-group 6.

Equation (3) in the appendix shows the result of a further analysis which was undertaken to investigate the nature and statistical significance of the apparently increased attack rate among smokers as a whole. At both the second and third surveys, miners had been asked how many cigarettes they smoked per day. For two of the collieries concerned these data were incomplete with respect to the second surveys. The number smoked per day at the time of the later (third) surveys was used therefore to see whether the apparent smoking effect increased with increasing tobacco consumption. Expressed in this way, smoking appeared to have no noticeable effect on the attack rate of CWP. The fitted equation (3) was statistically indistinguishable from equation (1) which includes no variable reflecting smoking habits ($\chi_1^2 = 0.08$).

3. CWP PREVALENCE AND ATTACK RATES IN ANOTHER GROUP OF COAL MINERS

3.1. *Men Studied*

In ten of the collieries studied by the Pneumoconiosis Field Research a series of fourth medical surveys were completed approximately 5 years after the third surveys. The following analyses relate to a sub-group of men who were X-rayed on at least three occasions (at the second, third and fourth surveys) who replied consistently to the questions on smoking at all these three surveys and for whom there was no radiological evidence of complicated pneumoconiosis at any survey. Men whose results contributed to the analyses described in Section 2 were excluded.

3.2. *Radiological Classifications*

Film classifications available for men considered refer to the four major categories of CWP only (I.L.O., 1959). Results from X-rays made at the second and fourth surveys are used here. All films made at the second surveys were classified soon after the surveys by any one of four medical officers in the research team. The films were then examined again, independently, within 5 years of the original readings by at least one other doctor in the team. Where classifications agreed, this was taken as "definitive". Where there was disagreement, the films concerned were re-examined in concert by at least three of the readers. After discussion, an agreed classification was obtained in each case. Films made at the fourth surveys were classified for clinical purposes soon after the surveys by any one of five medical officers, of whom only one had participated in the classification of the second survey films. In all cases, earlier X-rays from the same man were available for inspection when these clinical assessments were made.

3.3. *Smoking Habits and Phlegm Production*

The same respiratory symptoms questionnaire used at the second and third surveys was applied again at the fourth surveys. "Smokers" and "non-smokers" were defined on the basis of consistent replies at all three surveys to the questions recorded in Section 2.3. "Persistent phlegm" at any one survey was defined in the same way as for the preceding analysis.

3.4. *Dust Exposures*

For each of the men considered here there was available (a) a dust exposure during the period between the third and fourth surveys based on measurements of mass concentrations in occupational groups (using the MRE Gravimetric Sampler, Type 113A) and the time worked in those groups; (b) a similar figure for the period between second and third surveys, based on particle count concentrations converted to mass concentration units (see Section 2.3); (c) an exposure for at least part of the period between the first and second surveys, based on similar data as used for (b); (d) an estimate of exposure from the time that a man joined the industry up to the time that research measurements relevant to him began. The latter estimates were based on detailed records of occupational histories from which the number of years spent in any one of six broad categories of coal-mining activities was extracted. The exposures (d) were calculated as the product of these times and the means of concentrations measured in occupational groups corresponding to the relevant categories during the first 10 years of the research. Attack rates of CWP during the 10-year periods between the second and fourth surveys were analysed in relation to the sum of (a) and (b). Prevalence rates at the fourth surveys were analysed in relation to the sum (a) + (b) + (c) + (d).

3.5. *Results*

3.5.1. *Prevalence of CWP*

There were 2689 men who replied consistently to the questions on smoking at the second, third and fourth surveys, for whom there was no radiological evidence of complicated pneumoconiosis and for whom records were available for calculating dust exposures. The bottom row of Table 4 shows the prevalence of CWP among smokers

TABLE 4. PREVALENCE OF CWP (%), CATEGORY 1 OR HIGHER, AT FOURTH SURVEYS, BY CUMULATIVE DUST EXPOSURE, REPORTS OF PHLEGM AND SMOKING HABITS

	Cumulative dust exposure			
	Low (< 120 gh/m^3)		High ($\geqslant 120$ gh/m^3)	
	NS	S	NS	S
No phlegm at any of three surveys	2.7 (264)	2.3 (875)	17.3 (104)	20.5 (513)
Variable reports of phlegm	5.7 (35)	4.1 (364)	26.9 (52)	26.9 (360)
Phlegm at all three surveys	100.0 (1)	2.0 (51)	60.0 (5)	43.1 (65)
All men	3.3 (300)	2.8 (1290)	21.7 (161)	24.5 (938)

(Figures in brackets are the number of men in the group concerned. S = smokers; NS = non-smokers.)

and non-smokers in two broad cumulative dust-exposure groups. These groups correspond approximately to the numbers of men with less and with more than the median cumulative dust exposure estimated from the time that they started work in the coal industry up to the time of the fourth medical surveys. The median of these estimates is roughly twice the value calculated for the 10-year period between the first and third medical surveys—see Table 2. The higher prevalence among smokers (24.5%) as compared with non-smokers (21.7%) in the high dust-exposure group is not statistically significant ($P > 0.4$).

Only 5% of the men reported phlegm production at all three surveys, and nearly all of them were smokers. However, 933 men (35%) reported phlegm at least at one of the three surveys, and it appears from Table 4 that these men had, on the whole, a higher prevalence of CWP than men who denied producing phlegm at all three surveys. Figure 1 shows that at least some of this difference can be attributed to different mean cumulative dust exposures between sub-groups. Nevertheless, it will be seen that in the high dust-exposure group, men who sometimes reported phlegm had considerably higher prevalence than men who denied producing phlegm, although the estimated mean dust exposures in the latter groups were only marginally lower. Whatever the explanation for this result there is certainly no evidence from Fig. 1 of any difference in prevalence between smokers and non-smokers depending on whether or not they report phlegm.

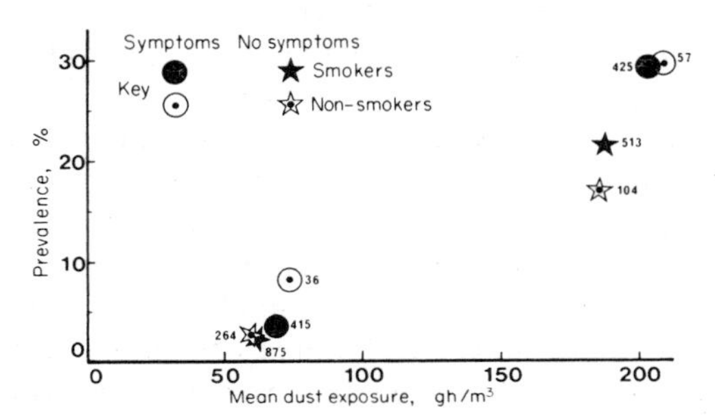

FIG. 1. Prevalence (category 1 +); data from Table 4.

3.5.2. *Attack rate of CWP*

Among 2488 men whose X-rays were classified as category 0 at the second surveys, 125 (5.0%) developed CWP during the ensuing 10 years. Table 5 shows the attack rates for smokers and non-smokers. The small differences between smokers and non-smokers are of no statistical significance. The pattern of results by reports of phlegm production is similar to that observed for prevalence at the fourth surveys (Table 4).

TABLE 5. ATTACK RATE OF CWP (%), CATEGORY 1 OR HIGHER, OVER 10 YEARS, BY DUST EXPOSURE, REPORTS OF PHLEGM AND SMOKING HABITS

	Dust exposure over 10 years			
	Low (< 40 gh/m³)		High (≥ 40 gh/m³)	
	NS	S	NS	S
No phlegm at any of three surveys	2.3 (177)	2.5 (644)	4.0 (175)	4.5 (662)
Variable reports of phlegm	10.0 (30)	5.9 (306)	10.2 (49)	8.4 (344)
Phlegm at all three surveys	75.0 (4)	7.0 (57)	0.0 (1)	15.4 (39)
All men	4.7 (211)	3.8 (1007)	5.3 (225)	6.2 (1045)

(Figures in brackets are the number of men in the group concerned. S = smokers; NS = non-smokers.)

4. DISCUSSION

The results reported in Sections 2 and 3 are intended to complement one another. The sophistication of radiological data quoted in Section 2 (averages of eight readers' classifications on a 12-point scale) justifies the use of fairly elaborate statistical methods to quantify the relationship between radiological response and dust exposure, and this permits detailed exploration of hypotheses concerning possible effects of smoking on the development of CWP. A deficiency in these data is that the information on smoking history is restricted to one 5-year period. To be convincing, any conclusions based on these results should be consistent, in a general way, with the pattern which emerges from the independent data set with less reliable radiological classifications, but more information both on smoking habits and dust exposure.

The analysis of attack rate in Section 2 appears to suggest that smokers may be at greater risk of developing CWP than non-smokers. The effect was seen only at higher dust exposures. The probability that the result is due simply to random variation is high ($P \approx 0.09$) and would not normally be regarded as convincing in epidemiological situations fraught with possibilities of unidentifiable biases that might distort results from formal probability calculations. The failure to demonstrate a clear and significant overall effect of smoking is not due to conflicting patterns of response depending on whether or not smoking is accompanied by persistent expectoration; nor is it attributable to the use of the dichotomy smoker/non-smoker to summarize smoking habits. Indeed, the null result obtained when smoking is expressed as the number of cigarettes smoked per day [equation (3)] reduces further the plausibility of the weak evidence suggesting that smokers are more likely to develop CWP (unless it is supposed that smoking as such, irrespective of the quantity of tobacco smoked, increases the probability of developing CWP, or that a susceptibility to CWP is associated in some way with a craving for nicotine). The analysis of independent data in Section 3 also shows no effect attributable to smoking (see Fig. 1).

There remains only the curiously suggestive picture revealed by the rearrangement, in Table 1, of results reported previously by RAE *et al.* (1971): non-smokers who reported persistent cough and phlegm had higher prevalence of CWP than smokers with the same symptoms. The contrast between this result and those reported in Section 2 appears particularly puzzling since the analyses reported in Section 2 are based on a sub-set of the data considered by RAE *et al.* (1971). Figure 2 resolves the

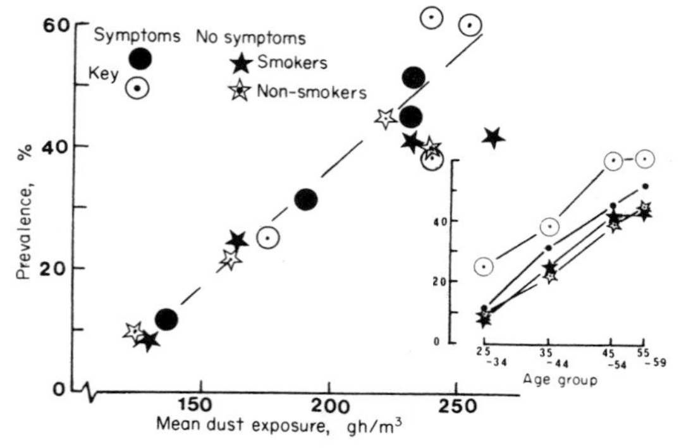

FIG. 2. Relation between prevalence (category 0/1 +) and mean dust exposure. *Inset:* The same prevalences by age group, data from Table 1.

enigma. Shown there are the prevalences in various sub-groups defined in Table 1 plotted against the mean cumulative dust exposures of the sub-groups concerned. (These cumulative exposures have been calculated in precisely the same way as that described by RAE *et al.*, 1971.) Inset in Fig. 2 are the same data plotted against the age-groups defined in Table 1. In so far as the age of a coal miner may be regarded as a crude indicator of his dust exposure the results in Table 1 might be taken to suggest that there may be real differences in the dose–response curves. However, the mean dust exposures actually relevant to the various sub-groups, shown in Fig. 2, demonstrate that such a conclusion would be wrong. It is clear that the differences are due to variations of dust exposures between sub-groups. The use of age as an indirect measure of dust exposure is thus shown to be potentially misleading in investigations concerned with *comparisons* of dose–response relationships.

It is concluded that there is no convincing evidence that smoking affects the probability of developing radiological signs of CWP. ROGAN *et al.* (1973), who showed that exposure to airborne dust reduces ventilatory function, were unable to demonstrate a potentiating interaction between dust exposure and smoking. The same authors pointed out that the results reported by RAE *et al.* (1971) are equally inconsistent with the suggestion (MINETTE, 1971) that coal-mine dust and tobacco smoke potentiate each other in their individual tendencies to produce symptoms indicative of chronic bronchitis. It seems, therefore, that while smoking must be regarded as deleterious to the health of coal miners as it is to others, there is no reason to believe that the habit influences the equally undesirable effects of inhaling airborne coal-mine dust.

APPENDIX

The model used for the analysis described in Section 2 was the linear logistic equation

$$Y = \log\left(\frac{P}{1-P}\right) = a_0 + \Sigma a_i x_i$$

where P = probability of radiological change; the x_i are explanatory variables; and the a's are constants to be estimated. For the analyses reported here the constants were estimated from the data iteratively, using the method of maximum likelihood.

Table 6 shows the means and ranges of variables contributing to the equations quoted in the paper, the estimated constants in the equations and corresponding "t" statistics. The latter were calculated as the ratios of the estimates ($\hat{a}$) to their approximate standard errors.

It will be noted that the approximate values of t associated with the coefficients for kaolin and mica exposures are of dubious statistical significance. Nevertheless, inclusion of this variable together with its interaction with quartz exposure yields significantly increased values of the log likelihood when compared with those obtained from alternative models involving other combinations of exposure variables. These matters are discussed further in another paper to this Symposium (WALTON *et al.*, pp. 669–688). The analysis in Table 2 of the present paper is concerned essentially with a study of residuals; equation (1) was used because it provided the most satisfactory "fit" of the data to the logistic model.

The standardized mean residuals for sub-groups, shown in Table 3, were calculated as

$$n^{-1/2} \sum^{n} \left\{ (P - \hat{P}) \left[\hat{P}(1 - \hat{P}) \right]^{-1/2} \right\}$$

where P is a binary variable taking the values 0 for no radiological change and 1 for some

TABLE 6. RESULTS FROM FITTING LOGISTIC EQUATIONS

Variable	Units	Mean	Range	Equation (1)		Equation (2)		Equation (3)	
				$\hat{a}$	t	$\hat{a}$	t	$\hat{a}$	t
* *Exposures*									
Mixed dust	gh/m^3	67.3	(8.7, 309.2)	0.0164	8.22	0.0168	8.36	0.0165	8.22
Quartz dust	gh/m^3	2.53	(0.23, 14.04)	0.1686	2.15	0.1625	2.06	0.1683	2.14
Kaolin and mica	gh/m^3	10.53	(1.47, 88.88)	0.0036	0.17	0.0029	0.14	0.0037	0.18
(Quartz) × (Kaolin and mica)	$(gh/m^3)^2$	45.46	(0.05, 1141.09)	−0.0044	2.02	−0.0043	1.97	−0.0044	2.02
Age at first survey	years	35.5	(16.0, 55.0)	0.0297	3.23	0.0289	3.12	0.0298	3.23
Smoking	Dummy	0.8575	(0, 1)	—	—	0.4039	1.62	—	—
	No. of cigarettes per day	13.6	(0, 55.5)	—	—	—	—	0.0025	0.27
Constant (a_0)				−5.2278		−5.5601		−5.2665	
			Log likelihood (λ)	−637.93		−636.51		−637.89	

* Exposures refer to 10 years between first and third medical surveys.

radiological change over 10 years; $\hat{P}$ is the estimate of P from (1) for an individual; and the summation is over the n individuals in the sub-group concerned.

Test for improvements in fit as a result of adding smoking variables to (1) were made using the statistic $-2(\lambda_1 - \lambda_j)$, where λ_1, λ_j are the log likelihoods associated with equations (1) and (j) respectively (j = 2, 3). Under the null hypothesis of no improvement in fit this statistic is distributed as χ_1^2.

A detailed exposition of the logistic model and its applications is given by Cox (1970).

REFERENCES

BUNDY, M. (1971) *Inhaled Particles III* (edited by WALTON, W. H.) vol. II, p. 919. Unwin Bros., Old Woking, Surrey.

COX, D. R. (1970) *The Analysis of Binary Data*, Methuen, London.

DODGSON, J., HADDEN, G. G., JONES, C. O. and WALTON, W. H. (1971) *Inhaled Particles III* (edited by WALTON, W. H.) vol. II, pp. 757–781. Unwin Bros., Old Woking, Surrey.

HAMILTON, R. J. and WALTON, W. H. (1961) *Inhaled Particles and Vapours* (edited by DAVIES, C. N.) pp. 465–475. Pergamon Press, Oxford.

INTERNATIONAL LABOUR OFFICE (1959) *Occup. Saf. Hlth* **9**, 63–72.

JACOBSEN, M., RAE, S., WALTON, W. H. and ROGAN, J. M. (1971) *Inhaled Particles III* (edited by WALTON, W. H.) vol. II, pp. 903–919. Unwin Bros., Old Woking, Surrey.

LIDDELL, F. D. K. and LINDARS, D. C. (1969) *Br. J. ind. Med.* **26**, 89–100.

MINETTE, A. (1971) *Inhaled Particles III* (edited by WALTON, W. H.) vol. II, p. 895. Unwin Bros., Old Woking, Surrey.

RAE, S., WALKER, D. D. and ATTFIELD, M. D. (1971) *Inhaled Particles III* (edited by WALTON, W. H.) vol. II, pp. 883–896. Unwin Bros., Old Woking, Surrey.

ROGAN, J. M., ATTFIELD, M. D., JACOBSEN, M., RAE, S., WALKER, D. D. and WALTON, W. H. (1973) *Br. J. ind. Med.* **30**, 217–226.

DISCUSSION

J. C. GILSON: The possible importance of the smoking pattern in relation to work is shown by the findings in a survey of foundry workers in the U.K. made by Dr Lloyd Davies and his colleagues. In this survey there was clear evidence of a positive relationship between severity of simple pneumoconiosis and smoking, but of course in foundry work men may smoke while they are being exposed to the dust.

M. BUNDY: I want to thank you for the fine job on the assessment of the effect of smoking on the risk of developing simple CWP. Having asked the original question I appreciate the answer.

A. G. HEPPLESTON: Could the results be explained by the fact that coal miners do not smoke underground during dust exposure but only after they leave the pit?

Mr JACOBSEN: We have no data on the effects of smoking while coal-mine dust is actually being inhaled. Our results reflect the reality under mining conditions in this country.

R. ALBERT: Smoking while at work (in contrast to smoking after work) may increase the risk of pulmonary disease if the cigarette is held between the lips because this would increase the likelihood of mouth breathing and hence the access of dust to the lung.

D. LIDDELL: Do miners smoke in total as much as other workers, bearing in mind that they are not allowed to smoke while at work?

Mr JACOBSEN: In Table 6 of the paper we show the average number of cigarettes smoked per day as 13.6. This figure was calculated as an average over all men contributing to that analysis, including the non-smokers. The average number of cigarettes smoked by the smokers was nearly 16 per day.

W. T. ULMER: You refer in your paper to the work by RAE *et al.* (1971) and by ROGAN *et al.* (1973), and in your verbal presentation you suggested that their results demonstrate linear relationships between dust exposure and respiratory symptoms and dust exposure and FEV_1. Our results lead us to believe that dust related pulmonary effects (e.g. symptoms, reductions in FEV_1) occur within the first few years of dust exposure, and that no further changes are observable after about 7 years. Are you really sure that the effect of dust exposure is additive, as is suggested by your linear model?

Mr JACOBSEN: We are not sure that the additive linear model is correct. We claim only that this model gives a simple and useful representation of the observed results. Other relationships can, no doubt, be fitted. The important point we wish to emphasize in the present context is that, assuming a linear model, we cannot detect a difference in slopes depending upon whether men smoke or do not smoke. Even if the linear model is not entirely correct we would expect any real interaction between dust exposure and smoking to be reflected in a difference in slopes of fitted straight lines.

J. SATISH: Your "non-smoker" group was well defined. However, the "smoker" group will have included occasional smokers as well as heavy smokers. Might this have been the reason why the difference between the groups was not well pronounced?

Mr JACOBSEN: We think this unlikely. If this were the explanation then one might have expected that an effect associated with smoking would increase with increasing tobacco consumption. We report in the paper that no such dose–response relationship was detectable [equation (3)].

R. WOLFF: Was any consideration taken of the "drop-out" population, that is, the workers who left the mines between the two surveys?

Mr JACOBSEN: No; the data refer to the survivor population only. We are conscious of the fact that this may have biased our estimates of effects attributable to dust but we have no reason to believe that the omission has influenced our results with regard to smoking. In the continuing research we are examining miners who have left the collieries.

POSSIBLE SYNERGISM OF EXPOSURE TO AIRBORNE MANGANESE AND SMOKING HABIT IN OCCURRENCE OF RESPIRATORY SYMPTOMS*

MARKO ŠARIĆ and SLAVICA LUČIĆ-PALAIĆ

Institute for Medical Research and Occupational Health, Yugoslav Academy of Sciences and Arts, Zagreb, Yugoslavia

Abstract—The possible combined action of manganese exposure and smoking on the rate of respiratory symptoms was studied in three groups of male workers at various levels of exposure to manganese: occupational exposure (369 workers), relatively high ambient exposure (190 workers) and low ambient exposure (204 workers).

The study was carried out by means of the standard epidemiological method.

Between non-smokers in the different groups there was no difference in the prevalence of respiratory symptoms. In smokers the prevalence was significantly higher in workers occupationally exposed to manganese than in those with a low ambient exposure. The tendency of the prevalence of respiratory symptoms to increase with the extent of the smoking habit was also most pronounced in the groups of occupationally exposed workers.

Since other relevant factors under control in the compared groups were more or less uniform, the results indicate that manganese exposure and smoking might have a possible synergistic effect on the occurrence and rate of respiratory symptoms.

IN THE study of a possible role of occupational exposure or some other ecological factors in the occurrence and rate of chronic non-specific lung disease, smoking habit is always found to interfere. Smoking, as a rule, shows a strong association with the prevalence of respiratory symptoms.

A possible synergistic effect of smoking and some other noxious agents to which a person may be exposed presents an interesting problem.

ŠARIĆ *et al.* (1974) suggested that occupational exposure to manganese may contribute to the development of chronic bronchitis. The present paper deals with the problem of interaction of exposure to airborne manganese and smoking habit in the occurrence of respiratory symptoms.

SAMPLE AND METHODS

The study was carried out in three groups of workers comparable by age and other characteristics but with different levels of exposure to manganese: a group of 369 workers employed in the production of manganese alloys, a group of 190 workers from

* This study was supported by Environmental Protection Agency agreement No. 02–513–6.

the electrode production without occupational exposure to manganese but working within the same plant as manganese alloy workers and a group of 204 workers from the aluminium rolling mill which is situated at a distance of about 5 km from the manganese alloys and electrode plants.

Tables 1 and 2 show general characteristics of examined workers.

TABLE 1. GENERAL CHARACTERISTICS OF COMPARED WORKERS

		Age (years)		Height (cm)		Weight (kg)	
	no.	$\bar{x}$	s.d.	$\bar{x}$	s.d.	$\bar{x}$	s.d.
1. Manganese alloy production	369	37.8	8.8	173.3	6.6	76.6	10.4
2. Electrode production	190	35.8	9.4	172.8	7.1	75.2	11.3
3. Aluminium rolling mill	204	36.8	8.7	173.6	6.3	75.2	10.4

Age: 1–2 $P < 0.01$

TABLE 2. DISTRIBUTION OF COMPARED WORKERS ACCORDING TO SMOKING HABIT

	I. Manganese alloy production		II. Electrode production		III. Aluminium rolling mill	
	no.	%	no.	%	no.	%
1. Non-smokers	169	45.9	102	53.7	81	39.7
2. Past smokers	57	15.4	19	10.0	29	14.2
3. Light smokers	51	13.8	35	18.4	41	20.1
4. Moderate smokers	73	19.8	25	13.2	42	20.6
5. Heavy smokers	19	5.1	9	4.7	11	5.4
6. Smokers, total	143	38.8	69	36.3	94	46.1

Table 3 illustrates the level of manganese exposure for examined groups of workers.

The examination was performed with the standard epidemiological technique. The *Questionnaire on Respiratory Symptoms* of the Committee on the Aetiology of Chronic Bronchitis of the British MEDICAL RESEARCH COUNCIL (1965) was used; forced expiratory volumes were measured, consistency and volume of the early morning sputum were determined, clinical and radiographic examinations of the lungs were done.

TABLE 3. LEVEL OF MANGANESE EXPOSURE FOR EXAMINED GROUPS OF WORKERS

Group	Exposure level
Manganese alloy production	0.391–16.347 mg/m^3
Electrode production	5–40 μg/m^3
Aluminium rolling mill	0.05–0.07 μg/m^3

Phlegm part–day was defined as bringing up phlegm in the morning or during the day and/or night for longer than 3 months in the last year. Regular wheezing in the chest was defined as wheezing independent of chest cold. Chronic bronchitis was defined as bringing up phlegm in the morning and during the day and/or night for at least three winter months in the last 2 years or longer.

According to smoking habit the workers were divided into the following categories:

1. non-smokers who never smoked or smoked not more than one cigarette a day;
2. past smokers who smoked more than one cigarette a day, but stopped smoking at least one month prior to examination; and
3. present smokers divided according to number of cigarettes smoked in their lifetime into:
   (a) light smokers if the product of the average number of cigarettes smoked per day and the number of years of smoking was less than 200,
   (b) moderate smokers if the product was between 200 and 600, and
   (c) heavy smokers if the product was higher than 600.

The categorization of the present smokers was done according to the criteria used by Brinkman and Coates (1963).

The statistical examination of data was carried out with the use of the *t*-test to determine the significance of differences.

RESULTS

The prevalence of the symptom of phlegm part-day in compared groups of workers is presented in Table 4.

Table 4. Prevalence of Phlegm Part-Day in Compared Groups of Workers by Smoking Habit

	I. Manganese alloy production		II. Electrode production		III. Aluminium rolling mill		Significance of difference
	no.	%	no.	%	no.	%	
1. Non-smokers	10	5.9	11	10.8	6	7.4	NS
2. Past smokers	2		3		1		NS
3. Light smokers	9	17.6	4		1		NS
4. Moderate smokers	11	15.1	6	24.0	7	16.7	NS
5. Heavy smokers	3		2		0		NS
6. Smokers, total	23	16.1	12	17.4	8	8.5	NS
Total	35	9.5	26	13.7	15	7.4	
Significance of difference	1–3 $P < 0.05$ 1–4 $P < 0.05$ 1–6 $P < 0.05$		NS		NS		

Note: In this and in the following tables the per cents were not calculated for less than five observations.

The prevalence of the symptom of regular wheezing in the chest is given in Table 5.

TABLE 5. PREVALENCE OF SYMPTOM OF REGULAR WHEEZING IN THE CHEST IN COMPARED GROUPS OF WORKERS ACCORDING TO SMOKING HABIT

	I. Manganese alloy production		II. Electrode production		III. Aluminium rolling mill		Significance of difference
	no.	%	no.	%	no.	%	
1. Non-smokers	9	5.3	6	5.9	5	6.2	NS
2. Past smokers	2		4		2		NS
3. Light smokers	3		0		3		NS
4. Moderate smokers	15	20.5	3		9	21.4	NS
5. Heavy smokers	7	36.8	0		2		NS
6. Smokers, total	25	17.5	3		14	14.9	I–II $P < 0.01$ I–III $P < 0.05$
Total	36	9.8	13	6.8	21	10.3	
Significance of difference	1–4 $P < 0.01$ 1–5 $P < 0.01$ 1–6 $P < 0.01$		NS		NS		

Table 6 shows the prevalence of chronic bronchitis and Table 7 combinations of this syndrome with some objective findings in the compared groups. Owing to relatively low rates data in Table 7 are shown by groups only for non-smokers and smokers and not by categories of smokers.

TABLE 6. PREVALENCE OF CHRONIC BRONCHITIS IN COMPARED GROUPS OF WORKERS ACCORDING TO SMOKING HABIT

	I. Manganese alloy production		II. Electrode production		III. Aluminium rolling mill		Significance of difference
	no.	%	no.	%	no.	%	
1. Non-smokers	14	8.3	11	10.8	4		NS
2. Past smokers	4		3		4		NS
3. Light smokers	6	11.8	5	14.3	5	12.2	NS
4. Moderate smokers	29	39.7	8	32.0	9	21.4	I–III $P < 0.05$
5. Heavy smokers	11	57.9	1		3		NS
6. Smokers, total	46	32.2	14	20.3	17	18.1	I–III $P < 0.05$
Total	64	17.3	28	14.7	25	12.3	
Significance of difference	1–4 $P < 0.01$ 1–5 $P < 0.01$ 1–6 $P < 0.01$ 3–4 $P < 0.01$ 3–5 $P < 0.01$ 4–5 $P < 0.01$		1–4 $P < 0.01$		NS		

TABLE 7. PREVALENCE OF SYMPTOMS OF CHRONIC BRONCHITIS IN COMBINATION WITH CERTAIN OBJECTIVE FINDINGS IN COMPARED GROUPS OF WORKERS ACCORDING TO SMOKING HABIT

	Manganese alloy production		Electrode production		Aluminium rolling mill	
	Non-smokers $n = 169$	Smokers $n = 143$	Non-smokers $n = 102$	Smokers $n = 69$	Non-smokers $n = 81$	Smokers $n = 94$
Chronic bronchitis with mucopurulent or purulent sputum	2	15 (10.5)	3	6 (8.7)	2	6 (6.4)
Chronic bronchitis with physical signs of bronchitis	7 (4.1)	28 (19.6)	4	4	0	7 (7.4)
Chronic bronchitis with reduced FVC% (79% or less)	0	7 (4.9)	0	1	1	1
Chronic bronchitis with reduced $FEV_{1.0}$% (79% or less)	0	7 (4.9)	2	1	1	4

Note: The numbers in parentheses are per cents. The obtained values of forced expiratory volumes are expressed as percentage of the values expected with regard to age and height of subjects (MORRIS *et al.*, 1971).

DISCUSSION

The analysis of data shows that the compared groups of non-smokers do not significantly differ as regards the prevalence of respiratory symptoms. In past smokers the differences are also negligible.

Among smokers the rate of respiratory symptoms was highest in the manganese alloy production, then in the electrode production, while in the aluminium rolling mill it was usually lowest. The prevalence increases with categories of smokers (light—moderate—heavy). The tendency of the rate of symptoms to rise with the extent of the smoking habit is most pronounced in the group of workers occupationally exposed to manganese, i.e. those working in the production of manganese alloys. This is particularly true for symptoms defined as chronic bronchitis.

As far as combination of the symptoms of chronic bronchitis and certain objective findings is concerned it is also interesting that differences between compared groups with regard to exposure were again more pronounced in smokers, the syndromes being more frequent in smokers from the manganese alloy production than in smokers from the other two groups of workers.

Owing to relatively low rates it has not been possible to elaborate the differences in the prevalence of these syndromes statistically or to analyse them from the point of view of smoking categories.

Since other relevant factors under control in compared groups of workers were more or less uniform. the results indicate a synergistic action of manganese exposure and smoking habit in the occurrence and rate of respiratory symptoms.

REFERENCES

BRINKMAN, G. L. and COATES, E. O. (1963) *Am. Rev. resp. Dis.* **87**, 684–693.

MEDICAL RESEARCH COUNCIL, Committee on the Aetiology of Chronic Bronchitis (1965) *Lancet* **1**, 775–779.

MORRIS, J. F., KOSKI, A. and JOHNSON, L. C. (1971) *Am. Rev. resp. Dis.* **103**, 57–67.

ŠARIĆ, M., LUČIĆ-PALAIĆ, S., PAUKOVIĆ, R. and HOLETIĆ, A. (1974) *Arh. Hig. Rada* **25**, 15–26.

DISCUSSION

C. E. ROSSITER: The smokers were divided into three groups by cigarette-years, so that the heavy smokers will probably have been much older than the light smokers, with moderate smokers intermediate. How much of the difference in symptom prevalences should be attributed to age effects only and how much to the manganese exposure?

Prof. ŠARIĆ: In the subdivision of smokers, age factor was taken into consideration. The compared groups did not differ markedly as to age or category of smokers. It is very difficult to separate the effect of age from that of smoking or of exposure to manganese. There is obviously an interference of age and other factors.

C.-J. GÖTHE: You talk about possible "synergism" between the effects of exposure to airborne manganese and smoking. Synergism means that the combined effect of two or more factors is stronger than a mere addition of the separate effects. It seems to me that most of the differences between the different exposure groups are not significant or on the borderline of statistical significance. Would it not be more adequate to speak about possible "additive" effects in the discussion of your results?

Prof. ŠARIĆ: There are some experimental studies in animals (RYLANDER *et al.*, 1971, *Inhaled Particles III*, pp. 535–541) suggesting a synergistic effect of MnO_2 particles and SO_2. The "irritation score" of infection-controlled guinea pigs exposed for several weeks to a combination of SO_2 and MnO_2 was higher than of animals exposed to the same concentration of SO_2 or MnO_2 only. I am referring to these data because they also support our findings. In our study non-smokers at different exposure levels to manganese did not differ as regards the prevalence of respiratory symptoms. However, in smokers—particularly with symptoms defined as chronic bronchitis—the rate was highest in the most exposed group, i.e. in those occupationally exposed to manganese. The rate also increased with categories of smokers. This suggests a possible synergistic effect of manganese and smoking habit rather than an additive effect.

R. AKSELSSON: Could you say anything about the chemical and physical properties of the manganese-containing particles? Are the properties the same for the three groups of workers?

Prof. ŠARIĆ: Our measurements were concerned with manganese concentrations only. We assume that manganese appears mainly as manganese dioxide both in the production of ferromanganese alloys and in the emissions from the factory.

M. G. HARRIS: Do manganese-alloy workers who smoke carry their cigarettes in their working clothes? If so, and if they smoke while at work, might not manganese dust on the cigarette produce fume on smoking, and the resultant compound be a factor in the production of bronchitis?

Prof. ŠARIĆ: I do not know whether this may happen. I can only say that workers in all three groups used to smoke at work.

G. V. COLES: Firstly, I agree that there is a possibility of increased manganese absorption from smoking materials carried in the pockets, etc. Secondly, I wonder whether you have investigated the effect of smoking habit on the neurological as well as the respiratory effects of absorption of manganese fume?

Prof. ŠARIĆ: Our study also included a neurological examination and collection of data on neurotoxic effects of manganese. Unfortunately, I cannot answer your question now because the relevant data have not yet been analysed.

PHYSIOLOGICAL CHANGES IN ASBESTOS PLEURAL DISEASE

K. P. S. LUMLEY

Medical Research Unit, H.M. Naval Base, Devonport, England

Abstract—This paper reports the findings of a study of lung function at rest and during progressive sub-maximal exercise in a group of men with varying degrees of asbestos-related pleural abnormality.

The results show that pulmonary fibrosis is accompanied by more adverse functional change than pleural abnormality, diffuse pleural thickening is associated with more functional abnormality than non-calcified pleural plaques, and pleural calcification is not associated with significant functional defects.

The relationship between lung function and asbestos exposure in this selected group is discussed. It is also suggested that $\dot{V}E_{1.0}$ is as useful an index of the ventilatory cost of exercise as $\dot{V}E_{1.5}$.

INTRODUCTION

In addition to pulmonary fibrosis those who have been exposed to asbestos dust may also develop pleural fibrosis. Apart from malignant disease of the pleura three types of asbestos-related pleural fibrosis are recognized radiologically. These are diffuse pleural thickening, which may involve the visceral and parietal pleura, localized non-calcified pleural plaques and pleural calcification, both of which occur on the parietal pleura. These pleural abnormalities are usually bilateral, which helps to distinguish them from pleural fibrosis or calcification resulting from other disease, and may be seen in the absence of radiological or clinical evidence of pulmonary fibrosis.

In a review of chest radiographs of asbestos workers in South Africa, HURWITZ (1961) reported that pleural abnormalities were more common than parenchymal fibrosis. Radiological surveys of dockyard employees (SHEERS and TEMPLETON, 1968; HARRIES *et al.*, 1972) also showed that pleural abnormalities were about ten times more prevalent than parenchymal fibrosis.

Localized pleural plaques are not thought to be associated with symptoms or abnormal physical signs (JONES and SHEERS, 1973), but BECKLAKE *et al.* (1970) found small but consistent adverse changes in lung function in those with pleural abnormalities and HARRIES (1970, pp. 198–199) also found that those with pleural abnormalities had worse lung function than those without. In these two studies pleural abnormalities were considered as a whole, but HARRIES (1970, p. 202) considered that some men with extensive pleural fibrosis were short of breath. This was an important observation because, in this country, compensation for pneumoconiosis due to asbestos under the National Insurance (Industrial Injuries) Act, 1965 is restricted to those with pulmonary fibrosis. In a report by the INDUSTRIAL INJURIES ADVISORY COUNCIL (1973) it was, however, recommended that the pleura should be taken into account when assessing disablement due to asbestosis. This recommendation has not been implemented.

It is therefore important to try to find out the amount of functional disability associated with these pleural abnormalities, and this paper reports the findings of a study of the pulmonary function at rest and during exercise in a group of men with varying degrees of asbestos-related parenchymal and pleural fibrosis.

METHODS

Selection of the Population

One hundred and eighty-six dockyard employees, two ex-dockyard employees and six Royal Naval personnel, aged between 28 and 64 years, were selected on the basis of chest radiographs taken in 1972. Men known to have diffuse pleural thickening were selected first, and these men were matched fairly closely by age and occupation with groups of men who had non-calcified pleural plaques, pleural calcification and normal chest radiographs.

Procedure

Each subject was interviewed and the presence or absence of symptoms determined from answers to a respiratory questionnaire based on the MEDICAL RESEARCH COUNCIL *Questionnaire on Respiratory Symptoms* (1966). The presence or absence of physical signs, including rales, rhonchi, pleural rub, and finger clubbing, was determined by clinical examination, a 12-lead resting electrocardiograph (ECG) was recorded, and height and weight measured.

Pulmonary function at rest was assessed by measurements of forced expiratory volume, 1 s ($FEV_{1 \cdot 0}$), forced vital capacity (FVC), total lung capacity (TLC), residual volume (RV) and transfer factor, single-breath carbon monoxide (DCO). A value for the indirect maximum breathing capacity (IMBC) was determined from $FEV_{1 \cdot 0}$.

The response to exercise was assessed by measurements of the ventilatory and heart-rate response to progressive sub-maximal exercise seated on a static electromagnetically braked bicycle ergometer. After a trial period to familiarize the subject, he was asked to pedal the ergometer at 60 ± 5 rev.min^{-1} at a work load of 5 W for 1 min, 10 W in the next minute, after which the work load was increased by 10 W min^{-1} to a maximum of 120 W.

Inspired air was metered through a Parkinson and Cowan CD4 Dry Gas meter and delivered via flexible tubing (internal dia. 0.032 m) to a low-resistance perspex flap valve (dead space 0.06 l.). The subject breathed through a rubber mouthpiece and expired air was delivered via similar tubing to a mixing chamber (capacity 3.2 l.) from which representative samples were collected to determine the oxygen and carbon dioxide concentrations of mixed expired air during each minute of work. Respiratory rate was measured from signals generated by the movement of a light flap valve in the inspired air line. Heart rate was measured by counting the R waves on a continuous ECG paper trace.*

Minute volume inspired ($\dot{V}I$), respiratory rate (Rf), heart rate (Cf), and oxygen and carbon dioxide concentrations of mixed expired air were determined, and minute volume expired ($\dot{V}E$), oxygen uptake ($\dot{V}O_2$), carbon dioxide output ($\dot{V}CO_2$), and tidal volume (V_t) calculated for each minute of work. From these results the VE and Cf at oxygen uptakes of 1.0 $l.min^{-1}$ ($\dot{V}E_{1\cdot0}$ and $Cf_{1\cdot0}$) and 1.5 $l.min^{-1}$ ($\dot{V}E_{1\cdot5}$ and $Cf_{1\cdot5}$), and V_t at a minute ventilation of 30 $l.min^{-1}$ (V_{t30}) were obtained by interpolation (Cotes, 1972).

Exercise tests were carried out either in the morning or afternoon at least 1½ h after the last meal and subjects were asked not to smoke for 3 h before attending. Chest radiographs were taken within a few days of clinical and lung function assessment.

Safety of Subjects

Subjects known or found to be suffering from valvular heart disease, ischaemic heart disease and hypertension (defined as those on regular treatment with hypotensive drugs or with a diastolic blood pressure $\geqslant$ 110 mmHg) were excluded from the study.

Each subject was allowed to set his own limit to the test and was advised that he could stop if overtaken by chest or leg pain, or undue fatigue or breathlessness. Subjects were also instructed to stop on the appearance of ischaemic change or arrhythmia on the ECG which was monitored continuously throughout the test and for a minimum of 3 min after stopping work. Means for emergency resuscitation were available in the laboratory.

Classification of Subjects

Chest radiographs taken in 1974–5 were read independently by three readers (G. S.' P. G. H. and K. P. S. L.) using a slightly modified form of the I.L.O./U.C. *International Classification of Radiographs of Pneumoconioses* (1971). Using these readings the subjects were placed in one of the following seven groups:

(i) Those with a mean score for irregular small opacities $\geqslant$ 1/1 irrespective of pleural abnormality.
(ii) Those with at least one reading of diffuse pleural thickening.
(iii) Those with non-calcified pleural plaques with no readings for diffuse pleural thickening.
(iv) Those with calcified plaques with no readings for diffuse pleural thickening.
(v) Those with at least one reading of irregular small opacities $\geqslant$ 1/1 but with no readings for pleural abnormality.
(vi) Those with significant other disease not related to asbestos.
(vii) Those with a normal film scored by all readers.

RESULTS

The age distribution of the men in each radiological category is shown in Table 1.

* Full details of the exercise laboratory apparatus are available from the author.

TABLE 1. STUDY POPULATION DISTRIBUTION BY AGE AND RADIOLOGICAL ABNORMALITY

Age (years)	Pulm. fibrosis $\geqslant 1/1$	Diffuse pl. th.	Pleural plaques	Pleural calc.	Pulm. fib. $<1/1$ (no pl. th.)	Other diseases	Normal	Total
25–				1				1
30–		5	2	2			5	14
35–	1	8	7	—			5	21
40–	1	7	4	2		1	3	18
45–	3	7	12	12		3	8	45
50–	4	9	13	10	1	1	9	47
55–	1	9	5	9	1	—	6	31
60–64	1	3	3	4		1	5	17
25–64	11	48	46	40	2	6	41	194
Mean age (years)	50	47	48	51	55	51	48	48.5
Mean height (m)	1.72	1.74	1.71	1.71	1.71	1.74	1.74	1.73
Mean weight (kg)	71.5	78.0	71.0	76.0	72.0	73.0	79.0	75.5

The six men with other chest disease unrelated to asbestos and the two men with a mean score for pulmonary fibrosis of less than 1/1, but with no pleural abnormality, are not considered further in this study. The age distribution and the mean ages and heights of the other groups are similar. Only eleven men were found to have a mean score of or greater than 1/1 for pulmonary fibrosis because the subjects were selected on the basis of pleural abnormality.

With the exception of one man with rhonchi and another with early finger clubbing, the men with normal chest radiographs were free from abnormal physical signs in the chest and were considered to be reasonably representative of normal healthy men. They are therefore referred to as the normal group.

Table 2 shows the mean values for pulmonary function in each of the five main groups. The values for $FEV_{1 \cdot 0}$, FVC, TLC and DCO have been adjusted to the mean age and height of the study population. The results show that pulmonary fibrosis, diffuse pleural thickening and pleural plaques are all associated with significantly lower values for lung function at rest and higher values for the ventilatory cost of exercise than the normal group. Diffuse pleural thickening is accompanied by worse lung function than pleural plaques, but the results for those with pleural calcification are close to and not significantly different from the results for the normal men. The mean values for $Cf_{1 \cdot 0}$ are similar in each group.

Although the 194 men were all able to attain an oxygen uptake of 1.0 l. min^{-1}, 31 (15.9%) were unable to attain an oxygen uptake of 1.5 l. min^{-1}, so that $\dot{V}E_{1 \cdot 5}$ and $Cf_{1 \cdot 5}$ could not be obtained by interpolation for these men. It was, however, noted that for the men in each group who did attain $\dot{V}E_{1 \cdot 5}$, the ratios between the means for $\dot{V}E_{1 \cdot 0}$ and $\dot{V}E_{1 \cdot 5}$ were almost exactly 1 to 1.5. Because of this finding $\dot{V}E_{1 \cdot 5}$ and $Cf_{1 \cdot 5}$ have been omitted from these results.

TABLE 2. MEAN VALUES FOR LUNG FUNCTION BY RADIOLOGICAL ABNORMALITY

Test		Pulmonary fibrosis	Diffuse pl. th.	Pleural plaques	Pleural calc.	Normal
$FEV_{1\cdot0}$	l.	2.45***	2.71***	3.06**	3.31	3.39
FVC	l.	3.33***	3.78***	4.07**	4.37	4.41
FEV/FVC%		75	72*	75	76	77
TLC	l.	5.20***	5.37***	6.07*	6.22	6.35
DCO	mmol min^{-1} kPa^{-1}	6.60***	8.14***	9.08*	9.41	9.85
$\dot{V}E_{1\cdot0}$	l. min^{-1}	29.7***	26.8*	26.4*	24.3	24.4
V_{t30}	l.	1.18***	1.33***	1.35***	1.48	1.53
Dyspnoeic Index at $\dot{V}E_{1\cdot0}$%		37***	28***	26**	24	20
$Cf_{1\cdot0}$	min^{-1}	103	101	108	103	104
$n =$		11	48	46	40	41

$P < 0.001$ = ***, < 0.01 = **, < 0.05 = * — In comparison with the normal group.

In order to examine the possibility that deficiencies in lung function associated with pleural abnormality merely reflected the amount of underlying pulmonary fibrosis, the men in these groups were subdivided into those with either a mean score of 1/0 for pulmonary fibrosis, cyanosis, rales, or clubbing, who were considered to have possible pulmonary fibrosis, and those with none of these characteristics, who were considered to have no evidence of pulmonary fibrosis.

Table 3 shows, with only three exceptions, that those with possible pulmonary fibrosis have worse lung function at rest and on exercise than those with no evidence of

TABLE 3. MEAN VALUES FOR PLEURAL ABNORMALITY WITH (+) AND WITHOUT (−) EVIDENCE OF POSSIBLE PULMONARY FIBROSIS

Test		Diffuse		Plaques		Calcification		Normal
		+	−	+	−	+	−	
$FEV_{1\cdot0}$	l.	2.49	2.79	3.10	3.04	3.19	3.35	3.39
FVC	l.	3.69	3.81	3.96	4.10	4.15	4.46	4.41
TLC	l.	5.10	5.48	5.89	6.09	6.03	6.30	6.35
DCO	mmol min^{-1} kPa^{-1}	8.04	9.68	8.41	9.28	9.28	9.48	9.85
$\dot{V}E_{1\cdot0}$	l. min^{-1}	28.1	26.4	28.4	25.8	23.9	24.4	24.4
V_{t30}	l.	1.24	1.37	1.31	1.36	1.49	1.47	1.53
Dyspnoeic. Index at $\dot{V}E_{1\cdot0}$%		32	27	28	25	23	23	20
$Cf_{1\cdot0}$	min^{-1}	101	101	108	108	101	104	104
$n =$		13	35	10	36	12	28	41

pulmonary fibrosis. The positions are reversed in the cases of pleural plaques for $FEV_{1\cdot0}$ and pleural calcification for $\dot{V}E_{1\cdot0}$ and V_{t30}, but in each the corresponding values are very close. Diffuse pleural thickening without evidence of pulmonary fibrosis is still associated with more functional abnormality than pleural plaques, but the results for pleural calcification, with and without evidence of pulmonary fibrosis, are very similar to those for the normal group. $Cf_{1\cdot0}$ is again similar for each group.

Asbestos Exposure

The relationship between lung function and asbestos exposure was examined by correlating individual values for $FEV_{1\cdot0}$ and $\dot{V}E_{1\cdot0}$ with the numbers of years of asbestos exposure and the numbers of years since first exposure to asbestos.

TABLE 4. CORRELATIONS BETWEEN LUNG FUNCTION AND ASBESTOS EXPOSURE FOR PLEURAL ABNORMALITY WITH AND WITHOUT EVIDENCE OF PULMONARY FIBROSIS

Test	Exposure	Diffuse		Plaques		Calcification		Normal
		With	Without	With	Without	With	Without	
$FEV_{1\cdot0}$	Years of exposure	+0.29	+0.12	−0.50	−0.30	+0.74	−0.19	−0.37
	Years since first exposure	+0.36	+0.16	−0.69	−0.10	+0.58	−0.11	−0.16
$\dot{V}E_{1\cdot0}$	Years of exposure	−0.13	+0.64	+0.50	−0.04	−0.20	+0.31	+0.003
	Years since first exposure	−0.06	+0.21	+0.91	+0.07	−0.04	+0.32	+0.05
$n =$		13	35	10	36	12	28	41

Although the correlations in Table 4 vary in strength, the slopes of the relationships suggest that $FEV_{1\cdot0}$ tends to decline and $\dot{V}E_{1\cdot0}$ to increase with both years of exposure and years since first exposure to asbestos in those with pleural plaques, pleural calcification without pulmonary fibrosis and the normal group. In the cases of diffuse pleural thickening and pleural calcification with possible pulmonary fibrosis, however, these trends tend to be reversed. There is no evidence from these results to suggest that $FEV_{1\cdot0}$ is better correlated with exposure than $\dot{V}E_{1\cdot0}$.

DISCUSSION

The findings show, as expected, that pulmonary fibrosis is accompanied by more functional abnormality than any of the pleural changes, and this is supported by the comparison between pleural abnormalities with and without evidence of possible pulmonary fibrosis. The results also show that diffuse pleural thickening is associated with substantially more adverse functional change than pleural plaques, and that pleural calcification is not accompanied by any significant functional abnormality.

The mean values for $\dot{V}E_{1\cdot0}$ and $Cf_{1\cdot0}$ for the normal group are close to normal values reported elsewhere (COTES, 1968; ROSSITER and WEILL, 1974), and the constancy of the ratio between $\dot{V}E_{1\cdot0}$ and $\dot{V}E_{1\cdot5}$ also agrees with the findings of the latter study. It implies that $\dot{V}E_{1\cdot0}$ is just as valuable an index as $\dot{V}E_{1\cdot5}$, which is important because $\dot{V}E_{1\cdot0}$ has the advantages of being both easier and safer for the subject to attain, because the risk of developing a dangerous arrhythmia increases with the increase in cardiac frequency required to reach $\dot{V}E_{1\cdot5}$.

The correlations between $FEV_{1\cdot0}$ and $\dot{V}E_{1\cdot0}$ with asbestos exposure show an interesting reversal of the expected trends for those with diffuse pleural thickening. A dust-exposure relationship is likely to be found for abnormalities, such as pleural plaques and calcification, which tend to develop gradually. Diffuse pleural thickening, on the other hand, is likely to result from a pleural reaction. This is a relatively sudden event, sometimes occurring in younger men who have been exposed to asbestos, which may help to explain the trends of the correlations in this group.

It is considered that of the three types of non-malignant pleural abnormality, diffuse pleural thickening is more likely to be accompanied by functional abnormality than pleural plaques and that pleural calcification, which is the most easily recognized type of pleural abnormality, is also the least likely to be associated with functional impairment.

Acknowledgements—I am grateful for the permission of the Medical Director General (Naval) to submit this article for publication. I also wish to thank Dr J. Heath, Mrs C. Ferris, and Mrs V. Welford for carrying out the lung function tests, Surgeon Commander P. G. Harries and Dr G.Sheers for reading the chest radiographs, Mr C. E. Rossiter for statistical advice, Mrs P. Turner for typing the manuscript, and the subjects for their participation in the study.

REFERENCES

BECKLAKE, M. R., FOURNIER-MASSEY, G., MCDONALD, J. C., SIEMIATYCKI, J. and ROSSITER, C. E (1970) *Bull. Physiopath. resp.* **6**, 637–659.

COTES, J. E. (1968) *Lung Function*, 2nd edn., p. 390. Blackwell, Oxford and Edinburgh.

COTES, J. E. (1972) *Br. J. Dis. Chest* **66**, 169–183.

HARRIES, P. G. (1970) *The Effects and Control of Diseases Associated with Exposure to Asbestos in a Naval Dockyard.* M. D. Thesis, London.

HARRIES, P. G., MACKENZIE, F. A. F., SHEERS, G., KEMP, J. H., OLIVER, T. P. and WRIGHT, D. S. (1972) *Br. J. ind. Med.* **29**, 274–279.

HURWITZ, M. (1961) *Am. J. Roentgenol.* **85**, 256–262.

INDUSTRIAL INJURIES ADVISORY COUNCIL (1973) *Pneumoconiosis and Byssinosis*, p. 32. Cmmd. 5443. H.M.S.O., London.

I.L.O./U.C. (1971) *International Classification of Radiographs of Pneumoconioses*, Occupational Safety and Health Series No. 22. International Labour Office, Geneva.

JONES, J. S. P. and SHEERS, G. (1973) *Biological Effects of Asbestos* (edited by BOGOVSKI, P., GILSON, J. C., TIMBRELL, V. and WAGNER, J. C.) pp. 243–248. Scientific Publications No. 8. International Agency for Research on Cancer, Lyon.

MEDICAL RESEARCH COUNCIL Committee on Research into Chronic Bronchitis (1966) *Questionnaire on Respiratory Symptoms*, Medical Research Council, London.

ROSSITER, C. E. and WEILL, H. (1974) *Int. J. Epidemiol.* **3**, 55–61.

SHEERS, G. and TEMPLETON, A. R. (1968) *Br. med. J.* **3**, 574–579.

DISCUSSION

R. A. FRANCIS: Why did you use $\dot{V}E_{1\cdot0}$ instead of $\dot{V}E_{1\cdot5}$?

Surg. Cdr LUMLEY: Most of the subjects were able to attain $\dot{V}E_{1\cdot5}$ but thirty-one, or 15.9%, were not. However, for those who attained both levels of oxygen uptake, the ratios between the means were exactly 1 to 1.5 in each group with pleural abnormality. This implied that $\dot{V}E_{1\cdot0}$, which is easier and safer for the subject, was as useful an index as $\dot{V}E_{1\cdot5}$. I therefore decided to omit $\dot{V}E_{1\cdot5}$ from the results.

C.-J. GÖTHE: Have you noticed any correlation between diffuse pleural thickening and body weight and, if so, could obesity explain some of the physiological changes in the group with diffuse pleural thickening?

Surg. Cdr LUMLEY: We did look at this briefly but there was very little correlation. The measurement of exercise ventilation at standardized oxygen uptake is for practical purposes independent of body weight.

J. C. McDONALD: Our findings in Quebec chrysotile miners and millers were essentially the same as yours. However, I wonder whether parenchymal changes are equally visible in persons with diffuse pleural thickening as in those without. Have you any information on this?

Surg. Cdr LUMLEY: I agree that it can be difficult to assess parenchymal change in the presence of diffuse pleural abnormality. We did our best to cope with this problem. I can't say more than that.

G. L. LEATHART: It has been my experience that men with diffuse pleural fibrosis have a good prognosis. Serial measurements over periods of up to 15 years do not as a rule show any deterioration. What has been your experience in the follow-up of these men?

Secondly, since you raised the question of compensation, may I make the point that many members of the public regard the diagnosis of asbestosis as equivalent to a death sentence. In view of this, and the relatively good prognosis in diffuse pleural fibrosis, do you not think that the automatic award of compensation for pleural fibrosis might do more harm than good?

Surg. Cdr LUMLEY: My experience is that men with pleural reactions tend to have some functional impairment which tends to improve after the period of active pleural reaction has passed, but a small number are left with a persisting functional defect, and I think that there is a case for compensating these individuals.

J. C. GILSON: The I.L.O./U.C. classification does not separate diffuse and plaque-like thickening of the pleura. This is being done in the modified classification now being used in a survey of asbestosis in our dockyard population in the U.K. We hope the results of this survey will answer Dr McDonald's question.

DIFFERENCES IN LUNG EFFECTS RESULTING FROM CHRYSOTILE AND CROCIDOLITE EXPOSURE

H. WEILL, C. E. ROSSITER, C. WAGGENSPACK, R. N. JONES and M. M. ZISKIND

Tulane University Medical Center, New Orleans, La., U.S.A.

Abstract—Crocidolite asbestos exposure may carry a greater risk for the development of lung and pleural tumours than chrysotile exposure, although differences in regard to lung fibrosis have not previously been demonstrated. Clinical, radiographic and physiological indicators of lung disease were related to qualitative and quantitative estimates of past total dust exposure in two groups of workers who had spent 20 to 30 years in the asbestos cement industry. One group had exposure to chrysotile, silica and crocidolite in the pipe-making area; the other group had no crocidolite exposure. Crocidolite exposure was related to the prevalence of small irregular opacities and pleural thickening but not to small rounded opacities. The "crocidolite" group had significantly smaller lung volumes, lower forced expiratory flows, and reduced pulmonary diffusion. Finger clubbing was the only clinical finding significantly more prevalent in the crocidolite-exposed workers. It is suggested that crocidolite exposure has a greater fibrogenic effect on the lungs than a similar total exposure to chrysotile asbestos.

INTRODUCTION

In recent years, epidemiological studies have established dose–response relationships between asbestos exposure in various industrial processes and resulting health effects. These relationships have been demonstrated in mining and milling of asbestos (ROSSITER *et al.*, 1972), and in asbestos–cement product manufacture (WEILL *et al.*, 1975), where the indicators of an adverse biological response have included radiographic abnormalities and impaired pulmonary function in currently employed workers. Mortality statistics have demonstrated a dose-related excess risk for the development of malignant disease among individuals occupationally exposed to asbestos with variation between types of industry (ENTERLINE and KENDRICK, 1967; MCDONALD *et al.*, 1971). Fewer data are available concerning the possibility that differing fibre types may have qualitatively or quantitatively distinct effects in human exposure to asbestos. Available information suggests that crocidolite and perhaps other amphiboles constitute a greater exposure hazard in regard to the development of malignant tumours of the lung and pleura (ENTERLINE and HENDERSON, 1973). The influence of fibre type on the development of diffuse pulmonary fibrosis or asbestosis has not been determined. The primary problem in this regard has been the difficulty in identifying specific fibre exposures in workers. This report is addressed to the question of whether the addition of crocidolite exposure is more likely to result in diffuse lung and pleural changes when compared to similar total asbestos exposure to chrysotile alone.

POPULATION AND METHODS

The presented data are obtained from a larger study of the health effects associated with exposure to dust in the asbestos–cement products manufacturing industry. Components of this investigation include a prevalence study of over 900 currently employed workers, a cohort of 300 workers who are being studied longitudinally, and a mortality study of some 7000 past workers of this industry.

The workers in this investigation have had a mixed dust exposure, the primary components being chrysotile and crocidolite asbestos and free crystalline silica. Two exposed populations have been studied, one in a plant manufacturing only shingles, and a second in a plant producing shingles, flooring and asbestos–cement pipe. The pipe operation in the second plant was the primary source of exposure to crocidolite asbestos in that plant, this type of fibre being utilized in addition to chrysotile, silica and cement to constitute the final product. In the shingle manufacturing operation, crocidolite-containing pressure pipe regrind was at times added to the mix between 1960 and 1971, when crocidolite-free shingle or non-pressure pipe regrind was not available. The cumulative crocidolite exposure in the shingle plant cannot be quantitated but is considered to be quite low. Complete work histories on each study participant made it possible to identify those workers who had been engaged in asbestos–cement pipe manufacturing for specified varying portions of their time in the industry. Individual past dust-exposure indexes were reconstructed on the basis of this work history and dust sampling data, collected over 20 years by the industry and state and federal agencies. Past dust measurements were made primarily through the use of the midget impinger with results expressed in million particles per cubic foot (mppcf). Individual product formulation allowed estimates of component dust proportion to be made (e.g. crocidolite or silica). Total and constituent dust estimates were made for each of several hundred job titles at the two plants for different time periods. Temporal changes in dust levels were obtained from the past dust-sampling data and confirmed that dust-control measures resulted in reduced airborne dust levels. Using the detailed occupational history that had been abstracted for each worker, total dust and component exposures for an individual were calculated by multiplying the dust-exposure level of each job by the time spent in the job. The individual results were totalled for all jobs and expressed in mppcf-years. It was therefore possible to identify two groups of workers who had spent 20 to 30 years in the industry; one group containing individuals who had worked for at least 75% of their time in the pipe area, and another group comprising workers who had never worked in that area. Biological indicators of diffuse pulmonary disease were assessed for inter-group differences and correlated with dust-exposure characteristics.

Chest X-ray films were classified according to the I.L.O. U/C International Classification for Pneumoconiosis by three experienced readers, resulting in a consensus reading.

Pulmonary function measurements included determination of lung volumes, expiratory flow rates, alveolar gas transfer and ventilation at standardized levels of exercise. Expiratory flows and volumes were determined with a water-sealed spirometer with calculations of vital capacity (VC), forced vital capacity (FVC), forced expiratory volume in 1 second (FEV_1), FEV_1/VC, and forced expiratory flow 25–75%

(FEF 25–75%). Functional residual capacity (FRC) was determined by a closed-circuit helium dilution method with calculation of residual volume (RV) accomplished by subtraction of the expiratory reserve volume obtained during the equilibration procedure, and of total lung capacity (TLC) by addition of VC to RV. Pulmonary diffusing capacity (D_{CO}) was measured by the breath-holding carbon monoxide technique using an automated apparatus for timing of events and valve sequencing by which inspired, alveolar, and washout volumes as well as breath-holding time are pre-set. Diffusion constant (K_{CO}) was calculated as a ratio of D_{CO} to alveolar volume (V_A) obtained by dilution of the inert gas during the single breath manoeuvre. Ventilation during two levels of exercise was corrected to standardized levels of oxygen uptake (V_{O_2}) of 1.0 and 1.5 litres per minute.

A standardized interviewer-administered questionnaire and limited physical examination provided clinical data.

RESULTS

TABLE 1. EXPOSURE AND OTHER CHARACTERISTICS OF MEN EMPLOYED IN ASBESTOS CEMENT PLANT FOR 20–30 YEARS

	75% or more in pipe area	Never worked in pipe area
Number	108	100
Age	49	52
Years of exposure	22.8	23.0
Total dust*	324	290
Crocidolite*	7.7	0.6
Chrysotile*	48	52
Silica*	120	78
Smoking prevalence (%)	51	51

* In mppcf-yr.

Table 1 indicates exposure and other characteristics of two groups of workers having maximum and minimum exposure to crocidolite in the plant containing the pipe area. These groups are comparable in regard to years of employment, total dust and chrysotile exposure, and smoking prevalence. The pipe-area employees were significantly younger. In addition to the differing crocidolite exposure, which was 13 times as high in the first group, this group had one and one-half times the silica exposure, a difference which will be discussed again later. Table 2 demonstrates selected radiographic findings in these two groups. While there was no significant difference in the prevalence of small rounded opacities, category 1/1 or above, a significantly higher prevalence of small irregular opacities of the same category was found in workers who had been employed in the pipe area for over 75% of their time in the industry. Similarly, pleural thickening of grade 1 or above was twice as prevalent in the "crocidolite" group as in those who had never worked in the pipe area. These differences in prevalence of small irregular opacities and pleural thickening are statistically significant and cannot be explained by their distribution in total dust, chrysotile or silica groups or years of exposure.

In order to determine if a dose–response relationship exists between crocidolite

TABLE 2. RADIOGRAPHIC CHARACTERISTICS

	75% or more in pipe area (108)	Never worked in pipe area (100)	
Small rounded opacities 1/1+	6 (5.6%)	4 (4%)	N.S.
Small irregular opacities 1/1+	11 (10.2%)	2 (2%)	$P = 0.02$
Pleural thickening 1+	34 (31%)	15 (15%)	$P = 0.006$

exposure and radiographic abnormalities, as well as to assess the possibility that the higher silica exposure in the pipe area accounted for the differences in prevalence of radiographic abnormalities, the groups have been expanded to four, with decreasing crocidolite exposure but with an increase in silica exposure in the last group. Figure 1 illustrates the exposure characteristics of these four groups: (a) more than 75% of time in the pipe area, (b) less than 75% in the the pipe area, (c) maintenance workers with minimal intermittent exposure to crocidolite, and (d) employees never in the pipe area or engaged in maintenance and who were considered to have minimal crocidolite exposure. The overall exposure pattern indicates steadily decreasing crocidolite

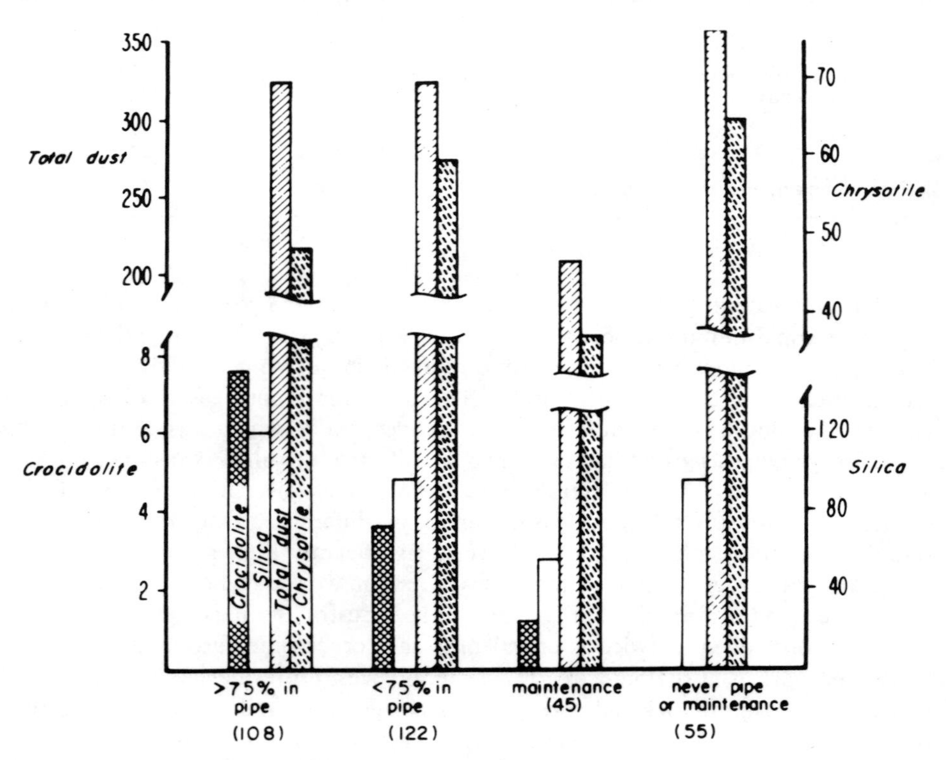

FIG. 1. Dust exposures (mppcf-yr).

exposure from the first to the fourth group, while the lowest total dust, chrysotile and silica exposures occur in the third group with an upturn of these exposures in group 4. It is this fourth group which will allow the separation of silica and crocidolite effects on the type of small opacity seen on the chest X-ray film. Average years of dust exposure was constant in the four groups while average age was lowest in the first group with highest crocidolite exposure.

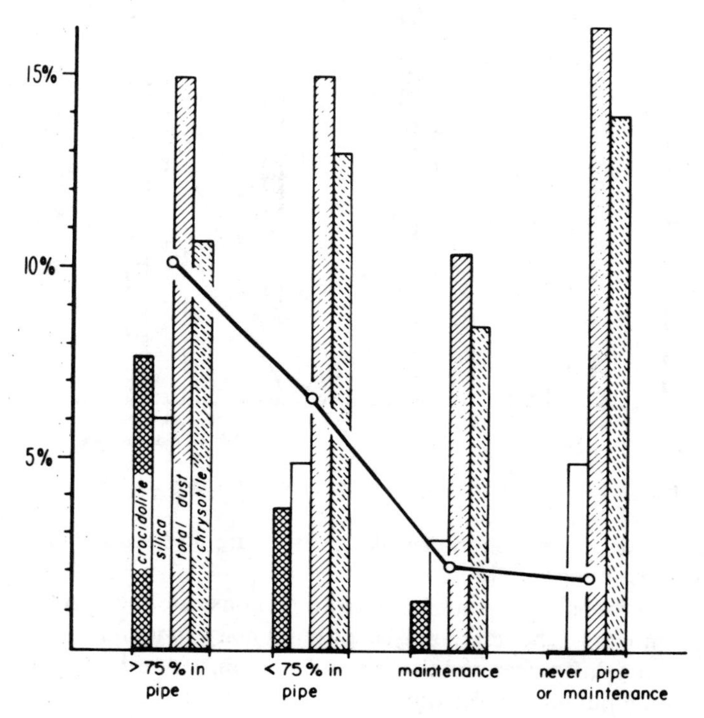

FIG. 2. Prevalences of small irregular opacities (Category 1/1 +).

Figure 2 displays the prevalence of small irregular opacities category 1/1 or above, for these four groups, with the group exposure characteristics shown as background. It seems clear that small irregular opacities relate best to level of crocidolite exposure and less impressively to total dust, chrysotile and silica. This finding is particularly significant since on separate analysis of the entire study population, prevalence of small irregular opacities correlates significantly with increasing age. Therefore, the younger crocidolite-exposed group would be expected to have a lower, not higher prevalence of this type opacity on the basis of age alone. A similar plot in Fig. 3 indicates that small rounded opacities, category 1/1 or above, correlate best with total dust, chrysotile and silica but not with extent of crocidolite exposure. Attention is directed to the fourth group where the lowest prevalence of small irregular opacities is associated with minimal crocidolite exposure, while an increase in prevalence of small rounded opacities is associated with an upturn in the levels of total dust, silica and chrysotile exposure. These analyses indicate that the differences shown in Table 2 are indeed

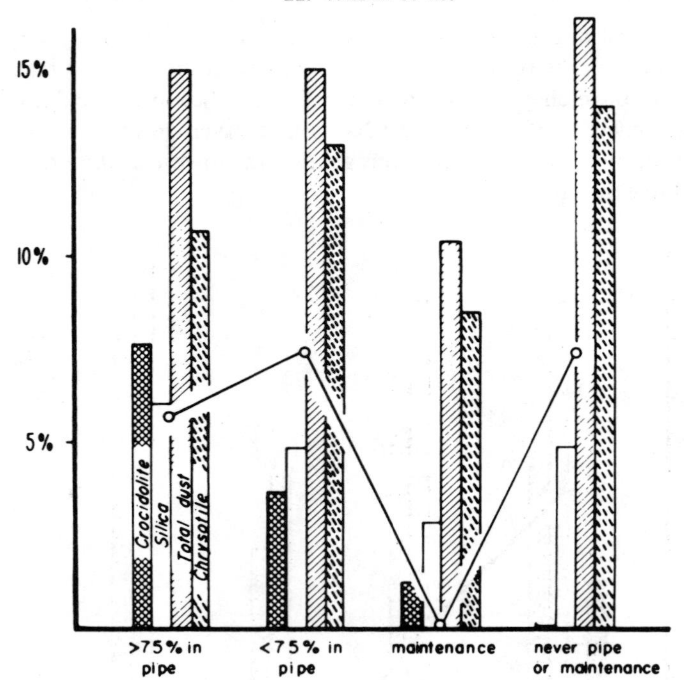

FIG. 3. Prevalences of small rounded opacities (Category 1/1 +).

related to the marked difference in crocidolite exposure and are not likely to be the result of the modest difference in exposure to silica.

The two initial groups are again employed to demonstrate the effect of crocidolite exposure on pulmonary function. Analysis of pulmonary function took into account demonstrated ethnic differences and the effect of smoking. In order to assess the effect of dust exposure on pulmonary function, a "standard group" comprised 244 workers who had minimal exposure to dust and who had no major respiratory symptoms or radiographic changes. Average lung function values in the various exposure groups

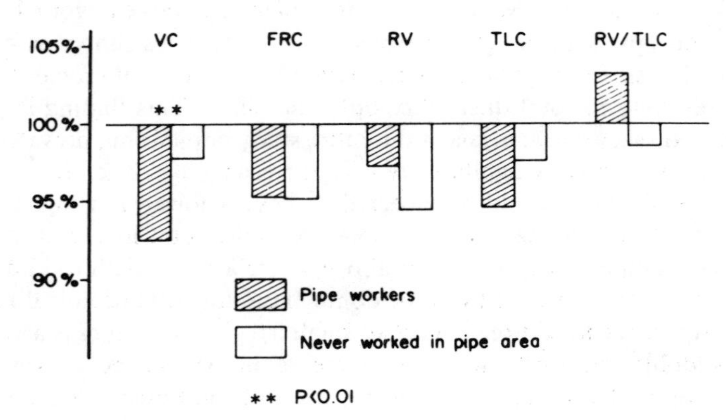

FIG. 4. Lung volumes (percentage of standardized values).

are compared to average values in the standard group, the latter always having average standardized values of 100% with the expected value for any other group similarly being 100%. This standard group also provided regressions for age and height, with all individual values being corrected for these variables.

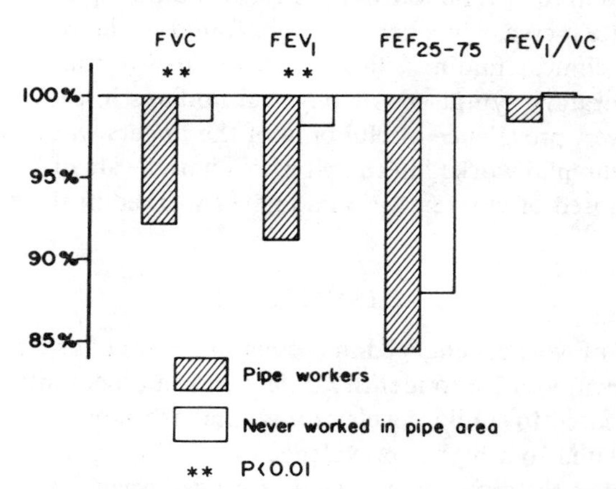

FIG. 5. Expiratory flow rates (percentage of standardized values).

Figure 4 reveals that the average vital capacity is significantly lower in the workers with past employment in the pipe area than in those who had never worked in that area. Total lung capacity is marginally lower in the "crocidolite" group, with residual volume and residual volume to total lung capacity ratio being slightly higher in the pipe area workers.

Figure 5 demonstrates that forced vital capacity and forced expiratory volume in 1 second are significantly lower in the crocidolite-exposed workers, while forced expiratory flow 25–75%, and the forced expiratory volume/vital capacity ratio, reveal the same trend, indicating greater maximum expiratory flow limitation in the crocidolite-exposed individuals. Figure 6 reveals that the pulmonary diffusing capacity (transfer factor) is significantly lower in the pipe-area workers but that this reduction is

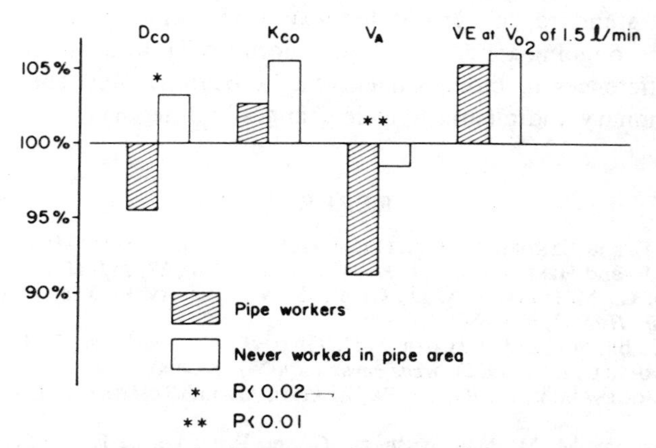

FIG. 6. Gas transfer (percentage of standardized values).

primarily the result of a significantly lower alveolar volume and is less related to the diffusion constant. No difference in total ventilation at a standardized oxygen uptake of 1.5 litres per minute was noted between the groups. Further analyses again indicated that the differences in lung function were related to differing crocidolite exposure and not to the moderate increase in silica exposure found in the pipe area.

On analysis of clinical findings, little correlation was found between crocidolite exposure and respiratory symptoms or physical findings in the chest, including rales. In contrast, however, prevalence of clubbing of the fingers was significantly higher in those employees who had worked in the pipe area with a rate of 11% compared to 3% in the group composed of workers who had never worked in the pipe area.

DISCUSSION

In a population of workers engaged in the manufacture of asbestos–cement building products, it has been possible to identify differences in crocidolite exposure in groups who have been exposed to similar levels of total and asbestos dust. Increasing crocidolite exposure is related to a higher prevalence of small irregular opacities and pleural thickening, but not to the prevalence of small rounded opacities. Reduction in average values of lung volumes, flow rates and gas transfer (primarily volume effect) was detected in the crocidolite-exposed workers. These differences in radiographic and pulmonary functional changes were attributed to crocidolite exposure after separate analyses had excluded the possibility that these findings were associated with differing age, years of exposure, total dust, chrysotile or silica. The clinical differences were limited to the finding that clubbing was more prevalent in the crocidolite–exposed group. This study confirms our earlier finding that small irregular opacities are associated with a more profound effect on lung function than are small rounded opacities (WEILL *et al.*, 1973), and seems to demonstrate for the first time that these indicators of a diffuse fibrogenic effect in the lungs are more likely to result in crocidolite-exposed workers than in those with an equivalent exposure to only chrysotile fibre. In addition to the evidence of a greater hazard for the development of malignant disease in crocidolite-exposed workers, these data support a separate and more stringent occupational standard for crocidolite exposure, limiting its use for commercial purposes. The ongoing longitudinal and mortality studies will provide further data regarding differences in biological effect of crocidolite and chrysotile exposure as regards pulmonary and pleural fibrotic changes and neoplasia.

REFERENCES

ENTERLINE, P. E. and KENDRICK, M. A. (1967) *Archs envir. Hlth* **15,** 181–186.
ENTERLINE, P. E. and HENDERSON, V. (1973) *Archs envir. Hlth* **27,** 312–317.
MCDONALD, J. C., MCDONALD, A. D., GIBBS, G. W., SIEMIATYCKI, J. and ROSSITER, C. E. (1971) *Archs envir. Hlth* **22,** 677–686.
ROSSITER, C. E., BRISTOL, L. J., CARTIER, P. H., GILSON, J. G., GRAINGER, T. R., SLUIS-CREMER, G. K. and MCDONALD, J. C. (1972) *Archs envir. Hlth* **24,** 388–400.
WEILL, H., WAGGENSPACK, C., BAILEY, W., ZISKIND, M. and ROSSITER, C. (1973) *J. occup. Med.* **15,** 248–252.
WEILL, H., ZISKIND, M. M., WAGGENSPACK, C. and ROSSITER, C. E. (1975) *Archs envir. Hlth* **30,** 88–97.

DISCUSSION

J. C. McDonald: Exposures were primarily measured in particle counts by midget impinger. Have you any information on fibre counts in the two areas?

Dr Weill: All our environmental information is based on total particles using the impinger method. I have no clue at this time concerning possible differences in proportion of fibrous dust in the two areas.

S. Holmes: You state that individual product formulation allowed estimates of component dust proportions to be made. This is unacceptable—proportions of different components in the airborne dust cloud often bear no relation to those in the original products.

Dr Weill: I accept that it makes the analysis less precise than one would have liked, but it's all we had and there is some correlation I would think.

D. F. K. Liddell: How was a "consensus reading" defined?

Mr Rossiter: The "consensus reading" was in fact the median of the three readings for each feature of the classification. The term is perhaps incorrect and one of the problems of translation from American to English.

P. D. Oldham: The word "consensus" in this context suggests a discussion among readers and an eventual agreed decision, but you have used it to imply a statistical average of the individual readings. I feel we should be very watchful in epidemiological work and ask what, in a particular instance, this somewhat emotive word actually means.

D. F. K. Liddell: You have described results separately for rounded and for irregular small opacities. How did you treat cases with combined opacities?

Dr Weill: When both types of opacities are present, both are read and counted and the profusion is related to the specific type of opacity reported. If there was a category 2 of irregular and category 1 of rounded they would be reported as such. However, there are undoubtedly difficulties in X-ray reading when both types are present as they are likely to be in the industry which we have studied.

K. Robock: What can you say about the absorption of X-rays by different types of asbestos fibres and the consequent influence on the X-ray picture? I remember the research of SMRE, Sheffield, on the absorption of X-rays by coal-mine dust and the great influence of iron on the X-ray picture.

Secondly, can you exclude the influence of different mechanical treatments of the silica in groups 1 and 4. Our experiments show that such treatment can lead to a marked change in the fibrogenic activity of silica.

Dr Weill: Thank you for those comments. I don't have any evidence or information on the points you have mentioned. I wouldn't think it very likely that they have much influence on the differences that we have seen, but it is a fascinating point.

H. Ayer: Asbestos textile workers studied by the National Institute for Occupational Safety and Health showed losses in FVC_{obs}/FVC_{pred} as shown in Fig. D1. The differences caused by smoking may

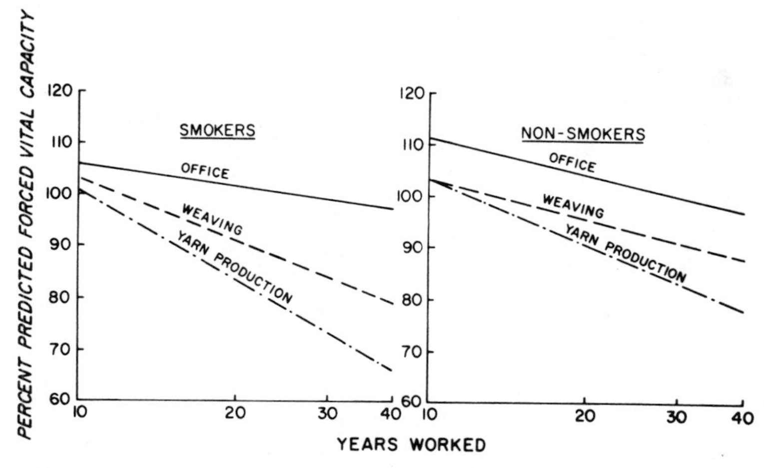

Fig. D1. Percentage of predicted forced vital capacity *vs*. years worked. Five asbestos textile mills.

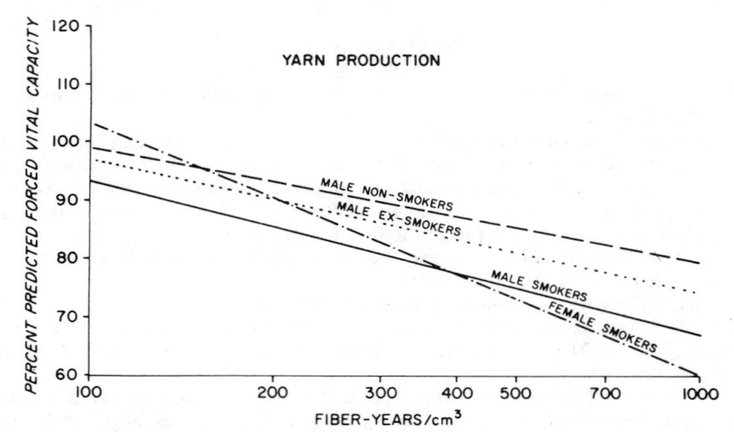

FIG. D2. Percentage of predicted forced vital capacity *vs.* cumulative asbestos dust exposure. Yarn production workers in five asbestos textile mills.

be seen from the relatively non-exposed office workers. Only workers with more than 10 years experience are shown. The regression on cumulative exposure (log scale) is shown in Fig. D2. Are these losses of 5 to 10% in fraction of predicted FVC for each doubling of exposure consistent with your observations on asbestos cement workers exposed to chrysotile only?

Dr WEILL: I don't think the losses we found were quite that great. Doubling the exposure caused a drop in FEV_1 of about 200 ml, and the figure for FVC would be about the same.

R. G. LOVE: Do you have any comment on the fact that there were no significant differences in the $FEF_{25-75}\%$ in your study groups, whereas there were such differences in VC_1, FVC and FEV_1, since it has been mentioned that the former measurement is a more sensitive indicator of deterioration of lung function?

Dr WEILL: I don't know how to interpret it. Perhaps it is related to the level of airways response, but I would not want to make a judgement on the limited data here.

RADIOLOGICAL CHANGES OVER 20 YEARS IN RELATION TO CHRYSOTILE EXPOSURE IN QUEBEC

DOUGLAS LIDDELL, GAIL EYSSEN, DUNCAN THOMAS and CORBETT McDONALD

Department of Epidemiology and Health, McGill University, Montreal, Canada

Abstract—Radiological changes in 267 male Quebec chrysotile mine and mill workers, each with five chest films spanning an average of 20 years, were related to age, smoking habit, mining area, duration of employment and average dust concentration before and between films.

(1) Abnormality in the earliest film was related mainly to the time since first employment. (2) In 45 (30%) of the 150 men completely normal at earliest film, some radiological abnormality developed during the period of observation: incidence was weakly related to age; in Asbestos, the risk of developing small opacities was lower in smokers than in non-smokers. (3) There was an irregular pattern of correlation, more evident in Thetford Mines than in Asbestos, between radiological progression and various stimulus variables.

That associations between radiological responses and measures of asbestos exposure were, as always, weak, despite powerful methodology, indicates that effects are obscured by other factors (including susceptibility) uncorrelated with exposure.

1. INTRODUCTION

The chest X-ray is an important tool in epidemiological studies of the pneumoconioses (WEILL and JONES, 1975), but in surveys of asbestosis its use has usually been cross-sectional. Thus, the type and severity of radiological abnormality in persons with varied occupational histories have been related to duration of exposure to asbestos and to other factors. The correlations have not been high, but there has generally been a fairly definite gradient in prevalence of various abnormalities in relation to indices of past exposure. For example, our own group reported (ROSSITER *et al.*, 1972) on 6127 male asbestos production workers in Quebec aged 36 to 65. In one of the two mining areas (Thetford Mines), the age-standardized prevalence of irregular small opacities (grade 1/0 or more) showed a strictly monotonic relationship with an index of total dust exposure; the prevalence was 1.8% in men with the least exposure and 17.2% in those with the highest. However, the coefficient of correlation between radiological score and exposure was only 0.27 (although the largest recorded).

The present study aimed to investigate relationships between radiological change assessed over approximately 20 years and exposure to chrysotile asbestos. It formed part of a comprehensive programme of epidemiological research into the health of workers in Quebec's chrysotile-producing industry, where presently some 6000 miners and millers are employed in two areas, Asbestos and Thetford Mines.

2. MATERIALS

Workers in the Quebec asbestos-producing industry have been subject to annual postero-anterior chest radiography since 1936 in Asbestos and since 1946 in Thetford Mines. The most recent film, to 1966, for each of the 13021 men ever X-rayed was studied by ROSSITER and his colleagues (1972). For the present investigation, these men were stratified by place of work, length of employment and whether there was evidence of radiological abnormality or not. A random sample, with large sampling fraction, was drawn from each stratum containing abnormal films; a small random sample was drawn from the other strata. For each of the 283 men selected in this way, we collected the most recent film available, to 1971, together with four earlier films taken at intervals of about 5 years, to form a quinquennial pentad (LIDDELL, 1974). In what follows, the term *earliest film* relates to the earliest included in the study and is not necessarily the man's first X-ray in the industry.

Each pentad was assessed, side-by-side in known temporal sequence, by an international panel of four readers.† The scales of abnormality of the I.L.O. U/Ç 1971 classification (I.L.O., 1972) were extended by four-fold elaboration for the following five features: rounded and irregular small opacities (50 points to each scale), width and extent of pleural thickening (14 points each), ill-defined cardiac outline (18 points); the remaining radiographic features were assessed using the scales of the international classification (EYSSEN, 1975). In addition, the four readers examined the films after they had all been intermixed into a single random order: here, assessment was on the (complete) I.L.O. U/C 1971 scales.

Each man's history of employment in the Quebec asbestos industry had been collected

TABLE 1. CRITERIA OF NORMALITY AND OF ATTACK

Feature	Normality	Attack
	All four readers agreed:	*At least three readers agreed:*
Small opacities	both rounded and irregular scored no more than 9* (upper limit of 0/0)	either rounded or irregular scored 13* or more (lower limit of 1/0)**
Pleural thickening	both width and extent scored 0* (not present)	either width or extent scored 2* or more (lower limit of width b or extent 1)
Ill-defined cardiac outline	scored no more than 2* (upper limit of "not present")	scored 5* or more (lower limit of Grade 1)
Obliterated costophrenic angle	absent	present
Ill-defined diaphragm	absent	present
Pleural calcification	absent	present

* On scales elaborated four-fold over the I.L.O. U/C classification; equivalents on the I.L.O. U/C scales are given in brackets.

** For a further study, the criterion was that at least three readers agreed either rounded or irregular small opacities scored 25* or more (lower limit of 2/1).

† Dr L. J. Bristol (U.S.A.), Dr P. H. Cartier (Canada), Dr J. C. Gilson (U.K.), Dr G. K. Sluis-Cremer (South Africa).

from company personnel files. Each job had been identified, together with its starting and ending dates, while estimates of the concentration of airborne respirable dust job by job and year by year had been made by GIBBS and LACHANCE (1972). Estimates of a man's dust exposure could therefore be calculated for any defined period of time. No information could be obtained about experience outside the Quebec asbestos industry. This could have had serious repercussions on the dose–response relationships in twelve cases (including some where even the reported history appeared unreliable); these and four where radiographic information was incomplete were excluded. This left 137 men from Asbestos and 130 from Thetford Mines. For all but three of the subjects, information on whether or not a man had ever smoked cigarettes was obtained from the man himself, from his relatives, or from the records of the local industrial medical clinics. These three were treated as smokers, because only 12% of known histories were of non-smokers. We also knew each man's date of birth.

3. METHODS

The analysis took place in three phases. Phase 1 was a "cross-sectional" study of all 267 men, to relate the X-ray status of the earliest film to potential stimuli. The men were then classified into two "cohorts". The first consisted of 150 men whose earliest film studied contained no evidence of abnormality (by the criteria listed in Table 1) by either method of reading; and Phase 2 was a study of "attacks" in this cohort. The second cohort consisted of the other 117 men; and Phase 3 was a study of progression of radiographic abnormality in these men. The radiographic variables for Phases 1 and 3 are defined in Table 2.

TABLE 2. RADIOGRAPHIC VARIABLES FOR CORRELATION STUDIES

Single film (Σ indicates summation over four readers for each film)

Small opacities: $R(\text{so}) = \{(\Sigma \text{ higher score* of profusion}) \cdot (\Sigma \text{ zones recorded as affected†})\}^{\frac{1}{2}}$
Pleural thickening: $\{(\Sigma \text{ width score*}) \cdot (\Sigma \text{ extent score*})\}^{\frac{1}{2}}$
Ill-defined cardiac outline: {Σ score*}
Obliterated costophrenic angle: no. of readers recording its presence
Ill-defined diaphragm: no. of readers recording its presence
Pleural calcification: no. of readers recording its presence

Change from earliest to latest film

Change in a specific feature was determined per unit time by differencing the variables defined above and dividing by t, the interval between the films. For example, for small opacities the variable used was: $\{R(\text{so})_5 - R(\text{so})_1\}/t$ where the subscript indicates the serial order of the film.

* On scales elaborated four-fold over the I.L.O. U/C classification.
† Each zone was counted only once for each reader; for scores* of 9 or less, it was assumed that the opacities were seen in one zone.

All phases were carried out for Asbestos and Thetford Mines separately. They were repeated without such separation; also with replacement of some of the exclusions, and with different combinations of variables. None of these additional studies threw extra light on the subject, and so they are not reported here.

Phase 1. A regression analysis (SOKAL and ROHLF, 1969) was carried out for each of the radiographic variables in the earliest film, relating the degree of abnormality to the following potential stimuli: age at first employment in the Quebec industry; years from first employment to the earliest film; average dust concentration in this period, measured in millions of particles per cubic foot* (Mp/cf); and whether a cigarette smoker or not. Canonical analysis (KENDALL and STUART, 1966) was also carried out on the same variables.

Phase 2. For the 150 men whose earliest films were considered normal, a study was made of the relationships between attacks of abnormality on each feature (as defined in Table 1) and certain stimulus variables. In four cases, the relevant criterion for two or more features was reached simultaneously; these cases were counted as attacks on both features. Once attacked, a man was withdrawn from the cohort so that later attacks of a different type were ignored. However, in a subsequent analysis of "definite" small opacities (profusion of grade 2/1 or more), only attacks of this nature led to withdrawal.

Each man was admitted to the study at the time of his earliest film and followed either until a film showed evidence of an attack or to his last available film. At each attack, the man concerned was compared with all men who had been under observation for at least as long without being attacked. Relative risks for high and low values of each stimulus variable were obtained by the method of MANTEL and BYAR (1974). For discrete stimulus variables no additional problem arose, but for continuous variables it was necessary to dichotomize: the split was made at a point chosen to obtain as equal as possible numbers of expected attacks. Because the exact point of dichotomy can influence significance testing, this purpose was achieved by the method of Cox (1972).

The stimulus variables which were considered for the present purposes were age at the time of the film showing attack, whether a cigarette smoker or not, and dust concentration (Mp/cf) averaged over the period of employment up to 5 years before the presumed point of attack, i.e. up to $7\frac{1}{2}$ years before the point of comparison. Logarithmic transformations were applied to the continuous variables, to fit Cox's postulate of an exponential relationship between a stimulus and the risk of attack.

Phase 3. For those men whose earliest film failed to meet the criteria of normality, regression analysis was used to explore the relationship between change in radiographic abnormality, assessed for the individual from the earliest to the latest film in the pentad, and factors which might have caused the changes. In addition to the potential stimulus variables for Phase 1, we included the average dust concentration (Mp/cf) in the earliest period of employment, of up to about 5 years, and the average concentration in the interval between the first and the penultimate film in the pentad. For six men whose earliest film was pre-employment neither of these last variables had meaning and their records were deleted from this phase, leaving 111 men for study.

A regression analysis was carried out separately for each of the six variables of radiographic change (see Table 2). The stimulus variables included were the six discussed in the preceding paragraph, together with the status of the earliest film in terms of the specific feature being examined. The material was also subject to canonical analysis.

* The SI equivalent of 1 Mp/cf is roughly 35 particles/cm^3.

4. DESCRIPTIVE FINDINGS

Table 3 describes the two cohorts in both mining areas. Workers in Asbestos were, on average, a little older at first employment, and had had shorter intervals from then until the earliest radiograph in the study. About the same proportion in each area were non-smokers, but dust levels were considerably lower at Asbestos than at Thetford Mines, particularly in the periods before the first films. The complete "cross-section" at Thetford Mines had more abnormality due to small opacities and considerably more pleural changes of all types except obliteration of the costophrenic angle.

TABLE 3. DESCRIPTION OF SUBJECTS

	Earliest film normal		Others	
	Asbestos	Thetford Mines	Asbestos	Thetford Mines
No. of men in cohort	86	64	51	66
Averages:				
Age at first employment (years)	25.2	22.7	25.7	21.9
Age at earliest film (years)	32.9	32.0	35.3	37.0
Period from first employment to earliest film (years)	7.6	9.3	9.6	15.1
Dust concentration in this period (Mp/cf)	13.1	24.5	16.6	21.4
Percentage of non-smokers	14	9	8	15
Abnormality in earliest film				
Percentage of readings at stated scores* or above				
Small opacities (13)*	0	0	4.4	6.1
Pleural thickening (2)	0	0	2.5	8.0
Ill-defined cardiac outline (5)	0	0	0.0	0.8
Obliterated c/p angle (Present)	0	0	37.7	24.6
Ill-defined diaphragm (Present)	0	0	0.5	1.5
Pleural calcification (Present)	0	0	1.5	13.3
	Numbers of attacks†		Average annual change§ (111 subjects)	
Small opacities	14 (16.2)	8 (12.5)	0.64	0.37
Pleural thickening	4 (4.7)	4 (6.2)	0.13	0.18
Ill-defined cardiac outline	—	—	0.05	0.20
Obliterated c/p angle }	9 (10.4)	3 (4.7)	0.02	0.03
Ill-defined diaphragm }			0.001	0.013
Pleural calcification	2 (2.3)	6 (9.4)	0.013	0.035
	25 (29.1)	20 (31.2)		
Period from earliest to latest film (yr)			19.4	19.1
Dust concentration in this period (Mp/cf)			4.7	6.7

* See Table 1.

† Figures in brackets are percentages of the specific cohort. Attacks appearing in the same film on two or more features were counted as attacks of each separately.

§ See Table 2 for definitions of variables.

TABLE 4. CORRELATION MATRICES FOR STUDY OF EARLIEST FILMS

Coefficients of correlation between earliest radiographic variables (see Table 2) and stimulus variables (see Section 3, Phase 1)
The upper value in each cell relates to Asbestos, the lower to Thetford Mines.

	Small opacities	Pleural thickening	Ill-defined cardiac outline	Obliterated c/p angle	Ill-defined diaphragm	Pleural calcification	Age at first employment	Years before earliest film	Concentration in prior period	Smoker or not
Earliest film										
Small opacities	1 1	0.100 0.105	0.361 0.284	0.174 0.076	−0.025 −0.042	−0.045 0.136	−0.072 −0.022	0.349 0.332	0.089 0.065	0.021 −0.116
Pleural thickening		1 1	−0.020 0.062	0.424 0.493	0.209 0.021	0.043 0.123	−0.006 −0.144	0.080 0.259	−0.048 −0.104	0.036 0.106
Ill-defined cardiac outline			1 1	0.112 0.049	−0.072 −0.061	−0.097 −0.044	−0.020 0.043	0.250 0.227	0.009 −0.041	0.025 −0.359
Obliterated c/p angle				1 1	0.232 0.096	0.009 −0.094	0.057 −0.114	0.039 0.020	0.059 −0.094	0.089 0.083
Ill-defined diaphragm					1 1	−0.010 −0.153	0.117 −0.053	−0.002 −0.034	−0.047 −0.018	−0.236 0.054
Pleural calcification						1 1	0.100 −0.152	−0.005 0.190	−0.029 −0.053	0.042 −0.018
Stimuli										
Age at first employment							1 1	−0.375 −0.418	−0.193 −0.052	−0.071 −0.180
Years before earliest film								1 1	0.262 0.128	−0.075 −0.028
Concentration in prior period									1 1	−0.032 0.011
Smoker (1) or not (0)										1 1

In both areas, those whose earliest film was considered normal (86 and 64) when compared with the others (51 and 66) had had a shorter period since first employment in the industry (2 years shorter in Asbestos, 6 in Thetford Mines), while that film had been taken at a younger age on average (2½ years at Asbestos, 5 at Thetford Mines). However, there were more attacks of small opacities and of obliterated costophrenic angle or ill-defined diaphragm at Asbestos than at Thetford Mines.

In the other cohort, the average annual change of all pleural radiological features was less at Asbestos than at Thetford Mines. However, there was more progression of small opacities at Asbestos, although the earliest films showed less abnormality on average, while dust concentrations both before the earliest film and in the interval studied were lower.

5. THE "CROSS-SECTION" (Phase 1)

In the cross-section, certain of the responses were related, as shown in the correlation matrix of Table 4. In both areas, pleural thickening was associated with obliteration of the costophrenic angle, while small opacities and ill-defined cardiac outline tended to occur together. Among the potential stimuli, the period between entry to the industry and the earliest film was negatively correlated with the age of entry. There was also a slight tendency for those who had longer in the industry before the earliest film to have been exposed to higher dust concentrations.

TABLE 5. RELATIONS OF EARLIEST FILM RADIOGRAPHIC VARIABLES TO STIMULUS VARIABLES
The largest crude correlation coefficient is given first, in each cell. Any "significant" partial correlations are entered step-wise, together with the coefficient of multiple correlation.

Radiographic variable on earliest film	Asbestos		Thetford mines	
	Stimulus variable		Stimulus variable	
Small opacities	Years before earliest film	0.349****	Years before earliest film	0.332****
Pleural thickening	Years before earliest film	0.080	Years before earliest film	0.259***
			Smoker or not	—0.359****
Ill-defined cardiac outline	Years before earliest film	0.250***	Years before earliest film	0.232***
			Multiple	0.419****
Obliterated c/p angle	Smoker or not	0.089	Age at employment	−0.114
Ill-defined diaphragm	Smoker or not	—0.236***	Smoker or not	0.054
Pleural calcification	Age at employment	0.100	Years before earliest film	0.190**

Asterisks indicate statistical significance which would be obtained in independent tests, on assumptions of normality:

* $P < 10\%$. ** $P < 5\%$. *** $P < 1\%$, **** $P < 0.1\%$.

The regression studies are summarized in Table 5. There is some evidence that the status of the earliest film was affected by long exposure as shown by the coefficients of correlation, in both areas, for small opacities and ill-defined cardiac outline and, in Thetford Mines, for pleural thickening and calcification. The only other variable appearing to make a contribution was smoking: those who were reported as not smoking cigarettes had worse diaphragm thickening in Asbestos and a greater prevalence of ill-defined cardiac outline in Thetford Mines.

TABLE 6. RELATIVE RISKS OF ATTACKS

		Age at film showing attack (Older *cf.* younger)†	Dust concentration averaged to approx. 5 years before film showing attack (Higher *cf.* lower)†	Cigarette smoking (Non-smoker *cf.* smoker)
Small opacities‡				
All 150 subjects				
Asbestos	(14 of 86)§	1.3	0.7	2.1
Thetford Mines	(8 of 64)	7.0	1.6	2.7
132 smokers				
Asbestos	(11 of 74)	1.2	0.6	—
Thetford Mines	(7 of 58)	5.9	2.5*	—
Small opacities (profusion 2/1 agreed by at least three readers)				
All 150 subjects				
Asbestos	(8 of 86)	1.6	1.7	5.0**
Thetford Mines	(1 of 64)	∞	∞*	0
Thickening of pleural walls‡				
All 150 subjects				
Asbestos	(4 of 86)	0	1.0	0
Thetford Mines	(4 of 64)	3.0	0.3	0
Obliterated costophrenic angle‡ *or ill-defined diaphragm*‡				
All 150 subjects				
Asbestos	(9 of 86)	1.2	2.0	0.9
Thetford Mines	(3 of 64)	2.0	0	0
Pleural calcification‡				
All 150 subjects				
Asbestos	(2 of 86)	∞	∞*	0
Thetford Mines	(6 of 64)	∞**	0.2	2.2
All types‡				
All 150 subjects				
Asbestos	(25 of 86)	1.1	1.1	1.4
Thetford Mines	(20 of 64)	5.6***	0.7	1.6
132 smokers				
Asbestos	(21 of 74)	1.1	0.9	—
Thetford Mines	(18 of 58)	3.5**	0.8	—

* See Table 5.

† The comparison is between two parts of the population, divided to give as equal as possible numbers of *expected* attacks in the two groups.

‡ As defined in Table 2.

§ Figures in brackets indicate the number of attacks and the number at risk.

The first canonical correlations were 0.400 and 0.512, both slightly larger than any reported in Table 5, but, although confirmatory of the findings from that table, provided no new insight.

6. ATTACKS ON NORMAL FILMS (Phase 2)

A total of only 45 men were attacked, 25 of them at Asbestos, 20 at Thetford Mines. Preliminary studies suggested the need to examine each type of attack separately, while as usual distinguishing the two areas. The number of attacks in any one analysis was, therefore, very small; see Table 3. As a result, little confidence can be placed in many of the relative risks given in Table 6, despite the advanced methodology described in Section 3.

The positive findings appear to be as follows:

Small opacities: when an attack was considered as agreement that the profusion was at least grade 1/0, older men tended to have higher risks than younger men, and there was some evidence of "protection" by smoking, and a suggestion that those attacked at Thetford Mines had been exposed to higher dust concentrations; with attack defined in terms of profusion of at least 2/1, there were rather more attacks than expected at Asbestos, and the risk for non-smokers there was 5 times that for smokers.

Pleural calcification: this was, as had been expected from our previous studies (ROSSITER *et al*., 1972), more common at Thetford Mines; attacks appeared also to be age-related there.

Other changes: there were indications of age-related effects, but little that could be considered of practical significance.

7. PROGRESSION IN LESS-THAN-NORMAL FILMS (Phase 3)

Table 7 gives the two correlation matrices (for Asbestos and Thetford Mines), each in three parts, dealing with (a) response variables, i.e. rates of progression; (b) potential stimuli; and (c) their relationships. Part (a) reveals certain inter-relationships in the degree of change, in particular between increased pleural thickening and obliteration of the costophrenic angle (both areas); thickening of wall and diaphragm (both areas); progression of small opacities and both onset of ill-defined cardiac outline and ill-defined diaphragm (Thetford Mines). Part (b) shows, as in the first cohort (Table 4), marked negative association between age at entry and the period from then to the earliest film: further, the non-smokers tended to have entered the industry comparatively late in life. All the dust concentrations were positively related, so that there was a considerable degree of redundancy in these variables. The upper section of part (c) shows how the progression variables were related to the status of the earliest film. In the regression analysis, only the italicized correlations were taken into account; many others can be observed and must not be ignored in the overall assessment of findings. The lower section of part (c) relates the responses to those variables which can most reasonably be considered as potential stimuli; there is little evidence of any consistent pattern.

The regression analyses are summarized in Table 8. The status of the earliest film appears an important variable for several responses, but not with the same sign

TABLE 7. CORRELATION MATRICES FOR STUDY OF PROGRESSION

Coefficients of correlation between variables of radiographic change (see Table 2) and stimulus variables (see Section 3, Phase 3)

The upper value in each cell relates to Asbestos, the lower to Thetford Mines.

(a) *Response variables*

Change in	Small opacities	Pleural thickening	Ill-defined cardiac outline	Obliterated c/p angle	Ill-defined diaphragm	Pleural calcification
Change in						
Small opacities	1 1	0.118 0.143	0.085 0.645	−0.137 0.142	0.021 0.427	−0.036 −0.189
Pleural thickening		1 1	0.191 0.048	0.588 0.402	0.293 0.403	0.264 0.219
Ill-defined cardiac outline			1 1	−0.058 0.038	0.154 0.419	0.041 −0.218
Obliterated c/p angle				1 1	0.417 0.152	0.187 0.298
Ill-defined diaphragm					1 1	0.362 0.069
Pleural calcification						1 1

(b) *Stimulus variables*

	Age at first employment	Years before earliest film	Concentration in prior period	Smoker or not	Concentration in earliest period	Concentration between films
Age at first employment	1 1	−0.368 −0.541	−0.209 0.017	−0.269 −0.403	−0.335 −0.095	−0.004 0.167
Years before earliest film		1 1	0.013 −0.042	−0.026 0.083	0.148 0.087	−0.129 −0.045
Concentration in prior period			1 1	0.090 −0.082	0.894 0.794	0.439 0.707
Smoker (1) or not (0)				1 1	0.107 −0.109	0.027 −0.350
Concentration in earliest period					1 1	0.239 0.524
Concentration between films						1 1

(c) *Response and stimulus variables*

Change in	Response variables: Small opacities	Pleural thickening	Ill-defined cardiac outline	Obliterated c/p angle	Ill-defined diaphragm	Pleural calcification
Earliest film variables						
Small opacities	*0.245* *0.415*	−0.023 0.017	0.070 0.433	−0.069 0.011	0.004 0.117	−0.093 0.025
Pleural thickening	−0.131 −0.167	*0.230* *−0.013*	−0.048 −0.083	0.076 −0.088	−0.186 −0.121	0.093 −0.076
Ill-defined cardiac outline	0.218 0.395	0.124 0.006	*0.030* *0.360*	0.136 0.231	0.357 0.076	−0.048 −0.110
Obliterated c/p angle	−0.255 −0.331	−0.192 −0.225	−0.065 −0.242	*−0.340* *−0.190*	−0.271 −0.282	−0.045 −0.145
Ill-defined diaphragm	−0.089 0.067	−0.111 0.056	−0.062 −0.054	−0.061 0.255	*−0.580* *0.003*	−0.042 −0.117
Pleural calcification	0.003 0.081	0.024 0.184	−0.083 −0.019	0.122 0.152	−0.018 0.158	*−0.040* *−0.072*
Stimulus variables						
Age at first employment	0.135 0.218	0.059 0.157	−0.001 0.225	−0.193 0.207	−0.125 0.137	−0.070 0.142
Years before earliest film	−0.028 0.126	0.090 0.205	−0.035 0.172	0.177 0.149	0.147 0.047	−0.012 0.079
Concentration in prior period	−0.058 0.224	0.112 −0.109	0.285 0.250	0.137 −0.090	0.102 0.056	0.222 −0.043
Smoker (1) or not (0)	−0.115 −0.206	−0.027 −0.088	0.096 −0.212	−0.119 −0.172	0.320 −0.071	0.086 −0.134
Concentration in earliest period	−0.023 0.071	0.074 0.039	0.295 0.147	0.160 −0.037	0.000 0.003	0.055 0.009
Concentration between films	0.140 0.177	0.132 −0.105	0.275 0.276	0.115 −0.109	0.295 0.015	0.333 −0.038

throughout: small opacities (positive, both places); pleural thickening (positive, Asbestos); ill-defined cardiac outline (positive, Thetford Mines); pleural change affecting the costophrenic angle and the diaphragm (negative, Asbestos). At Thetford Mines, the combination of age at entry and period between entry and earliest film (roughly equivalent to age at earliest film) was a leading variable for all radiographic features, although only marginally for ill-defined diaphragm and pleural calcification.

Dust concentrations were associated with radiographic change as follows: concentration over the earliest period of employment with increase in ill-defined cardiac outline at Asbestos; dust concentration in the period between the first and penultimate film with increase of pleural calcification (Asbestos), with increase of ill-defined diaphragm (Asbestos), and of ill-defined cardiac outline (Thetford Mines).

TABLE 8. RELATIONS OF PROGRESSION TO STIMULUS VARIABLES

The largest crude correlation coefficient is given first in each cell. Any "significant" partial correlations are entered step-wise (except that age at first employment and years before earliest film were always treated in combination), together with the coefficients of multiple correlation.

Variable of radiographic change	Asbestos: Stimulus variable		Thetford Mines: Stimulus variable	
Small opacities	Small opacities on earliest film	0.245*	Small opacities on earliest film	0.415****
			Age at first employment	0.248 } *
			Years before earliest film	0.179 }
			Concentration in prior period	0.218*
			Multiple	0.533****
Pleural thickening	Pleural thickening on earliest film	0.230	Years before earliest film	0.205 } ***
			Age at first employment	0.326 }
			Multiple	0.379***
Ill-defined cardiac outline	Concentration in earliest period	0.295**	I-d cardiac outline on earliest film	0.360***
			Concentration between films	0.301**
			Age at first employment	0.191 } **
			Years before earliest film	0.270 }
			Multiple	0.542****
Obliterated c/p angle	Obliterated c/p angle on earliest film	−0.340**	Age at first employment	0.207 } **
			Years before earliest film	0.317 }
				0.373**
Ill-defined diaphragm	Ill-defined diaphragm on earliest film	−0.580****	Age at first employment	0.137 }
	Concentration between films	0.308**	Years before earliest film	0.145 }
	Multiple	0.632****		0.199
Pleural calcification	Concentration between films	0.333**	Age at first employment	0.142 }
			Years before earliest film	0.187 }
				0.233

* See Table 5.

The first canonical correlations were 0.824 (Asbestos) and 0.802 (Thetford Mines). Although considerably larger than any reported in Table 8, they are accounted for mainly by the large number of variables (18) included. As in Phase 1, they provided no new insight.

8. DISCUSSION

Clinically and radiologically asbestosis is a reasonably distinct disease entity. Its occurrence is virtually confined to those who have been exposed at work to airborne asbestos fibre, often in heavy concentrations. There seems no reasonable doubt that asbestosis is caused in this way and that the risk is related to the amount of exposure; indeed, control measures and safety standards are based on this concept.

Most previous X-ray inquiries of asbestos workers (including that by our own group; ROSSITER *et al.*, 1972) have been essentially cross-sectional. Correlations have not been high, but the prevalence of various abnormalities has generally shown a gradient when men have been grouped *a priori* by indices of past exposure. Our present study incorporated a cross-sectional element (Phase 1), but was mainly longitudinal (Phases 2 and 3). The methods of reasoning were *a posteriori*, i.e. from effects back to causes. Our study is also unusual in that it included measures of exposure to asbestos and to cigarette smoking. So far as we are aware, it is the first to consider rates of attack and of progression separately.

The highest correlations in the cross-sectional study of earliest films were rather higher than have appeared previously. However, although several of them rated three or even four asterisks in Table 5, the problems of simultaneous inference have to be borne in mind as well as the fact that the highest coefficient in that table (0.419) indicates that only 17.6% of the total variation in this feature at Thetford Mines could be accounted for by the stimulus variables.

Only a few of the relative risks of attack quoted in Table 6 were "significant"; the probability levels should be adjusted upwards to take account of the large number of simultaneous inferences being drawn.

In the progression study, multiple correlations as high as 0.632 in Asbestos and 0.542 in Thetford Mines were recorded; even so, the stimulus variables only accounted for 39.9% and 29.4%, respectively, of the total variation in these responses. Further, the "stimulus" variable accounting for most of the total variation was usually the status of the first film and not a measure of exposure.

It is disappointing that, despite its refinements over earlier studies, ours has provided so little evidence of the relationship between risk and exposure, either for attacks or progression. The nature of the basic hypothesis and the implication of our findings must therefore be examined. Several possibilities require consideration.

First, the response and stimulus variables chosen for analysis may be inappropriate or inaccurate. Changes visible on a chest X-ray are indirect manifestations of disease and their assessment is seriously hampered by observer error and by changes in radiographic technique over time. Environmental measurements with imperfect instruments at a limited number of work places may reflect poorly the amount of dust which a worker inhales. Moreover, some of the earlier assessments of dust concentrations could be little more than educated guesses. Fibre counts, rather than dust concentrations would have been preferable, but these were more scanty and even less reliable. We did what we could to minimize errors from these sources, but their elimination is impossible.

Secondly, problems arise from differences in the modes of progression of chronic occupational disease. Asbestosis is relatively insidious and probably progressive. Thus, advanced changes tend to be found in men with long duration of employment even in the absence of any occupational cause for either their occurrence or progression. On the other hand, the causes of attack and of progression may be different and so obscured by analyses which do not distinguish between them. Our methods should have reduced these problems, but are unlikely to have eliminated them.

Finally, there is the possibility that in asbestosis the cause-and-effect relationship is complicated by variation in a number of qualities of the individual which collectively might be referred to as "susceptibility". This term covers a wide range of social, psychological, behavioural and physiological characteristics which may modify extent of exposure, amount of fibre inhaled, amount retained and nature of the pathological response. There is much evidence for the existence of these factors in all disease. So far as the pneumoconioses are concerned, dust-clearance mechanisms are usually highly effective and little is known of why and when they fail.

In the present study, 80% of the men exposed for over 30 years, often to heavy concentrations, remained completely unaffected, whereas others were attacked after quite short periods of employment. The causes of this variation are a mystery but its effects are almost certainly sufficient to explain the unconvincing levels of correlation with exposure so regularly found by investigators of dust disease. Nevertheless, we plan to analyse the data in other ways. For example, the records of each reader can be taken separately rather than averaged, and different criteria for defining an attack can be tried, while other measures of exposure can be introduced. The findings will eventually be integrated with those from the several other facets of the full investigation of the health effects of chrysotile.

Acknowledgement—This study was supported in part by the Institute of Occupational and Environmental Health of the Quebec Asbestos Mining Association.

REFERENCES

COX, D. R. (1972) *Jl R. statist. Soc. B* **34**, 187–220.

EYSSEN, G. E. (1975) *Methods of Assessing Radiographic Progression in the Pneumoconioses.* Ph.D. thesis, McGill University, Montreal.

GIBBS, G. W. and LACHANCE, M. (1972) *Archs envir. Hlth* **24**, 189–197.

INTERNATIONAL LABOUR OFFICE (1972) *I.L.O. U/C Classification of Radiographs of the Pneumoconioses. 1971.* Occupational Safety and Health Series no. 22. International Labour Office, Geneva.

KENDALL, M. G. and STUART, A. (1966) *The Advanced Theory of Statistics*, Vol. 3: *Design and Analysis, and Time-Series*, pp. 285–311. Hafner, New York.

LIDDELL, F. D. K. (1974) *Br. J. ind. Med.* **31**, 185–195.

MANTEL, N. and BYAR, D. P. (1974) *J. Am. statist. Ass.* **69**, 81–86.

ROSSITER, C. E., BRISTOL, L. J., CARTIER, P. H., GILSON, J. C., GRAINGER, T. R., SLUIS-CREMER, G. K. and MCDONALD, J. C. (1972) *Archs.envir. Hlth* **24**, 388–400.

SOKAL, R. R. and ROHLF, F. J. (1969) *Biometry*, pp. 404–490. Freeman, San Francisco.

WEILL, H. and JONES, R. (1975) *Archs envir. Hlth* **30**, 435–439.

DISCUSSION

D. C. F. MUIR: Can you tell me whether there was reasonable agreement between the radiological assessments of the different readers or were you averaging widely different values?

Prof. LIDDELL: Observer variation in our study was neither better nor worse than in other studies. However, our statistical methods have attempted to minimize its effects. In the correlation studies (Phases 1 and 3), different levels of reading (whether of single films or of progression) were not important. In the study of attacks (Phase 2), we used what can reasonably be called consensuses. A subject only entered this phase if there was complete agreement among the readers that his earliest film was normal; an attack was counted as such only if at least three readers of the four recorded fairly definite change (as fully defined in the paper).

J. C. GILSON: The effects of technique as you say are important but they were not included in the analysis you present.

I think it important to realize that the X-rays on which this study is based were not taken for research purposes and varied greatly. In the future it should be possible to do much better by standardization of the technique.

K. ROBOCK: I wonder if anybody has any information on the connection between the results or findings from X-ray pictures and those from pathological–anatomical examinations post-mortem?

C. E. ROSSITER: In coalworkers' simple pneumoconiosis the correlation between X-ray change and lung dust burden is very high (0.8–0.9) probably because the radiographic response is largely just the resultant of absorption of X-rays by lung dust.

In asbestos workers, such correlations are inevitably lower because the radiographic response is the resultant of X-ray absorption not by asbestos, but rather by the tissue responses to the asbestos exposure. The inherent variation of individual responses leads to the lower correlations observed in studies of asbestos workers.

Prof. LIDDELL: In this context, the rather negative findings in Phase 2 (despite the sophisticated methods used) are to my mind of great importance.

LIST OF DELEGATES

ABRAHAM, R. P., C.F. Cassella & Co. Ltd, Regent House, Brittania Walk, London N1 7ND.
ADAMIS, Z., State Inst. of Occup. Hlth, 1450 Budapest IX, Nagyvárad tér. 2, Hungary.
AGHDAIE, N., University of Strathclyde, Dept of Environmental Engineering, Glasgow G1 1XJ.
AHARONSON, E., Israel.
AKSELSSON, K. R., University of Lund, Dept of Environmental Hlth, Box 2009, S-22002 Lund, Sweden.
ALANKO, K., Institute of Occupational Health, Department of Oulu, Kajaanintie 46C, SF-90100 Oulu 10, Finland.
ALBERT, R. E., New York University Medical Center, 550 First Avenue, New York, U.S.A. 10016.
ANTWEILER, H., Med. Institut f. Lufthygiene u. Silikoseforschung a.d. Universität Düsseldorf, D-4 Düsseldorf, Gurlittstrasse 53, Fed. Rep. Germany.
ARCHIBALD, R. McL., N.C.B. Medical Service, Hobart House, Grosvenor Place, London SW1X 7AE.
ARYANPUR, J., National Iranian Oil Co., P.O. Box 3094, Tehran, Iran.
ASKERGREN, A., Marie Hallsvagen 44, S-161 71 Bromma, Sweden.
ÅSTRÖM, A., Saab Scania, S15187 Södertälje, Sweden.
ATHERTON, R. S., Programmes Analysis Unit, Chilton, Didcot, Oxon OX11 0RF.
ATTFIELD, M., Institute of Occupational Medicine, Roxburgh Place, Edinburgh EH8 9SU.
AXELL, K. J., Ljungbyföretagens Hälsovårdscentral, Kyrkogatan 9, 341 00 Ljungby, Sweden.
AYER, H., Kettering Laboratory, University of Cincinnati, Cincinnati, U.S.A. 45267.

BAILEY, M. R., C.E.G.B., Berkeley Nuclear Laboratories, Berkeley.
BARRACLOUGH, N., Health and Safety Executive, H.M. Factory Inspectorate, 403–405 Edgware Road, London NW2 6LN.
BAUER, H. D., Silikose-Forschungsinstitut der Bergbau-Berufsgenossenschaft, 463 Bochum, Hunscheidtstr. 12, Fed. Rep. Germany.
BAUNACH, F., N.R.I.O.D., P.O. Box 4788, Johannesburg, R.S.A.
BAXTER, P. J., Employment Medical Advisory Service, Baynard's House, Chepstow Pl., London W2 4TY.
BEARD, R. R., Stanford Medical Center, Stanford, California, U.S.A. 94305.
BECKETT, S., Institute of Occupational Medicine, Roxburgh Place, Edinburgh EH8 9SU.
BEIGBEDER, R., 1 Rue Saint-Gorgon, 57710 Aumetz, France.
BELL, K. A., Environmental Health Lab., Racho Los Amigos Hospital, 7601 E. Imperial Highway, Downey, California, U.S.A. 90242.
BENNETT, J. G., N.C.B. Radiological Service, Cinderhill Road, Bulwell, Nottingham NG6 8RG.
BERLIN, M. H. H., Dept of Environmental Health, Box 2009, S-220 02 Lund, Sweden.
BERRY, G., M.R.C. Pneumoconiosis Unit, Llandough Hospital, Penarth, S. Glam. CF6 1XW.
BEVERLEY, W. H. A., BBA Group of Companies, Cleckheaton, Yorks.
BIANCO, A., Comitato Nazionale Energia Nucleare, Laboratorio Fisica Sanitaria, Via Mazzini 2, 40318 Bologna, Italy.
BIGNON, J., Clinique de Pneumophtisologie, Hôpital Laënnec, 42 Rue de Sèvres, 75007 Paris, France.
BINGHAM, E., University of Cincinnati College of Medicine, Dept of Environmental Health, Cincinnati, Ohio, U.S.A. 45267.
BJÖRLING, M., Saab Scania, 461 01 Trollhättan, Sweden.
BLACKETT, N. T., Hazelton Laboratories Europe Ltd., Otley Road, Harrogate, Yorks.
BLOOMFIELD, G. W., Occup. Hlth Labs, Health and Safety Executive, 403–405 Edgware Rd, London NW2 6LN.
BLOOR, J. R., Roussel Laboratories, Kingfisher Drive, Covingham, Swindon, Wilts.
BOECKER, B. B., Inhalation Toxicology Research Inst., Lovelace Foundation, P.O. Box 5890, Albuquerque, U.S.A. 87115.
BOLTON, R. E., Institute of Occupational Medicine, Roxburgh Place, Edinburgh EH8 9SU.
BOSMAN, P. H., Chamber of Mines of South Africa, P.O. Box 809, Johannesburg, R.S.A.
BOULEY, G., I.N.S.E.R.M., U. 122, Centre Pharmaceutique, 92290 Chatenay-Malabry, France.
BOWRA, G. T., The Boots Co. Ltd., Occup. Health Service, Station Street, Nottingham.

BRADLEY, A., Institute of Occupational Medicine, Roxburgh Place, Edinburgh EH8 9SU.
BRADLEY, P. C. B., Unilever Australia Pty Ltd, 1–35 Macquarrie Street, Sydney, N.S.W., Australia.
BRAIN, J. D., Dept of Physiology, Harvard School of Public Health, 665 Huntington Avenue, Boston, Mass, U.S.A. 02115.
BRIGHTWELL, J., National Radiological Protection Board, Harwell, Didcot, Oxon. OX11 0RQ.
BROADBENT, D. S., J. Crosfield & Sons Ltd., P.O. Box 26, Warrington WA5 1AB.
BRÖNDUM, F., A.B. Landskronaindustriens, Hälsovårdsceetral, Sweden.
BRUCE, C. F., Proctor and Gamble Ltd, St Nicholas Ave, Gosforth, Newcastle-upon-Tyne 3.
BRUCH, J., Institut für Lufthygiene, D–4 Düsseldorf, Gurlittstrasse 53, Fed. Rep. Germany.
BRUCKMANN, E., Silikose-Forschungsinstitut der Bergbau-Berufsgenossenschaft, 463 Bochum, Hunscheidtstr. 12, Fed. Rep. Germany.
BRYCE, D. M., The Boots Co. Ltd., Station Street, Nottingham NG2 3AA.
BUCH, S. A., Inveresk Research International, Inveresk Gate, Musselburgh, Scotland.
BUCHWALD, H., Industrial Health Division, Alberta Labour, 10523–100 Avenue, Edmonton, Canada T5J 0A8.
BEUHLER, E. V., Proctor and Gamble Ltd, Miami Valley Labs, P.O. Box 39175, Cincinnati, U.S.A. 45247.
BUNDY, M., United States Steel Corp., 600 Grant Street, Pittsburgh, Pa., U.S.A. 15230.
BURGESS, C., Health and Safety Executive, H. S. G. Dl Baynard's House, Chepstow Pl., London W2 4TY.
BURNS, J., Institute of Occupational Medicine, Roxburgh Place, Edinburgh EH8 9SU.
BURRELL, R., Dept of Microbiology, W.V.U. Medical Center, Morgantown, W.V., U.S.A. 26506.
BUTTERWORTH, R., British Nuclear Fuels Ltd., Capenhurst Works, Chester.

CAIRNS, A. L., Fisons Ltd., 12 Derby Road, Loughborough, Leics.
CAMERON, J. D., Medical Centre, Pilkington Bros. Ltd, St Helens, Merseyside.
CARNEY, I. F., I.C.I. Ltd, Central Toxicology Lab., Alderley Park, Nr Macclesfield, Cheshire.
CARTER, R. F., M.O.d. (P.E.) A.W.R.E., Aldermaston, Reading, Berks. RG7 4PR.
CARTON, B., I.N.R.S., Route de Neufchateau, 54500 Vandoeuvre, France.
ČERNÝ, I., Czechoslovak Rubber & Plastic Indust. Ltd, General Directorate, Gottwaldov, Czechoslovakia.
CHAU, S. T., 34-F Ylian Ching Road, Singapore 22.
CHEW, P. K., c/o The British Council, 3/4 Bruntsfield Crescent, Edinburgh EH10 4AD.
CLARK, D. G., Inveresk Research International, Inveresk Gate, Musselburgh, Scotland.
CLARK, G. C., Huntingdon Research Centre, Huntingdon, Cambridge.
COATE, W. B., Hazelton Laboratories America Inc., Vienna, Virginia, U.S.A.
COENEN, W., Staubforschungsinstitut, D53 Bonn, Langwartweg 103, Fed. Rep. Germany.
COLE, P., Host Defence Unit, Cardiothoracic Institute, Fulham Road, London SW3.
COLES, M. K., Pneumoconiosis Medical Panel, Hill Street, Stoke-on-Trent.
COLES, G. V., TUC Centenary Inst. of Occup. Hlth, London School of Hygiene and Tropical Medicine, Keppel Street (Gower Street) London WC1E 7HT.
CONNING, D. M., I.C.I. Ltd, Central Toxicology Lab., Alderley Park, Nr Macclesfield, Cheshire.
COOPER, W. C., Tabershaw/Cooper Assocs Inc., 2180 Milvia St, Berkeley, Calif., U.S.A. 94704.
CORN, M., Grad. School of Public Health, University of Pittsburgh, Pittsburgh, Pa., U.S.A. 15261.
COWAN, C. B., Fisons Ltd, Pharmaceutical Div., Research and Development Laboratories, Bakewell Road, Loughborough, Leics.
COWEN, R. A., Reckitt and Colman, Sinfin Lane, Sunnydale, Derby.
COX, G. A., Boehringer Ingelheim Ltd., Southern Industrial Estate, Bracknell, Berks.
CRAIG, D. K., Battelle, Biology Dept, Battelle North West, P.O. Box 999, Richland, WA, U.S.A. 99352.
CRAWFORD, N. P., Institute of Occupational Medicine, Roxburgh Place, Edinburgh EH8 9SU.
CREASEY, J. M., Physics Division, Chemical Defence Establishment, Porton Down, Salisbury.
CRITCHLOW, A., Health and Safety Executive, S.M.R.E., Red Hill, Sheffield S3 7HQ.
CUNDY, E. K., Research and Development Dept., English Clays Lovering Pochin & Co. Ltd., John Keay House, St Austell, Cornwall.

DAHLGREN, E. H., Boliden AB, S-93050, Boliden, Sweden.
DANIEL, H., Cerchar—BP 27—60103 Creil, France.
DAVIES, C. N., Dept of Chemistry, University of Essex, Wivenhoe Park, Colchester, Essex.
DAVIES, J. E., Health Centre, U.M.L. Ltd., Lever House, Bebington, Wirral, Merseyside.
DAVIS, J. M. G., Institute of Occupational Medicine, Roxburgh Place, Edinburgh EH8 9SU.

DAYKIN, K., Colgate-Palmolive Ltd., 371 Ordsall Lane, Salford, Manchester 5.
DEMPSEY, A. N., Pneumoconiosis Medical Panel, Albertbridge House West, Bridge St, Manchester.
DEVIR, S. E., Israel Institute for Biological Research, P.O. Box 19, Ness-Ziona, Israel.
DEWELL, P., 17 Brotherton Avenue, Webheath, Redditch, Worcs.
DICK, J. A., N.C.B. Radiological Centre, Golden Smithies Lane, Wath-upon-Dearne, Rotherham, Yorks.
DILLEN, R., S.A. Eternit, 2920 Kapelle O/D BOS, Belgium.
DIXON, E. M., Celanese Corp., 1211 Avenue of the Americas, New York, N.Y. U.S.A. 10036.
DOBSON, T. E., Workmans Compensation Board of Nova Scotia, P.O. Box 1150, Halifax, N.S., Canada.
DODGSON, J., Institute of Occupational Medicine, Roxburgh Place, Edinburgh EH8 9SU.
DOLPHIN, G. W., National Radiological Protection Board, Harwell, Didcot, Oxon OX11 0RQ.
DOUGLAS, R. B., Dept of Applied Physiology, London School of Hygiene and Tropical Medicine, Keppel Street (Gower Street), London WC1E 7HT.
DOWSETT, D. J., Physics Dept, University College Hospital, Shropshire House, Capper St, London WC1.
DUFMATS, H. E., Lung Clinic, Renströmska Hospital, University in Göteborg, Sweden.
DUFOUR, G., C.E.C., 37 Bd Saint Marcel, 75013 Paris, France.
DU TOIT, R. S. J., Dept. of Mines, P.O. Box 1132, Johannesburg 2000, R.S.A.

EDLIN, D. W., N.C.B. Regional Laboratory, 2 Station Street, Mansfield Woodhouse, Notts.
ELLISON, J. McK., D.H.S.S., Alexander Fleming House, Elephant and Castle, London SE1 6BY.
ENGER, N., Elkem-Spigerverket a/s, Postboks 4224, Nydalen, Oslo 4, Norway.
ESNAULT, A., B.P. 400, 44608 Saint-Nazaire, France.
EVANS, D. J., Health & Safety Executive, Baynard's House, Chepstow Place, London W2 4TY.
EVANS, J. C., Environmental and Medical Sciences Divn, A.E.R.E., Harwell, Didcot, Oxon OX11 0RQ.
EYSSEN, G. E., McGill University, Dept of Epidemiology and Health, 3775 University Street, Montreal, P.Q., Canada H3A 2B4.

FERGUSON, D. A., School of Public Health and Tropical Medicine, University of Sydney, Sydney, Australia.
FERIN, J., School of Medicine and Dentistry, University of Rochester, Rochester, N.Y., U.S.A. 14642.
FERNIE, J. M., Institute of Occupational Medicine, Roxburgh Place, Edinburgh EH8 9SU.
FJÄLLING, H., Uddevalla Företagshälsovård A. B., N. Drottningg 21, 45100 Uddevalla, Sweden.
FLETCHER, G. H., Employment Medical Advisory Service, Quay House, Quay Street, Manchester M3 3JE.
FOORD, N., Environmental and Medical Sciences Divn, A.E.R.E., Harwell, Didcot, Oxon OX11 0RA.
FORD, V. H. W., N.C.B., M.R.D.E., Ashby Road, Stanhope Bretby, Nr Burton-on-Trent, Staffs.
FRANCIS, R. A., TUC Centenary Institute of Occupational Health, London School of Hygiene and Tropical Medicine, Keppel Street (Gower Street), London WC1E 7HT.
FRANZ, H. c/o Boehringer Ingelheim Ltd., Southern Industrial Estate, Bracknell, Berks.
FRITH, H., Department of Toxicology, Fisons Pharmaceutical Division, Loughborough, Leics.
FROST, J., Clinic of Occupational Diseases, Rigshospitalet, Blegdamsvej, Copenhagen DK2100, Denmark.
FURNESS, E. A., N.C.B. Scientific Control, Lyon Road, Harrow HA4 9NF.

GAMBLE, S., Johnson and Johnson Ltd., 260 Bath Road, Slough, Berks.
GARLAND, R. P., N.C.B. Regional Laboratory, 2 Station Street, Mansfield Woodhouse, Notts.
GAZE, R., Cape Industries Ltd., 114/116 Park Street, London W1Y 4AB.
GEBHART, J., Abteilung für Biophys. Strahlenforschung der GSF, 600 Frankfurt/M. Paul-Ehrlichstr. 20, Fed. Rep. Germany.
GIACHINO, G. M., Institute Industrial Medicine, Via Zuretti 29, 10126 Torino, Italy.
GIBSON, H., Institute of Occupational Medicine, Roxburgh Place, Edinburgh EH8 9SU.
GILSON, J. C., MRC Pneumoconiosis Unit, Llandough Hospital, Penarth, Glam.
GILL, W. F., D.G.V. Soc. Affairs, Centre Louvigny, Luxembourg.
GLICK, M., Joint Coal Board, Box 3842, G.P.O. Sydney, N.S.W. 2001, Australia.
GLØMME, J. K., Kingosgt 9, Oslo 4, Norway.
GOELZER, B. I. F., Occupational Health Unit, W.H.O., 1211 Geneva 27, Switzerland.
GORE, D. J., M.R.C. Radiobiology Unit, Harwell, Didcot, Oxon OX11 0RA.
GORMLEY, I. P., Institute of Occupational Medicine, Roxburgh Place, Edinburgh EH8 9SU.

GÖTHE, C.-J., Clinic of Occupational Medicine, Södersjukhuset, S-100 64 Stockholm, Sweden.
GRADOLPH, P. L., The Ferndale Clinic, O'Donnell-Gradolph Assoc , 23338 Woodward, Ferndale, Michigan, U.S.A. 48220.
GREENOUGH, R. J., Department of Toxicology, Fisons Pharmaceutical Division, Loughborough, Leics.
GRIEBEN, C., C. H. Boehringer Sohn, 6507 Ingelheim am Rhein, Fed. Rep. Germany.
GRIMLUND, K., Husqvarna A.B., Husqvarna, Sweden.
GRÖNQVIST, B., Domnarvets Jernverk, Borlänge, Sweden.
GRÜNDORFER, W., 1020 Vienna, Böcklinstrasse 34, Austria.
GUTHE, T., Elkem/Spigerverket, Middelthunsgate 27, Oslo 3, Norway.

HACKENBERG, U., Inbifo Institut für Biologische Forschung, Germany.
HADDEN, G. G., Institute of Occupational Medicine, Roxburgh Place, Edinburgh EH8 9SU.
HAEGER-ARONSEN, B., Dept of Occupational Medicine, University Hospital, Lund, Sweden.
HAGLIND, J. A., Ö. Långgat. 29, 731 00 Köping, Sweden.
HAHN, F. F., Inhalation Toxicology Research Institute, Lovelace Foundation, P.O. Box 5890, Albuquerque, N.M., U.S.A. 87115.
HAIDER, B., Ges. Strahlen- u. Umweltforschung, Inst. f. Strahlenschutz, 8042 Neuherberg, Fed. Rep. Germany.
HAMILTON, R. I. C., Sydney City Council, Sydney, N.S.W., Australia.
HANKINSON, J. L., U.S. Department of Health, Education and Welfare, ALFORD, P.O. Box 4292, Morgantown, WV, U.S.A.
HANTZ, C. R. J., Section d'Etudes de Biologie et de Chimie, 91710 Vert le Petit, France.
HARDY, C. J., Huntingdon Research Centre, Cambs.
HARRIS, D. H., Martindale Protection Ltd., Neasden Lane, London NW10 1RN.
HARRIS, M. G., Chrysler Scotland Ltd, Linwood Road, Paisley, Renfrewshire.
HARRIS, R. L. Jr, Occupational Hlth Studies Group, School of Public Health, University of North Carolina, Chapel Hill, N.C., U.S.A. 27514.
HASSI, J. Institute of Occupational Health, Department of Oulu, Kajaanintie 46C, SF-90100, Oulu 10, Finland.
HAUCK, H., Inst. f. Med. Physik, Universität Wien, Währingerstr. 13, A-1090 Vienna, Austria.
HAYNES, R., Sartorius Instruments Ltd, 18 Avenue Road, Belmont, Surrey.
HEARD, M. J., A.E.R.E., Harwell, Didcot, Oxon, OX11 0RA.
HEDGECOCK, G. A., Medical Centre, Pilkington Bros. Ltd, Prescot Road, St Helens, Lancs.
HEGNELL, B. O., AB Pripps Bryggerier, Box 121, 72122 V. Frölunda, Sweden.
HEISE, E. R., Dept of Microbiology, Bowman Gray School of Medicine, Winston-Salem, N.C., U.S.A. 27103.
HEKMAT, M., Research and Training Centre for Labour Hygiene and Protective Measures, Tehran, Iran.
HENDERSON, W. J., Tenovus Institute for Cancer Research, Heath Park, Cardiff CF4 4XX
HEPPLESTON, A. G., University Department of Pathology, Royal Victoria Infirmary, Newcastle-upon-Tyne, NE1 4LP.
HEXT, P. M., Department of Biochemistry, University College, P.O. Box 78, Cardiff CF1 1XL.
HEYDER, J., Ges. f. Strahlen- u. Umweltforschung, D6 Frankfurt/Main, Paul-Ehrlich-Str. 20, Fed. Rep. Germany.
HIGGINS, R. I., Chloride Group Ltd, Wynne Avenue, Swinton, Manchester M27 2HB.
HILDICK-SMITH, G., Johnson and Johnson, 501 George Street, New Brunswick, N.J., U.S.A. 08903.
HILL, J. W., Pilkington Bros. Ltd, Prescot Road, St Helens, Merseyside.
HOLMES, S., T.B.A. Industrial Products Ltd., P.O. Box 40, Rochdale OL12 7EQ.
HOOPER, M. B., Natural Philosophy Dept, University of Strathclyde, Glasgow G4 0NG.
HORN, W., C.E.C., DGV/G/1-Centre Louvigny, Luxembourg.
HOUNAM, R. F., Environmental and Medical Sciences Division, A.E.R.E., Harwell, Didcot, Oxon. OX11 0RA.
HUMPHREY, J., Beecham Pharmaceuticals, Clarendon Road, Worthing, Sussex BN14 8QH.
HUNT, R. D., Industrial Health Unit, BBA Group Services Ltd., Cleckheaton, Yorkshire.
HUNTER, I. J., 11 Ada Avenue, Wahroonga, N.S.W. 2076, Australia.
HUNTER, L., 11 Ada Avenue, Wahroonga, N.S.W. 2076, Sydney, Australia.
HUTCHINSON, J. E., Pneumoconiosis Medical Panel, Arden House, Regent Farm Road, Gosforth, Newcastle-upon-Tyne NE3 3JN.

IRMSCHER, G., Zentralinstitut für Arbeitsmedizin der D.D.R., 1134 Berlin, Nöldnerstr. 40–42, G.D.R.
ISLES, K. D., Institute of Occupational Medicine, Roxburgh Place, Edinburgh EH8 9SU.

JACKSON, H. M., Health and Safety Executive, Occupational Health and Hygiene Laboratory, 403 Edgware Road, London NW2.

JACKSON, Mrs. Wickham Research Labs Ltd., Wickham, Hants.

JACOBSEN, M., Institute of Occupational Medicine, Roxburgh Place, Edinburgh EH8 9SU.

JACOBSEN, S. C. E., Munksiö AB, Box 624, S-551 02 Jönköping, Sweden.

JAHR, J., Yrkeshygienisk Institutt, P.O. Box 81 49, Oslo Dep., Oslo 1, Norway.

JAMES, A. C., Biology Department, National Radiological Protection Board, Harwell, Didcot, Oxon. OX11 0RQ.

JANSSON, C-D., Röhnskörsverken, 93200 Skellettehamn, Sweden.

JENSEN, A. M., IFO AB, S-29500 Bromölla, Sweden.

JOHANSSON, G. I., Dept of Nuclear Physics, Lund Inst. of Technology, Sölvegatan 17, S-22362 Lund, Sweden.

JOHNSTON, J. R., Institute of Occupational Medicine, Roxburgh Place, Edinburgh EH8 9SU.

JONES, A. T., N.S.W. Division Occupational Hlth, P.O. Box 163, Lidcombe, N.S.W. 2141, Australia.

JONES, C. O., Institute of Occupational Medicine, Roxburgh Place, Edinburgh EH8 9SU.

JONES, J. G., British Steel Corp., Ebbw Vale, Gwent, Wales.

JOSHI, S., Institute of Hygiene and Work Physiology, Swiss Federal Institute of Technology, Clausiusstr. 25, CH-8006 Zurich, Switzerland.

JUNIPER, C., Unilever Limited, Lever House, Bebington, Wirral, Merseyside.

KAGAN, E., N.R.I.O.D., P.O. Box 4788, Johannesburg, R.S.A.

KANG, B., Dept of Occupational Health, University of Manchester, Stopford Bldg, Oxford Rd, Manchester.

KARBE, E., Battelle Institut E.V., 6 Frankfurt/Main, AM Römerhof 35, Fed. Rep. Germany.

KAVOUSSI, N., Occupational Hlth Dept, School of Public Health, Tehran University, Tehran, Iran.

KIRKBY, W. W., Environmental Safety Division, Unilever Research Laboratory, Colworth House, Sharnbrook, Bedford.

KEELEY, C. R., Martindale Protection Ltd, Neasden Lane, London NW10 1RN.

KNIGHT, G., Elliot Lake Lab., Canada Centre for Mineral & Energy Tech. (Canmet), P.O. Box 100, Elliot Lake, Ont. P5A 2J6, Canada.

KONETZKE, G., Zentralinstitut für Arbeitsmedizin der D.D.R., 1134, Berlin, Nöldnerstr. 40–42, G.D.R.

KÖSTER, K., Battelle Institut E.V., 6 Frankfurt/Main, AM Römerhof 35, Fed. Rep. Germany.

KRATEL, R., Kratel S. A., 7 Avenue Eugene-Pittard, 1206 Geneva, Switzerland.

KREYLING, W., Institut für Strahlenschutz, 8042 Neuherberg bei München, Fed. Rep. Germany.

KRIEGSEIS, W., I. Physikalisches Institut Universität Giessen, D63 Giessen, Leihgesterner Weg 104, Fed. Rep. Germany.

KUSCHNER, M., School of Medicine, Health Sciences Center, State University of New York at Stony Brook, N.Y., U.S.A. 11794.

KYLIN, B., Sandvik Aktiebolag, Health Department, Sandviken, Sweden.

LAHAM, S., Inhalation Toxicology Unit, Environmental Health Directorate, Dept of National Health and Welfare, Ottawa, K1A 0L2, Canada.

LAING, J. G. D., Anglo-American Corp. of S.A. Ltd., P.O. Box 61587, Marshalltown, R.S.A.

LAPP, N. L., West Virginia University School of Medicine, Morgantown, W.V., U.S.A. 26506.

LARDEUX, P., I.N.R.S., 30 Rue Olivier Noyer, F-75680, Paris Cedex 14, France.

LEATHART, G. L., Dept of Industrial Health, Medical School, Newcastle-upon-Tyne NE1.

LEBERT, S., Max Planck Institut für Immunbiologie, 78 Freiburg i. Br., Fed. Rep. Germany.

LE BOUFFANT, L., Cerchar, B.P. 27, 60103 Creil, France.

LE POUTRE, J., S.A. Eternit, 2920 Kapelle op den Bos, Belgium.

LEVER, M. J., Physiological Flow Studies Unit, Imperial College, London SW7.

LEWINSOHN, H. C., T.B.A. Industrial Products Ltd., P.O. Box 40, Rochdale, Lancs.

LIDDELL, D., McGill University, Dept of Epidemiology and Health, 3775 University St., Montreal, P.Q., Canada H3A 2B4.

LIPPMANN, M., New York University Medical Center, Institute of Environmental Medicine, 550 First Avenue, New York, N.Y., U.S.A. 10016.

LLEWELLYN, O. P., Courtaulds Ltd., P.O. Box 5, Spondon, Derby DE2 7BP.

LOURENÇO, R. V., Section of Pulmonary Diseases, University of Illinois Medical Center, Chicago, Ill., U.S.A. 60680.

LOVE, R. G., Institute of Occupational Medicine, Roxburgh Place, Edinburgh EH8 9SU.

LUGTON, W. G. D., Group R. & D. Centre, British-American Tobacco Co. Ltd, Regents Pk Rd, Southampton.
LUMLEY, K. P. S., Medical Research Unit, H.M. Naval Base, Devonport, Plymouth, Devon.
LUNDGREN, K. M., Landskrona, Sweden.
LUNDQVIST, G. R., Hygienjnisk Institut, Aarhus Universitet, DK 8000, Aarhus, Denmark.
LYNCH, J., N.I.O.S.H., Post Office & Court House, Cincinnati, Ohio, U.S.A. 45202.
LYONS, J. P., Pneumoconiosis Medical Panel, 9 The Friary, Cardiff.

MCCALLUM, R. I., Dept of Industrial Health, The University, Newcastle-upon-Tyne.
MCCRAE, R. M., Research and Development Division, Nevendon Road, Basildon, Essex SS13 1BT.
MCDERMOTT, J. A., c/o Proctor & Gamble Ltd., Newcastle-upon-Tyne.
MCDERMOTT, M., Medical Research Council, Pneumoconiosis Unit, Llandough Hospital, Penarth, Glam. CF6 1XW.
MCDONALD, C., 505 Pine Avenue West, Montreal, P.Q., Canada.
MACFARLAND, H. N., Gulf Oil Corp., P.O. Box 1166, Pittsburgh, Pa., U.S.A. 15230.
MCINROY, D. D. R., 21 Malvern Street, Lithgow 2790, N.S.W., Australia.
MCLAREN, M. T., Department of Pathology, The University, Newcastle-upon-Tyne.
MCLEAN, A. S., National Radiological Protection Board, Harwell, Didcot, Oxon. OX11 0RQ.
MCLINTOCK, J. S., N.C.B., Medical Service, Hobart House, Grosvenor Place, London SW1X 7AE.
MCMAHON, T. A., Harvard University, Pierce Hall, 29 Oxford Street, Cambridge, Mass. U.S.A.
MAGOS, L., M.R.C. Toxicology Unit, Carshalton, Surrey.
MAGUIRE, B. A., Health and Safety Executive, S.M.R.E., Broad Lane, Sheffield S3 7HQ.
MAJOR, P. C., DHEW/USPHS/CDC/ALFORD, 944 Chestnut Ridge Road, Morgantown, W.V., U.S.A. 26505.
MALCOLM, D., Shandon, Dale Brow, Prestbury, Ches.
MALMQVIST, K. G., Dept of Nuclear Physics, Lund Institute of Technology, Sölveg 14, S-22362 Lund, Sweden.
MARTELL, E. A., National Center for Atmospheric Research, Box 3000, Boulder, Colorado, U.S.A. 80303.
MARTIN, C. F., Cone Mills Inc., 1201 Maple Street, Greensboro, N.C., U.S.A. 27405.
MARTIN, J.-C., Cerchar—BP 27, 60103 Creil, France.
MARTIN, R. B., Proctor and Gamble Ltd., St Nicholas Ave., Gosforth, Newcastle-upon-Tyne 3.
MELVILLE, A. W. T., Institute of Occupational Medicine, Roxburgh Place, Edinburgh EH8 9SU.
MERCHANT, J. A., DHEW/USPHS/CDC/NIOSH/ALFORD, P.O. Box 4292, Morgantown, W.V., U.S.A. 26505.
METIVIER, H. J., C.E.A. Laboratoire de Toxicologie Expérimentale, B.P. 61, 92120 Montrouge, France.
MEYER, P., Research Inst. for P.H. Eng., T.N.O, Schoemakerstraat 97, P.O. Box 214, Delft, N'Lands.
MIDDLETON, A. P., Institute of Occupational Medicine, Roxburgh Place, Edinburgh EH8 9SU.
MIDDLETON, K., Senior Service Ltd., Virginia House, Gregory Street, Hyde, Cheshire.
MIEDEMA, J., Hofwykstraat 73, Breda (Lethl), Netherlands.
MILLER, B. F., The Boots Co. Ltd., Station Street, Nottingham NG2 3AA.
MITCHELL, R. I., Battelle-Columbus Lab., 505 King Avenue, Columbus, Ohio, U.S.A. 43201.
MOLINA, C. M., Plan Nacional de Higiene y Seguridad del Trabajo, Torrelaguna, s/n Madrid 27, Spain.
MOORE, W. K. S., Occupational Health Service, The Boots Co. Ltd., Station Street, Nottingham.
MORÉN, F., AB Draco, Fack S-22101 Lund 1, Sweden.
MORENO, F., D.P.T.O. Quimica Inorganica, Facultad de Farmacia, Santiago de Compostela, Spain.
MORGAN, A., Environmental and Medical Sciences Division, A.E.R.E., Harwell, Oxon. OX11 0RA.
MORGAN, W. K. C., Division of Pulmonary Diseases, West Virginia University Medical Center, Morgantown, W.V. U.S.A. 26506.
MUIR, D. C. F., Institute of Occupational Medicine, Roxburgh Place, Edinburgh EH8 9SU.
MUNDER, P.-G., Max Planck Institut für Immunbiologie, 7800 Freiburg i. Br., Stübeweg 52, Fed. Rep. Germany.
MURPHY, D. C., TUC Centenary Institute of Occupational Health, London School of Hygiene and Tropical Medicine, Keppel Street (Gower Street), London WC1E 7HT.
MURPHY, R. L., Medical Center Library, West Virginia University, Morgantown, W.V., U.S.A. 26506.
MUSTAFA, M. G., Center for the Health Sciences, University of California School of Medicine, Los Angeles, California, U.S.A. 90024.

NAVRÁTIL, M., Institute of Hygiene and Epidemiology; Šrobárova 48, Prague 10, Czechoslovakia.
NELSON, K. W., ASARCO, 120 Broadway, New York, N.Y. U.S.A. 10005.
NETHERCOTT, A. S., Dept. of Health, Private Bag X54318, Durban 4000, R.S.A.
NICKOL, K. H., Medical Department, 9/330 Ford Motor Co. Ltd., Dagenham, RM9 6SA.
NILSSON, L., TRE Skåne Foretagshalsovård, Fack 213 01 Malmö, Sweden.
NOLIBÉ, D., C.E.A. Laboratoire de Toxicologie Expérimentale, B.P. 61, 92120 Montrouge, France.
NORDAHL, R., AB Tudor, 44041 Nol, Sweden.
NORINDER, B., AB Gotaverken, Fack S-40270 Göteborg 8, Sweden.

OBERHOLSTER, G., Dept of Health, Private Bag X88, Pretoria, R.S.A.
O'CONNOR, D. T., National Radiological Protection Board, Harwell, Didcot, Oxon. OX11 0RQ.
OGDEN, T. L., Institute of Occupational Medicine, Roxburgh Place, Edinburgh EH8 9SU.
OLDHAM, P. D., M.R.C. Pneumoconiosis Unit, Llandough Hospital, Penarth, Glam.
OREN, R., Israel Institute for Biological Research, Ness-Ziona, P.O.B. 19, Israel.
OTTERY, J., Institute of Occupational Medicine, Roxburgh Place, Edinburgh EH8 9SU.

PAGE-SHIPP, R. J., Industrial Hygiene, S.A. Iron & Steel Industrial Corp., P.O. Box 450, Pretoria, R.S.A.
PARKES, W. R., Pneumoconiosis Medical Panel, 194 Euston Road, London NW1.
PARNELL, P. M., Medical Dept, Comalco Prods P/L, Nelson Road, Yennora 2161, N.S.W., Australia.
PARROTT, W. M., Health & Safety Executive, Meldrum House, Drumsheugh Gardens, Edinburgh.
PATRICK, G., Medical Research Council, Radiobiology Unit, Harwell, Didcot, Oxon. OX11 0RQ.
PAVIA, D., TUC Centenary Institute of Occup. Hlth, London School of Hygiene and Tropical Medicine, Keppel Street (Gower Street), London WC1E 7HT.
PAYNE, L. R., Employment Medical Advisory Service, 4 Coptall House, Station Square, Coventry, CU1 2PP.
PEARCE, N. H., University of Bristol, 21 Woodland Road, Bristol BS8 1TE.
PELLENC, P., E.D.F. Service General de Medecine du Travail, 30 Ave. de Wagram, 75008 Paris, France.
PERRAUD, R., Commissariat Energie Atomique, Division de la Crouzille, B.P.1, 87640 Razes, France.
PHALEN, R., Community & Environmental Medicine, University of California, Irvine, Calif. U.S.A. 92664.
PHAM, Q-T., INSERM U14, Case Officielle No. 10, 54500 Vandoeuvre Annexe 2, France.
PHILLIPS, T. J. G., Branch M2 (Rm 125), D.H.S.S., 10 John Adams Street, London WC2.
PIGOTT, G. H., I.C.I. Ltd, Central Toxicology Lab., Alderley Park, Nr Macclesfield SK10 4TJ.
PIOLATTO, G., Institute of Industrial Medicine, Via Zuretti 29, 10126 Turin, Italy.
PLUNKETT, E. R., City of Hope Medical Center, 1500 E. Duarte Road, Duarte, CA, U.S.A. 91010.
POOLEY, F. D., Dept of Mineral Exploitation, University College, P.O. Box 97, Cardiff, CF1 1XP.
PORSTENDORFER, J., Institut für Biophysik der Justus Liebig Universität, Strahlenzentrum, D-63, Giessen, Fed. Rep. Germany.
PRIESTER, H., Battelle Institut E.V., 6 Frankfurt/Main, A.M. Romerhof 35, Fed. Rep. Germany.
PRODI, V., Comitato Nazionale Energia Nucleare, Lab. Fisica Sanitaria, Via Mazzini, 2, 40138 Bologna, Italy.
PRUEGGER, F. G., A-8010 Graz, Merangasse 23, Austria.
PULLINGER, D. H., Hazelton Labs (Europe) Ltd, Otley Road, Harrogate, Yorks.

RAABE, O. G., Inhalation Toxicology Research Institute, Lovelace Foundation, P.O. Box 5890, Albuquerque, New Mexico, U.S.A. 87115.
RABER, A., Allgemeine Unfallversicherungsanstalt, Weberg 2–6 1200 Vienna, Austria.
RADFORD, E. P., Johns Hopkins University School of Hygiene and Public Health, 615 N. Wolfe Street, Baltimore, Maryland, U.S.A. 21205.
RASCHE, B., Silikose-Forschungsinstitut der Bergbau-Berufsgenossenschaft, 463 Bochum, Hunscheidtstrasse 12, Fed. Rep. Germany.
RAXELL, R., AB Gustavsbergs Fabriker, 134 00 Gustavsberg, Sweden.
REGER, R., ALFORD, P.O. Box 4292, Morgantown, W. Va., U.S.A. 26505.
REICHEL, G., Silikose-Forschungsinstitut, 4630 Bochum, Hunscheidtstrasse 12, Fed Rep. Germany.
REISNER, M., Steinkohlenbergbauverein, D-43 Essen, Frillendorfer Str. 351, Fed Rep. Germany.
RENDALL, R. E. G., National Research Institute for Occupational Diseases, P.O. Box 4788, Johannesburg, R.S.A.
RESARE, D.C.-E., Stockholm, Sweden.

RHODES, N., T.B.A. Industrial Prods Ltd., P.O. Box 40, Rochdale, OL12 7EQ.
RICHARDS, R. J., Department of Biochemistry, University College, Cardiff CF1 1XL.
RICHARDS, S., Joseph Lucas Group, Research Centre, Dog Kennel Lane, Shirley, Solihull, B90 4JJ.
RICHARDSON, R. B., Group R & D Centre, British-American Tobacco Co. Ltd, Regents Pk Rd, Southampton.
RILEY, R. A., Imperial Chemical Industries Ltd, Central Toxicology Labs, Alderley Park, Macclesfield, Cheshire.
ROBERT, L., E.D.F. Service General de Medicine du Travail, 30 Avenue de Wagram, 75008 Paris, France.
ROBERTSON, A., Institute of Occupational Medicine, Roxburgh Place, Edinburgh EH8 9SU.
ROBERTSON, W. M., N.C.B. Yorkshire Reg. Lab., Golden Smithies Lane, Wath-upon-Dearne, Yorkshire.
ROBOCK, K., Wirtschaftsverband Asbestzement e.V., Arbeits- und Umweltschutz, 404 Neuss, Fed. Rep. Germany.
RODERICK, H., Tunstall Lab., Sittingbourne Research Centre, Sittingbourne, Kent ME9 8AG.
ROHL, A. N., Environmental Sciences Lab., Mt Sinai School of Medicine, Fifth Avenue & 100 Street, New York, N.Y. U.S.A. 10029.
ROLLE, R., Johnson and Johnson, West Research, Route 1, New Brunswick, N.J. U.S.A. 08873.
ROSS, D. S., Babcock & Wilcox (Operations) Ltd, Renfrew PA4 8DG.
ROSSCAMP, Dr.
ROSSITER, C. E., M.R.C. Pneumoconiosis Unit, Llandough Hospital, Penarth, Glam. CF6 1XW.
ROTEMARK, G., Lung Clinic, Centrallasarettet, 96119 Boden, Sweden.
ROTHENBERG, S. J., Dept of Chemistry, University of Essex, Wivenhoe Park, Essex.
RUPRECHT, L., Gesellschaft für Strahlen- u. Umweltforschung, 8042 Neuherberg bei München, Ingolstädter Landstrasse 1, Fed. Rep. Germany.

SANDERSON, D. M., Fisons Ltd, Chesterford Park Research Station, Nr Saffron Walden, Essex.
ŠARIĆ, M., Institute for Medical Research and Occupational Health, Moše Pijade 158, 41000 Zagreb, Yugoslavia.
SCANSETTI, G., Institute of Industrial Medicine, Via Zuretti 29, 101 26 Turin, Italy.
SCHARMANN, A., I. Physikalisches Institut Universität Giessen, D-63 Giessen, Leihgesterner Weg 104, Fed. Rep. Germany.
SCHÜTZ, A., Staubforschungsinstitut, D-53 Bonn, Langwartweg 103, Fed. Rep. Germany.
SCHÜTZ, A., Department of Occupational Medicine, University Hospital, S-221 85 Lund, Sweden.
SEBASTIEN, P., C.E.C., 37 Bd Saint-Marcel, 75013 Paris, France.
SEMPLE, B., Johnson and Johnson, Route 1, New Brunswick, N.Y., U.S.A. 08903.
SENEVIRATNE, P., Lever Bros (Ceylon) Ltd, P.O. Box 283, Colombo, Sri Lanka.
SHAND, P. A., N.C.B., Lauriston House, Lauriston Place, Edinburgh.
SHEERS, G., Plymouth General Hospital, Dept of Chest Diseases, Plymouth.
SHENTON-TAYLOR, T., Building A3.2, A.W.R.E., Aldermaston, Reading, Berks.
SHERWOOD, R. J., Colt International Ltd, Havant, Hants PO9 2LY.
SHORT, M. D., Dept of Medical Physics, University College Hospital, Gower St, London WC1.
SIMMONS, J. H., Occupational Health Lab., H & S.E., 403 Edgware Road, London NW2.
SIMONS, P. J., Hazelton Laboratories Europe, Otley Road, Harrogate, Yorkshire.
SJÖBERG, S. A., Boliden Aktiebolag, Kemidivisionen, Fack 251 00 Helsingborg, Finland.
SJÖHOLM, J., Läkarmottagningen, Höganäs AB, Fack 26301 Höganäs 1, Sweden.
SKIDMORE, J. W., M.R.C. Pneumoconiosis Unit, Llandough Hospital, Penarth, W. Glam.
SKURIC, Z., Andrija Stampar School of Public Heatlth, University of Zagreb, Yugoslavia.
SKYLLBERG, S., National Board of Occupational Health and Security, Fack 10360 Stockholm, Sweden.
SMIT, P., Chamber of Mines, Johannesburg, R.S.A.
SMITH, H., Biology Department, National Radiological Protection Board, Harwell, Didcot, Oxon. OX11 0RQ.
SMITHER, W., Cape Industries Ltd, 114 Park Street, London W1Y 4AB.
SNIEGOWSKI, A., Z.B.i.P.M. "Cuprum", Pl. I Maja 1/2, 50–136 Wroklaw, Poland.
SOETIDJO HARDJOSOEKATMO, R. M., Medical Div., Pertamina, Jakarta, Indonesia.
SPURLING, N. W., Dept of Pathology, Allen & Hanburys Research Ltd, Ware, Herts. SG12 0DJ.
SPURNY, K., Inst. Aerobiology, 5949 Grafschaft, Fed. Rep. Germany.
STAHLHOFEN, W., Abteilung für Strahlenforschung der G.S.F., Frankfurt/Main, Paul Ehrlichstr. 20, Fed. Rep. Germany.
STATHER, J. W., National Radiological Protection Board, Harwell, Didcot, Oxon. OX11 0RG.

STEEL, J., Department of Industrial Health, Medical School, University of Newcastle-upon-Tyne NE1 7RU.
STEVENSON, N. A., Fisons Ltd, Pharmaceutical Div., Research and Development Lab., Bakewell Rd, Loughborough, Leics.
STEWART, A. W. K., University of Strathclyde, Glasgow G1 1XJ.
STEWART, J. D., Personnel Department, Training Section, H.M. Dockyards, Portsmouth.
STEWART, P. S., Group R & D Centre, British-American Tobacco Co. Ltd, Regents Park Rd, Southampton.
STEYN, E. R., Dept of Health, Private Bag X 88, Pretoria, R.S.A.
STONE, D., Council for Tobacco Research—U.S.A., 110 E. 59th Street, New York, N.Y., U.S.A. 10022.
STOTT, N.B., A.E.R.E., Harwell, Didcot, Oxon.
SUDLOW, M., Dept of Medicine, The University, Edinburgh.
SUTARMAN, Prof., Pertamina Central Hospital, Jalan Melawi Raya 27, Kebayoranbaru, Jakarta-Selatan, Indonesia.
SVENSSON, K., Saab Scania, 46101 Trollhattan, Sweden.
SWENSSON, A., Dept of Occupational Health, National Board of Occupational Safety and Health, S-100 26 Stockholm, Sweden.
SWIFT, D. L., Johns Hopkins University, 615 N. Wolfe Street, Baltimore, MD. U.S.A. 21205.
SWINBURNE, L. M., Dept of Pathology, St James Hospital, Leeds.

TEGLBJAERG, D. S., Institute of Industrial Hygiene, Baunegaardsvej 73, 2900 Hellerup, Denmark.
TEJNING, S., Dept of Occupational Medicine, University Hospital, S-221 85 Lund, Sweden.
THOMAS, D. J., N.C.B. Radiological Services, Cwm Group Offices, Llantwit Fardre, Pontypridd, Glam.
THOMAS, R. G., Mammalian Biology H-4 MS 880 Los Alamos Scientific Labs, P.O. Box 1663, Los Alamos, N.M. U.S.A. 87545.
THOMSON, M. L., TUC Centenary Institute of Occupational Health, London School of Hygiene and Tropical Medicine, Keppel Street (Gower Street), London WC1E 7HT.
THORNE, M. C., M.R.C. Radiobiology Unit, Harwell, Didcot, Oxon.
THYSSEN, J., Bayer AG Institute of Toxicology, 56 Wuppertal 1, Fed. Rep. Germany.
TIMBRELL, V., M.R.C. Pneumoconiosis Unit, Llandough Hospital, Penarth, Glam. CF6 1XW.
TIMM, J., Företagshälsovården AB Felix, S-24100 Eslöv, Sweden.
TINSTON, D. J., Central Toxicology Labs (I.C.I.), Alderley Park, Macclesfield, Cheshire.
TOFANY, V. J., St Mary's Hospital, 89 Genesee Street, Rochester, New York U.S.A. 14611.
TOMENIUS, L. J., The National Swedish Environmental Protection Board, Dept of Environmental Hygiene, Fack S-104 01 Stockholm, Sweden.
TURNER-WARWICK, M., Cardio-Thoracic Institute, Brompton Hospital, London SW3.

ULMER, W. T., Silikose-Forschungsinstitut der Bergbau-Berufsgenossenschaft, Medizinsche Abteilung, 463 Bochum, Hunscheidtstr 12, Fed. Rep. Germany.

VALADARES, J. M., Ave. Brigadeiro Luíz Antônio 2344 (7° andar), 01402 São Paulo, Brazil.
VAN DE VATE, J. F., Reactor Centrum Nederland, Petten (N-H), Netherlands.
VAN DER WAL, J. F., TNO, Schoemakerstr. 97, Delft, Netherlands.
DE VRIES, J., Rijks Geneeskundige Dienst, N.W. Buitensingel 15, 's-Gravenhage, Netherlands.

WAGG, R. M., Health and Safety Executive, HM Factory Inspectorate, 403–405 Edgware Road, London NW2 6LN.
WAGNER, J. C., M.R.C. Pneumoconiosis Unit, Llandough Hospital, Penarth, S. Glam. CF6 1XW.
WALTON, W. H., Institute of Occupational Medicine, Roxburgh Place, Edinburgh EH8 9SU.
WANG, C. S., Dept of Chemical Engin., 232 Hinds Hall, Syracuse University, Syracuse, N.Y. U.S.A. 13210.
WARNER, C. G., 164 Redlands Road, Penarth, Glam. CF6 1QR.
WASHINGTON, J. S., N.C.B. Radiological Centre, Kemball, Fenton, Stoke-on-Trent.
WEBSTER, I., N.R.I.O.D., P.O. Box 4788, Johannesburg, R.S.A.
WEHNER, A. P., Biology Department, Battelle Pacific Northwest Labs, Richland, WA. U.S.A. 99352.
WEILL, H., Tulane University School of Medicine, 1700 Perdido St, New Orleans, Louisiana U.S.A. 70112.
WELLER, W., Silikose-Forschungsinstitut, 463 Bochum, Hunscheidtstr. 12, Fed. Rep. Germany.

WELLS, A. B., Unilever Research, Colworth/Welwyn Lab., Colworth House, Sharnbrook,Bedford MK44 1LQ.

WELLS, A. C., Environmental & Medical Sciences Division, A.E.R.E., Harwell, Oxon.

WHEELER, H. A., Yardley of London Ltd, Miles Gray Road, Basildon, Essex.

WILES, F. J., Medical Bureau for Occupational Diseases, P.O. Box 4584, Johannesburg, R.S.A.

WILTON, L. V., Group R & D Centre, British-American Tobacco Co. Ltd., Regents Park Rd, Southampton.

WOLFF, R. K., Respiratory Unit, St Joseph's Hospital, 50 Charlton Ave E., Hamilton, Ontario, Canada LN8 1YA.

WRIGHT, G. W., 460 South Marion Parkway, Denver, Colorado, U.S.A.

WULF, R. J., Carter-Wallace Inc., Carter Products Research, Cranbury, N.J. U.S.A. 08512.

YEATES, D. B., Institute of Environmental Medicine, New York University Medical Center, 550 First Avenue, New York U.S.A. 10016.

YRJANHEIKKI, E., Institute of Occupational Health, Dept of Oulu, Kajaanintie 46c, SF-90100 Oulu 10, Finland.

YU, C. P., Dept of Engineering Science, State University of New York at Buffalo, N.Y. U.S.A. 14214.

ZETTERQVIST, E., Esselte AB, Hälsovardsavdelningen, Vasagatan 11, 10 tr., 111–20 Stockholm, Sweden.

AUTHOR INDEX

SUBJECT INDEX